OXFORD MEDICAL PUBLICATIONS

Introduction to
OPHTHALMOLOGY

Introduction to Ophthalmology

Third edition

JOHN PARR

Emeritus Professor of Ophthalmology,
University of Otago Medical School,
Dunedin, New Zealand

OXFORD NEW YORK TOKYO
OXFORD UNIVERSITY PRESS
1989

Oxford University Press, Walton Street, Oxford OX2 6DP

OXFORD NEW YORK TORONTO
DELHI BOMBAY CALCUTTA MADRAS KARACHI
PETALING JAYA SINGAPORE HONG KONG TOKYO
NAIROBI DAR ES SALAAM CAPE TOWN
MELBOURNE AUCKLAND
and associated companies in
BEIRUT BERLIN IBADAN NICOSIA

© John Parr 1976, 1982, 1989

First Oxford edition 1978
Second edition 1982
Third edition 1989

ISBN 0-19-261743-5
British Library and
Library of Congress cataloguing
data available from the publisher

All rights reserved. No part of this publication may be reproduced, stored in a retrieval system or transmitted, in any form or by any means, electronic, mechanical, photocopying, recording, or otherwise, without the prior permission of Oxford University Press.

Published by arrangement with
University of Otago Press. This Oxford edition is not
available in New Zealand or Australia. The New Zealand edition
can be obtained from University of Otago Press, Dunedin.

Printed in New Zealand
by John McIndoe Limited, Dunedin

CONTENTS

Preface

Part one BASIC SCIENCES

1	Anatomy of the eye and visual system	1
2	Ophthalmic optics	41
3	Physiology of vision	53

Part two EXAMINATION AND INTERPRETATION

4	Eye examination by the general physician	92
5	Instrumental examination of the eye	111
6	Interpretation of ophthalmoscopic changes	129

Part three CLINICAL TOPICS

7	Retinal vascular disease	149
8	Optic disc oedema and optic atrophy	163
9	Glaucoma	173
10	Squint and amblyopia	181
11	Failing vision in old people	187

Part four CASUALTY OFFICER OPHTHALMOLOGY

12	Injuries	197
13	Painful red eyes	203
14	The watering eye	213
15	Sudden loss of vision	215
	Epilogue	222
	Objectives in undergraduate ophthalmology	
	Further reading	
	Index	226

Colour Illustrations   pages 121-128

PREFACE

For this edition I have made many small and a few larger changes. Some follow new understandings in physiology and pathology. Some are demanded by new clinical practices. Some are different and, I hope, clearer ways of writing about and illustrating old information. And some eliminate the unconscious sexism of the solely masculine third person pronoun.

I have not changed the overall balance of the book with its distinctive emphasis on the basic sciences and on the essential techniques of eye examination. I have continued to selectively limit the clinical section to what is needed by a non-ophthalmologist. But I have added notes on carotid insufficiency retinopathy, retinopathy of prematurity, ocular toxocariasis, central serous retinopathy and retinal pigment epithelial detachments, while the newer treatments with intraocular lenses, refractive corneal surgery, and trabeculoplasty, iridotomy and capsulotomy with lasers must now be mentioned. The book is bigger but only by 17 pages.

The new colour plates are from photographs taken by the photographers of our department of ophthalmology, Allan Cumming and Geoff Weston. The additional cost of these has been met by a grant from the Department of Ophthalmology of the University of Otago Medical School.

I thank my illustrator, Peter Scott for his genial collaboration and the twenty-five new illustrations, and Allan Cumming for figures 3-9 and 3-10. I greatly appreciate the easy co-operation with my joint publishers the two University Presses of Otago and Oxford, and in particular with Dr Bill Sewell, the former Editor at Otago.

PART ONE

BASIC SCIENCES

Chapter 1

ANATOMY OF THE EYE AND VISUAL SYSTEM

THE EYEBALL
Embryology

TISSUES OF THE EYE
Outer layer
  Sclera
  Cornea
  Canal of Schlemm
Middle layer
  Choroid
  Ciliary body
  Iris
Inner layer
  Pigment epithelium
  Neural retina
  Optic disc
  Central area of retina
  Retinal blood vessels
Optic nerve
Lens
Vitreous
Aqueous
Anterior chamber

ORBITS AND OCULAR APPENDAGES
Orbits
Eyelids
Conjunctiva
Tenon's capsule
Lacrimal apparatus
Extraocular muscles
  Muscles
  Movements
    Monocular
    Binocular

NERVOUS PATHWAYS
Intracranial visual pathway
  Optic chiasma
  Optic tract
  Lateral geniculate body
  Optic radiation
  Visual cortex
Pupillary pathways
Accommodation pathway
Motor pathways
  Functional systems of eye movements
  Ocular motor nerves
  Central organization
  Vertical eye movements

ANATOMY OF THE EYE

Terminology

Where anatomists and clinicians use different terms for the same part, the terminology chosen is usually that of the clinician.

In describing the eye itself the terms inner and outer relate respectively to the centre and the surface of the eyeball. Relationships of the eyes in situ and of their adnexae to the midline of the face are designated by the terms nasal or medial and temporal or lateral, while for anteroposterior relationships the terms superficial and deep are sometimes used. It can be confusing that the terms superficial and deep are commonly applied to the retina and here they refer to the inner and external surfaces respectively. This is because we think of the retina as seen by a clinician looking inside the eye with an ophthalmoscope and not as encountered by an anatomist dissecting the eye from its outer surface. A haemorrhage in the inner layers of the retina is called a superficial retinal haemorrhage because it is nearer to the surface seen with an ophthalmoscope, that is it is superficial. In a similar way we tend to think of the retina as overlying the choroid because that is the way we see these two layers clinically. The interior of the globe seen with an ophthalmoscope is called the fundus of the eye.

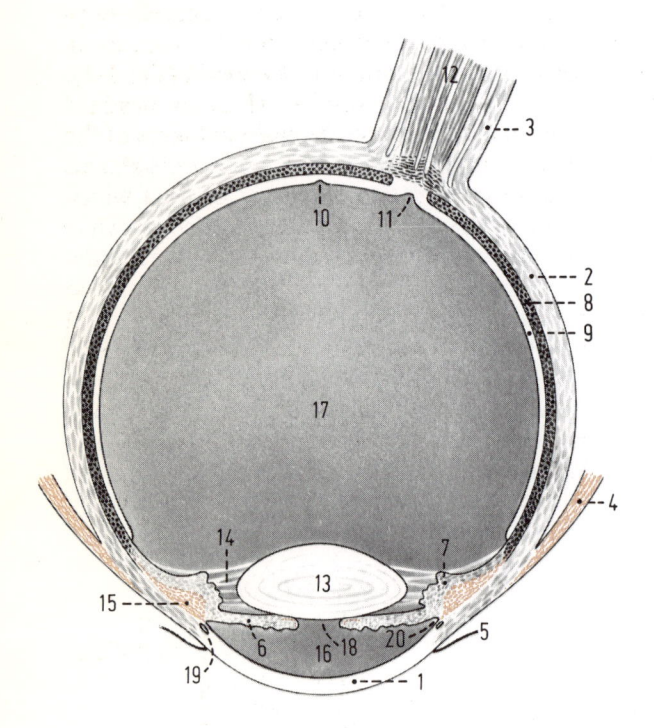

1	cornea	11	optic disc
2	sclera	12	optic nerve
3	optic nerve sheath	13	lens
4	extra-ocular muscle	14	suspensory zonule
5	conjunctiva	15	ciliary muscle
6	iris	16	anterior chamber
7	ciliary body	17	vitreous
8	choroid	18	pupil
9	retina	19	canal of Schlemm
10	fovea	20	angle of anterior chamber

Fig 1-1 Eye in horizontal section.

ANATOMY

THE EYEBALL

The vertebrate eye is both an image-forming device, of the camera obscura type, and an outlying piece of brain with light-sensitive cells enclosed in a protective and nourishing shell. It forms optical images, transduces these patterns of light into electrical changes, partially processes and gives meaning to the nervous excitations and then codes the resulting information for transmission to another part of the brain. These two primary functions, the optical and the neurosensory, determine the structure of the eye.

The human eyeball or globe is a hollow spheroid about 25mm in diameter; this adult size is almost reached by the age of three years.

It is composed of three layers and three internal zones (Fig 1-1). The three layers are an outer fibrous layer (the sclera and cornea), a middle vasculomuscular layer (the uvea or uveal tract comprising the choroid, ciliary body, and iris) and an inner neural layer (the retina). The three internal zones are those occupied by the aqueous, the lens and the vitreous.

The eye is not made of rigid tissues but is a pressurised chamber and it is this which preserves its shape and the stability of its optical surfaces. The outer coat of the eye is kept taut by an intraocular pressure which results from the secretion of fluid, the aqueous, into the eye and a controlled resistance to its outflow from the eye.

A clear mental picture of this basic design of the eye as revealed in a hemi-section of the globe is essential and this usually means the ability to draw a schematic diagram of the components in their right proportions and places. A horizontal section is most commonly illustrated because this can include both the optic nerve and the central foveal area of the retina. It is perhaps wise to orientate your diagram in a way that is most readily applicable to the eye of a patient in front of you, that is with the cornea nearest you towards the bottom of the page so that the picture represents the inferior half of a sectioned globe, with its cornea towards you, as seen from above (Fig 1-1).

The illustrations in this book are orientated in such a way for this reason and not, as one reviewer of an earlier edition suggested, because of its antipodean origin. In most ophthalmic books sections of the eyeball or portions of it, e.g. the retina, are shown with the anterior aspect directed upwards. However this conventional representation does not correspond so directly with the depths at which structures are encountered when looking at or into a patient's eye, e.g. with an ophthalmoscope.

Embryology of the Eye

Very early (three weeks) in embryonic development an outgrowth of neural ectoderm occurs on each side of the primitive forebrain (Fig 1-2). These are the optic vesicles which are destined to form the retina and the epithelial parts of the ciliary body and the iris. Each soon invaginates to form an optic cup, the inner layer of which will give rise to the neural part of the retina while the outer layer becomes the pigment epithelium of the retina. The stalk will become the optic nerve. Initially the cup is incomplete caudally and it is through this foetal fissure that blood vessels can enter the interior of the developing eye. Failure of proper closure of the foetal fissure gives rise to a permanent defect called a coloboma. When it affects the iris, for example, this results in a keyhole-shaped pupil.

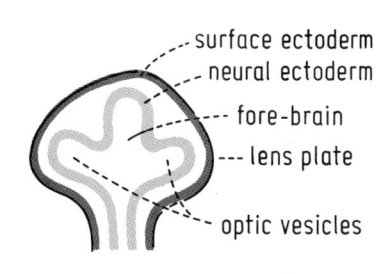

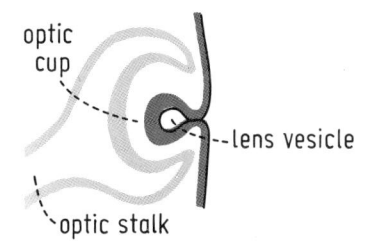

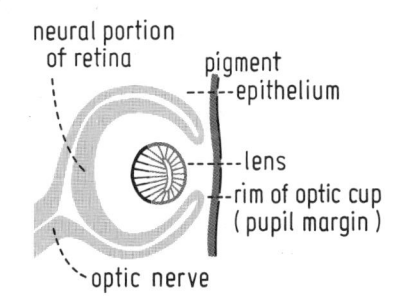

Fig 1-2 Early development of the eye.

The optic cup causes a vesicle to form from the overlying surface ectoderm which soon becomes detached to lie within the rim of the optic cup where it will eventually become the lens.

The sclera and cornea are formed from mesodermal tissue surrounding the developing optic cup; the corneal and conjunctival epithelium is derived from surface ectoderm. The anterior chamber first appears as a cavity in the mesoderm contributing to the formation of the iris and the cornea. For a time there is a complete layer of vascularized mesoderm which forms the stromal part of the iris in front of the anterior part of the optic cup and the anterior surface of the developing lens. The pupil forms in this with the disappearance of a central circular area. Failure of total absorption of this area with fine strands crossing the pupil is a common congenital anomaly of no significance (persistent pupillary membrane). Other common relics of this stage of development are small deposits of brown pigment on the anterior surface of the lens (epicapsular lens stars).

THE TISSUES OF THE EYE

The Outer Layer

Five-sixths of the circumference of the outer coat is the opaque sclera and the remaining one-sixth is the transparent cornea (Fig 1-3).

The **sclera** as seen through its overlying conjunctiva, is the white of the eye. Its radius of curvature is about 12mm; it is from 0.4 to 1.0mm thick. Being composed of obliquely arranged, interlacing bundles of collagen fibrils it is tough and resists stretching. There are few cells and consequently few blood vessels. This relative avascularity of the sclera has two surgical implications. It does not bleed when cut and repair depends on blood vessels from the tissues on either side of it, the choroid internally and the conjunctiva or Tenon's capsule externally.

The zone anteriorly where the sclera becomes continuous with the cornea is called the *limbus*.

Posteriorly, 3mm nasal and 1mm inferior to the posterior pole of the globe, there is an opening for the optic nerve fibres and retinal vessels called the *scleral foramen*. This is about 1.5 to 2.0mm in diameter internally and 3.0 to 3.5mm externally. It is bridged by a fenestrated network of collagenous and glial fibres called the *lamina cribrosa*. At the margin of the scleral foramen the outer part of the sclera is continuous with the dural sheath of the optic nerve.

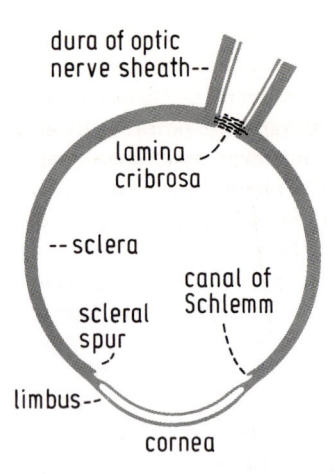

Fig 1-3 Outer fibrous coat of the eye, the corneosclera.

The **cornea** is covered by a thin (8 μm) film of tears and as a result has a perfect mirror surface. Reflections from this mirror are best seen against the black background of the pupil which derives its name from this fact. The word pupil comes from pupilla, a little girl, on account of the minified image as of a child an observer may see of him or herself in another's eye.

Its radius of curvature is about 8mm, but it is not truly spherical because the curvature is flatter at the periphery. This aspherical curvature of the corneal surface reduces spherical aberration. It is here that about two-thirds of the total refraction of light entering the eye occurs, the refractive power of the cornea being 43D, and the total refractive power of the eye being 60D. The diameter of the cornea is 11.5mm and it is 0.5 to 0.6mm thick.

Corneal Structure

In histological sections of the cornea there are five distinct layers, four of which can be distinguished in the living eye with the slit-lamp microscope (Fig 1-4). The five layers are epithelium, Bowman's membrane, stroma, Descemet's membrane, and mesothelium. With the slit-lamp microscope Descemet's membrane and mesothelium cannot be distinguished, but the tear film on the epithelial surface can be readily seen (Fig 5-3).

The *epithelium* is stratified squamous and since the surface cells do not keratinize it is perfectly transparent. Cells of the epithelium are able to slide on each other and the underlying Bowman's membrane and in this way promptly fill in small defects in this surface layer.

Bowman's membrane is a thin (12 μm) acellular layer of collagen fibrils, i.e. it is condensed stroma. It is tough, but if destroyed it does not regenerate and is replaced by scar tissue which is not transparent.

The *stroma* accounts for nine-tenths of the thickness of the cornea. It is tough and hard to puncture or cut. It is composed of regular layers of parallel collagen fibrils embedded in a dehydrated ground substance of acid mucopolysaccharides. This regular arrangement, together with the reduced hydration and absence of blood vessels, accounts for the transparency of the stroma. Scattering of light rays with consequent loss of transparency occurs if the regular structure is altered by mechanical stress (as in injury or when there is an abrupt increase in intraocular pressure) or if it is replaced with the irregularly disposed collagen fibrils of scar tissue, if the ground substance becomes hydrated in oedema of the stroma, if there is inflammatory infiltration with leucocytes, or if the stroma becomes vascularized as a result of injury or inflammation. The normal avascularity of the cornea is the basis for the greater success of corneal than most other tissue transplants (corneal grafting). The cornea is 'immunologically privileged' because of the difficult access for blood-borne cells which mediate immune reactions.

Between the lamellae are flattened connective tissue fibrocytes and a few leucocytes.

Descemet's membrane, although it is a thin (10 μm) layer, is an unusually thick basement membrane produced by the mesothelium. It is sufficiently tough and elastic to withstand the intraocular pressure when all overlying stroma is lost from a small area, as in deep ulceration. The bulging forwards of the membrane into the bottom of such a crater is called a descemetocoele.

The *mesothelium,* often called the corneal *endothelium,* is a single layer of flat cells which have an important metabolic function in abstracting water from the stroma. Damage or degeneration of the mesothelium therefore allows the water content of the stroma to increase with consequent increase in thickness and loss of transparency. A full-thickness corneal graft will not be clear unless there is viable mesothelium on the transplanted disc of cornea.

The *nerve supply* of the cornea is profuse,

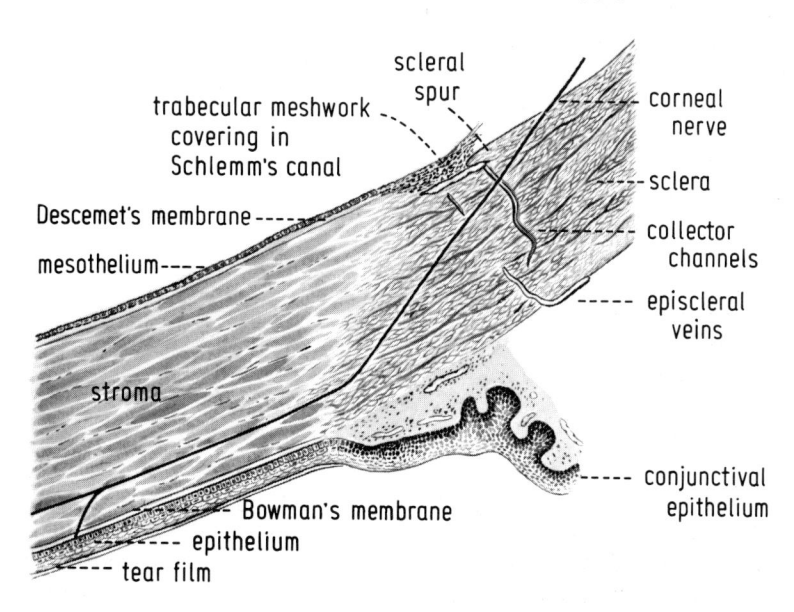

Fig 1-4 Cornea, conjunctiva and sclera.

making it one of the most sensitive parts of the body. Branches derived from the ophthalmic division of the fifth cranial nerve enter the mid stroma at the periphery and run more or less radially towards the centre. Much branching gives rise to plexuses at all levels and eventually naked axons ramify between the stromal lamellae and among the cells of the epithelium. For the first 0.5 to 1.0mm of their course in the cornea many corneal nerves retain their myelin sheaths and are visible with the slit-lamp microscope.

The **canal of Schlemm** is an irregular channel encircling the eye within the inner surface of the sclera at the limbus. It is formed by a small gutter in the sclera being bridged over internally by sieve-like layers called the *trabeculae* or *trabecular meshwork*. The posterior margin of the furrow projects forwards and internally and is called the *scleral spur;* to this some fibres of the ciliary muscle are attached. From the external aspect of the canal, small veins, called *collector channels*, pass through the sclera to join episcleral veins on the surface of the eye. The trabecular meshwork, canal of Schlemm, and collector channels constitute the pathway by which aqueous leaves the eye. Some collector channels still contain aqueous unmixed with blood after they have emerged on to the scleral surface where they can be seen with a slit-lamp microscope; these are called *aqueous veins*.

The Middle Layer

The word *uvea* is derived from uva, a grape, because this layer looks like the inside of a dusky grape skin. The word uveitis, inflammation in the layer, is in common usage.

Although it is a continuous layer it consists of three parts which differ in location and structure. From behind forwards these are the choroid, the ciliary body, and the iris (Fig 1-5).

The **choroid** is a vascular layer applied to the outer surface of the retina for which it serves a function comparable to that of the pia-arachnoid for the rest of the brain. It is essentially a meshwork of blood vessels in which the arteries and veins are external and a dense network layer of wide-bore capillaries, the *choriocapillaris*, is internal (Figs 1-6, 1-17). It is the indirect blood supply to the outer layers of the retina (the pigment epithelium, the rods and cones and their nuclei) which are themselves devoid of blood

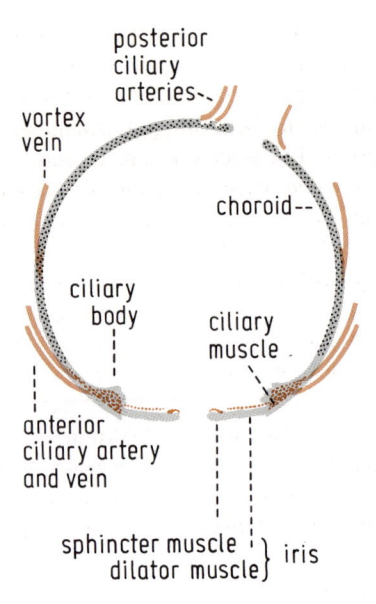

Fig 1-5 Middle vasculo-muscular coat of the eye, the uvea.

vessels. It is therefore the sole blood supply of the foveal part of the retina which has only these retinal components.

The blood to the choroid comes from the ciliary arteries which are branches of the ophthalmic artery. Half a dozen or more *posterior ciliary arteries* pass through the sclera around the optic nerve where they also supply the optic disc (Fig 1-5). The *anterior ciliary arteries* enter the globe in front of the insertion of each of the four rectus muscles and supply the ciliary body and iris as well as the anterior part of the choroid. Blood is drained from the choroid by the four *vortex veins* which pass quite obliquely through the sclera to emerge, one in each quadrant, behind the equator of the globe.

Cells containing melanin *pigment* occur throughout the choroid and are most concentrated in its outer part. These give the whole choroid its purplish-brown, grape-like colour. The intensity of pigmentation varies from individual to individual and with race and age and thus contributes to the normal variation in the colour and pattern of the fundus background seen with an ophthalmoscope.

On the inner surface of the choroid, between the choriocapillaris and the retinal pigment epithelium, is a thin (2-3 μm) two-layered sheet called *Bruch's membrane*. The inner layer is the basement membrane of the pigment epithelium and the outer layer is composed of collagen which is continuous with the collagen fibrils of the choroidal stroma. Localized thickenings commonly develop in this membrane, for example with age, and are visible with an ophthalmoscope as little spots called colloid bodies.

The **ciliary body** is a band between 4 and 6mm wide and roughly triangular in cross-section which lines the interior of the sclera just behind the limbus. The position of its anterior margin can usually be discerned in the living eye when the sclera is trans-illuminated. Functionally it has two components, the ciliary processes which secrete the aqueous and the ciliary muscle which provides the motive power for *accommodation* (the increase in the refractive power of the lens for near vision).

The *ciliary processes*, about seventy in number, are anteroposterior ridges with project from the inner aspect of the anterior part of the ciliary body (Fig 1-7). They are composed of vascular tissue covered by a double layer of epithelium derived from the embryonic optic cup. The outer layer is a continuation of the pigment epithelium of the retina and is also pigmented. The inner layer is continuous with the neural portion of the retina and is unpigmented. This epithelium, with its large surface area due to the folding and its rich underlying blood supply, is the source of the aqueous.

The suspensory zonule of the lens is attached to both the ciliary processes and the valleys between them.

The *ciliary muscle* lies in the anterior and outer part of the ciliary body. On contraction it causes the ciliary body to move forward and to thicken and thereby relaxes the suspensory zonule of the lens. It is non-striated muscle and is innervated by parasympathetic fibres from the third cranial nerve. It is therefore paralysed by parasympatholytic drugs (cholinergic blocking) such as atropine and cyclopentolate. These are effective in the form of eye drops and such drops are used, especially in children, to temporarily inhibit all accommodation while any refractive error is being determined.

CHOROID
pigment cells
Bruch's membrane
choriocapillaris
larger vessels
pigment epithelium (of retina)

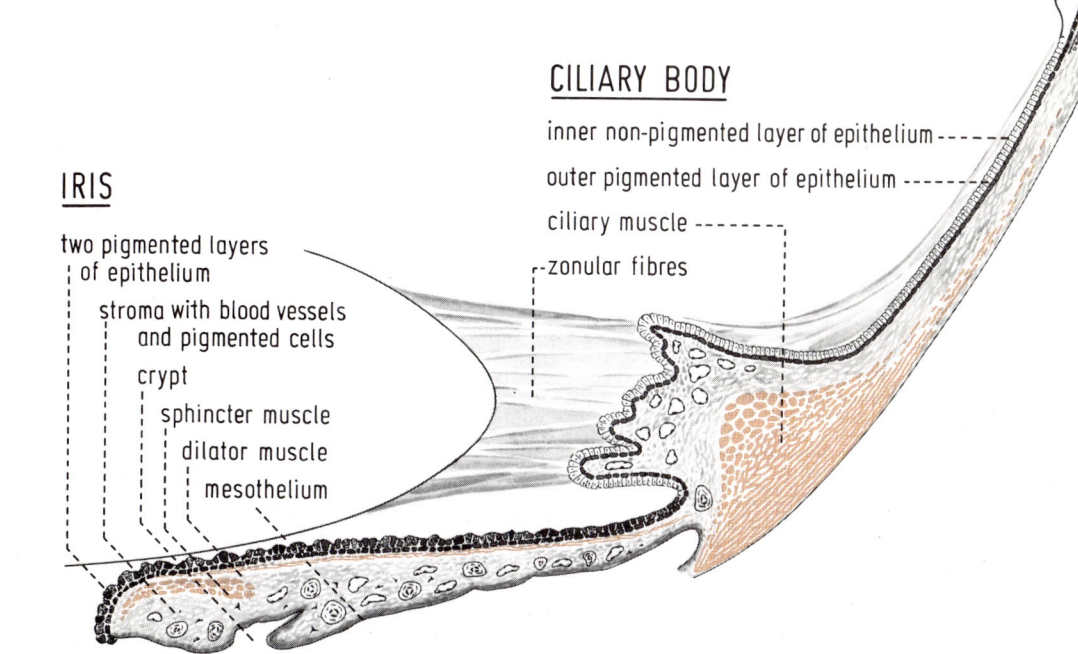

CILIARY BODY
inner non-pigmented layer of epithelium
outer pigmented layer of epithelium
ciliary muscle
zonular fibres

IRIS
two pigmented layers of epithelium
stroma with blood vessels and pigmented cells
crypt
sphincter muscle
dilator muscle
mesothelium

Anteriorly a slip of ciliary muscle is inserted into the scleral spur which forms the posterior lip of Schlemm's canal. It is thought that through this attachment contraction of the muscle enlarges the microscopic channels in the trabeculae between the anterior chamber and Schlemm's canal, thereby facilitating the outflow of aqueous. This may explain the beneficial effect of parasympathomimetic drops such as physostigmine and pilocarpine which are used in the treatment of some types of glaucoma (the condition in which the intraocular pressure is abnormally high).

Blood Supply

The arterial supply to the ciliary body (and to the iris) is derived from the anterior ciliary arteries and from two of the posterior ciliary arteries, the long posterior ciliary arteries, which run forwards inside the sclera one on each side in the horizontal meridian. The venous drainage from the ciliary body (and from the iris) is mainly into the vortex veins, but there are also small anterior ciliary veins which emerge through the sclera just posterior to the limbus to join episcleral veins.

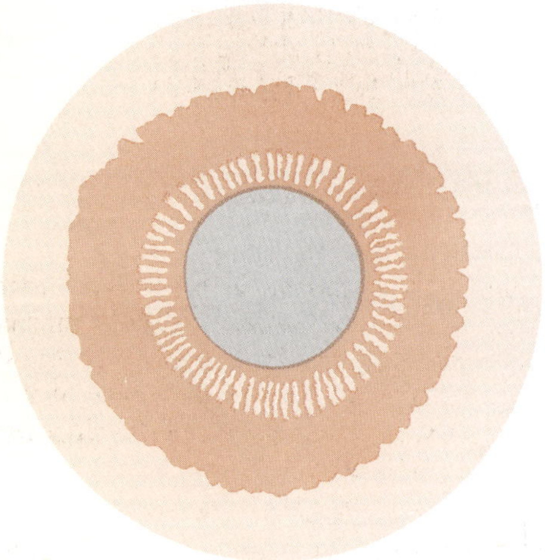

Fig 1-7 Ciliary body as seen from behind. The radial ridges are the ciliary processes. In the centre is the posterior surface of the lens. Between the lens equator and the ciliary processes is the posterior aspect of the periphery of the iris. The transparent fibrils of the suspensory zonule which bridge this annular gap are not shown. The outer circumferential notched line between retina and ciliary body is the ora serrata.

The **iris** is a diaphragm separating the anterior and posterior chambers. It has a central hole, the pupil, through which light rays pass on their way to the retina and through which aqueous passes from the posterior to the anterior chamber. Peripherally it is continuous with the anterior surface of the ciliary body and its central pupillary margin rests on the anterior surface of the lens. When inflamed (iritis) the iris may become adherent to the lens unless the pupil is fully dilated and thereby withdrawn from contact with the lens; these adhesions are called posterior synechiae. The iris appears to be a quite rigid structure, the only movement normally seen being the alteration in the size of the pupil. In fact it is a soft, floppy membrane which is supported and, because pushed forwards centrally, slightly taughtened by the lens. If the lens is dislocated or removed the iris trembles like a jelly with the normal eye movements (iridodonesis).

The iris consists of a vascular *stroma* covered on its sponge-like anterior surface by mesothelium and on its smooth posterior surface by two layers of epithelium derived from the embryonic optic cup. In contrast to the retina and ciliary body, both layers of *iris epithelium* are pigmented. The posterior layer curves forwards into the pupil to form the sharply outlined dark margin of the pupil where it then becomes continuous with the anterior layer of epithelial cells. The epithelial pupil margin therefore corresponds to the rim of the embryonic optic cup.

Within the stroma are numerous blood vessels, pigment cells and two non-striated muscles.

The *iris vessels* are unusual in that they normally bleed very little when cut, a great convenience in surgery of the iris. However when a vessel at the periphery of the iris is torn, as it may be by a blow on the eye, bleeding into the anterior chamber commonly occurs (hyphaema) (p. 201). Another unusual feature of the iris with surgical implications is that, when torn or cut, it does not heal.

The arterial supply and venous drainage of the iris is shared with that of the ciliary body which has already been described. When the iris or ciliary body is inflamed the anterior ciliary vessels are diluted. This hyperaemia is visible as a ring of redness around the limbus (ciliary injection; limbal hyperaemia). This distinctive type of 'red eye' is useful diagnostically in distinguishing intraocular or corneal inflammation from superficial conjunctival inflammation which gives rise to a more generalized hyperaemia of the conjunctival vessels (conjunctival injection or hyperaemia).

The number of melanin-containing *pigment cells* in the stroma varies from almost none to very many. The density of stromal pigmentation determines *the colour of the iris* (Fig 1-8). (The word iris means a rainbow.) In all irides (except those of an albino) the epithelial layers deep to the stroma are totally opaque with pigment. If, as in all babies of the white-skinned races, there is no stromal pigment, light which strikes the iris passes through the stroma. In the translucent stroma the light rays undergo diffraction and the shorter the wavelength the greater the scattering. Because of this, whereas most of the light of longer wavelength eventually reaches and is absorbed by the pigment in the epithelium, much of the light of shorter wavelength suffers multiple deflections and is reverted to emerge from the iris surface. As a consequence the iris looks blue. If, as the child grows, the stroma becomes heavily pigmented the iris becomes brown. With moderate stromal pigmentation the iris looks green because the scattered blue rays are absorbed by the stromal pigment, the unscattered red rays are absorbed in the epithelium and some of the green rays are scattered enough to avoid epithelial absorption but are not absorbed by the yellow-brown stromal pigment.

The muscles of the iris lie deeply, adjacent to the epithelium. *The sphincter,* which constricts the pupil, is a 1mm wide band surrounding the pupil. It is innervated by parasympathetic fibres from the third cranial nerve. The *dilator,* which dilates the pupil, consists of radial fibres in the periphery. It is innervated by sympathetic fibres. Of the two the sphincter is much the stronger so that when, as in iritis, the muscles are directly irritated it wins and the pupil becomes small.

To examine the interior of the eye properly it is necessary to dilate the pupil. Dilatation of the pupil (mydriasis) for this purpose is achieved with either a short acting parasympatholytic drug, e.g. tropicamide, or a sympathomimetic drug, e.g. phenylephrine, administered as eye-drops. To induce constriction of the pupil (miosis) drops containing a parasympathomimetic drug are used, e.g. pilocarpine.

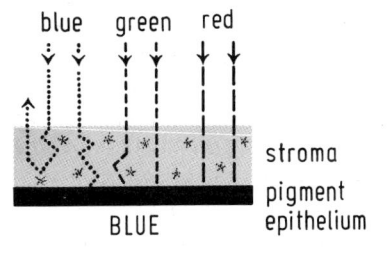

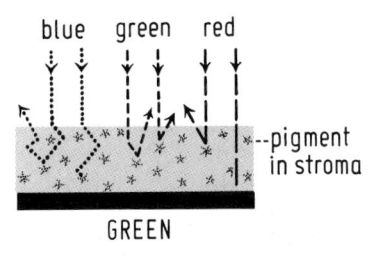

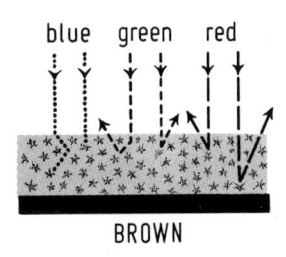

Fig 1-8 Colour of the iris.

The iris has pain receptors so that iritis for example can be very painful. This is relieved by paralysing the sphincter muscle with long acting parasympatholytic drops, e.g. atropine, which are also indicated to forestall the development of posterior synechiae.

The Inner Layer

The retina is a delicate, thin (0.4mm) layer which lines the interior of the posterior two-thirds of the globe; its anterior margin is about 8mm from the limbus (Fig 1-9).

Corresponding to the two layers of the embryonic optic cup it consists of two main parts, the transparent neural portion internally and the pigment epithelium externally. It is common usage to refer to the neural part as 'the retina'.

The neural retina is attached to the outer layer only at the optic disc and at its anterior margin (the ora serrata). Elsewhere the two parts are closely apposed but not adherent. As a consequence the neural part can become separated by fluid from the pigment epithelium, an important condition known as retinal detachment.

The **pigment epithelium** is a single layer of hexagonal cells which contain pigment granules (melanin) (Fig 1-10). Delicate villi projecting from the apical (internal) surface of these cells surround the external tips of the apposed photoreceptors.

In spite of its simple appearance the pigment epithelium has a surprising number of functions which are vital to the neural retina. Its pigment absorbs scattered light which would otherwise degrade the optical image; the absorbed light is converted to heat which is dissipated by the ample flow of blood through the choroid. (This same photothermal mechanism is deliberately overloaded when photocoagulation (p. 157) is used to focally destroy the tissues immediately in front of and behind the pigment epithelium.) It selectively transports metabolites between the choroidal circulation and the outer retina, but because there are 'tight' junctions between adjoining cells, it is an impermeable barrier to diffusion of even small unwanted molecules from the choroid into the retina (Fig 1-18). It pumps water outwards from the vitreous and neural retina to the choroid thereby helping to keep the neural retina in contact with the outer layers of the globe. It conveys vitamin A to the photoreceptors both for incorporation into newly-made visual pigments and for regeneration of these molecules after they have been split by the action of light (p. 56). It synthesizes an acid-mucopolysaccharide which fills the spaces among the outer tips of the photoreceptors. It synthesizes and renews its own melanin granules. It phagocytoses and digests the fragments which are continually being shed from the outer tips of the rods and cones (p. 13). And if there is tissue damage it can proliferate, become phagocytic or even form a sort of fibrous scar tissue.

The density of pigmentation varies from individual to individual; it tends to lessen with age. This variation is independent of the variation in the amount of pigment in the choroid (which tends to increase with age). The amounts of pigment in these two locations determine the

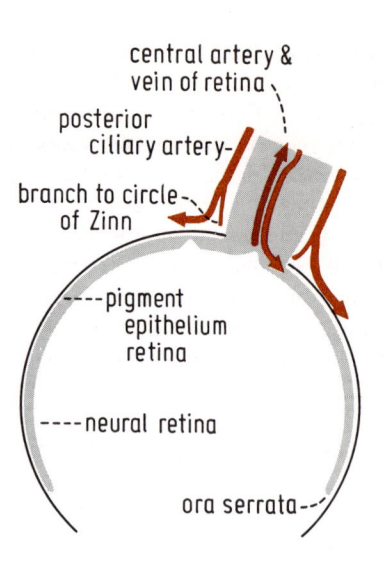

Fig 1-9 Inner neural coat of the eye, the retina.

ophthalmoscopic colour and pattern of the fundus background in the following manner.

The retina internal to the pigment epithelium is transparent, except for the blood contained in the retinal arteries and veins, and therefore reflects little light. Light is reflected from the blood in the larger choroidal vessels and this is modified in two ways by the overlying pigment epithelium. The pigment acts as a diffusing screen, which renders the discontinuous pattern of red vessels more or less uniform, and as a colour filter, which changes the colour to an orange-red (in the eyes of most Caucasians) (Fig 6-22a). When there is much pigment in this epithelium the colour is a uniform dusky red (Fig 6-22b). In the macular region the pigment epithelium is more heavily pigmented and this area is therefore slightly darker than the rest of the fundus. When there is relatively little pigment in both the pigment epithelium and in the choroid, the colour is a light red or, if the pigment in the epithelium is very sparse, the large choroidal vessels are discernible as red ribbons on a pale (scleral) background, the blonde type of fundus (Fig 6-22c). When there is little pigment in the pigment epithelium with much pigment in the choroid the appearance is that of the tessellated or tigroid fundus in which patches of choroidal pigment are seen more or less clearly outlined by the larger choroidal vessels (Fig 6-22d).

ANATOMY

The **neural part of the retina** is a most complex tissue (Fig 1-10). It contains photoreceptors (the rods and cones), five types of neurones (receptor nuclei, horizontal cells, bipolar cells, amacrine cells, and ganglion cells), a specialized type of glial cell (Müller's cells), and very many cell processes. In each eye there are about 120 million rods, 6 million cones and 1 million nerve fibres. One retinal neurone may have more than 200 connections to 20 or 30 other neurones.

In histological sections it is obviously layered, there being one layer of rods and cones, three dark cellular (nuclear) layers, two apparently structureless synaptic (plexiform) layers, and one nerve fibre layer.

The *outer nuclear layer* contains the nuclei of the rods and cones, the *inner nuclear layer* contains the cell bodies of bipolar, horizontal, amacrine, and Müller's cells, and the *ganglion cell layer* contains the ganglion cell bodies.

In each plexiform layer the processes of three cell types synapse; receptor, bipolar, and horizontal cells in the *outer plexiform layer*, bipolar, amacrine, and ganglion cells in the *inner plexiform layer*.

Functional Organization

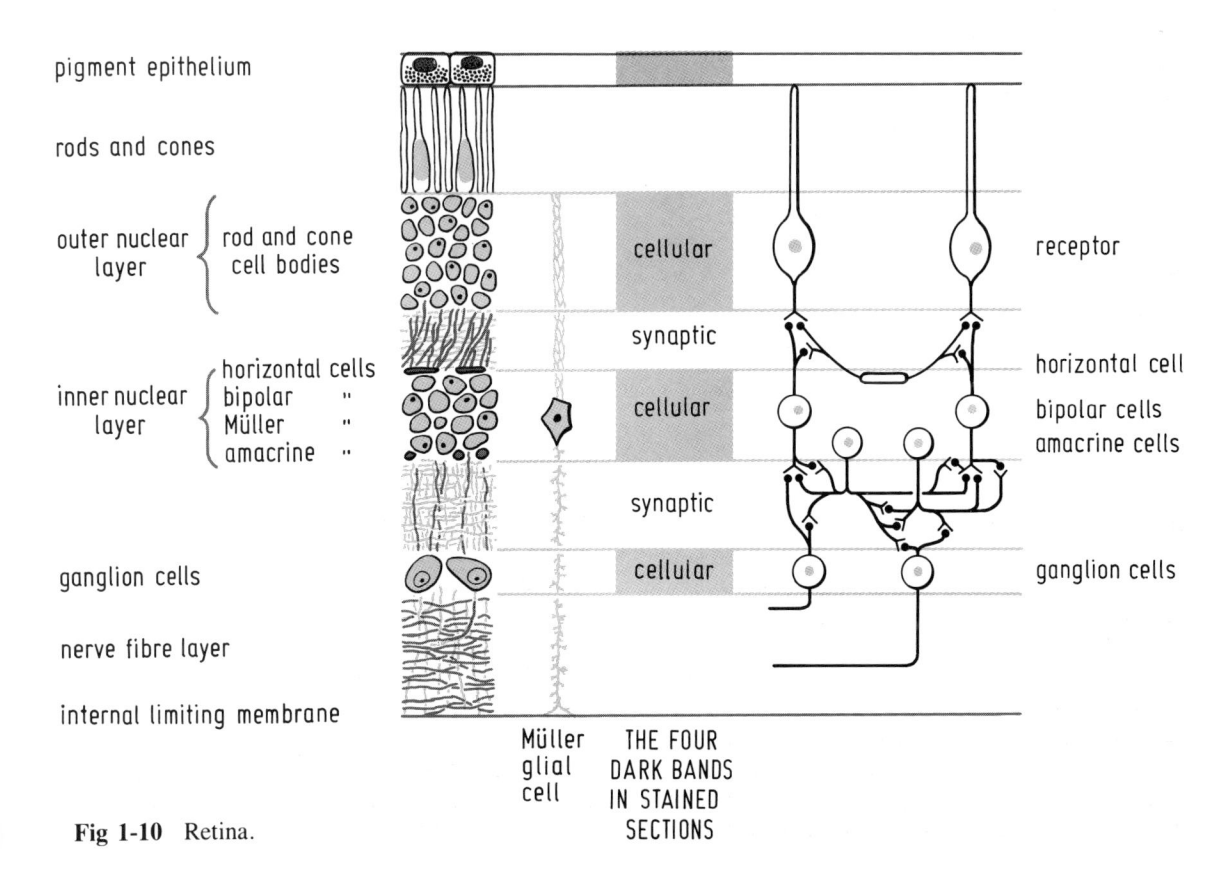

The classical interpretation is that there is a more or less direct pathway from the rods and cones and their nuclei externally to bipolar cells, and thence to ganglion cells and their nerve fibres internally. In this view the retina is vertically organized. While essentially true this is an over simplification because in fact almost 90% of nerve processes in the retina lie in the horizontal plane parallel to its surface with little more than 10% being in the vertical direction of the ultimate signal pathway. It is this most complex tangential nerve network which enables the retina to carry out, through neuronal interaction, its brain-like

Fig 1-10 Retina.

activity of property extraction, coding, and transmission.

Bipolar cell dendrites are activated directly by receptors with which they synapse, and indirectly through horizontal cells by more distant receptors. Ganglion cell dendrites are activated directly by bipolar cells with which they synapse, or indirectly through amacrine cells. An example of the effect of these alternative pathways is that when the centre of a bipolar cell's receptive field (p. 75) is stimulated the direct receptor-bipolar contact mediates an excitatory response, whereas when the periphery of the receptive field is stimulated the receptor-horizontal-bipolar contact mediates an inhibitory response. This is a mechanism for enhancing contrast. Discrete one-to-one pathways are available from the cones of the fovea to the cortex so that there can be discrimination of details and colour, but in the rest of the retina potential pathways from many receptors converge on to single ganglion cells and thus make possible increased sensitivity to weak stimuli.

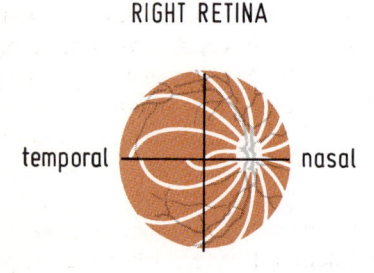

Fig 1-11 Directions of nerve fibres in the retina.

The axons of the ganglion cells form the innermost layer of the retina, the *nerve fibre layer*. Until they reach the optic disc these axons cannot be myelinated if they are to be transparent, as they must be for the retina to function. The nerve fibres in the retina all converge on the optic disc but only those from the nasal retina run a straight course. Fibres from the rest of the retina run a curved, arcuate course because they are displaced from the direct route by the large bulk of fibres from the macula (the *papillo-macular bundle*) (Figs 1-11, 15-3; Plate 7, p. 124). The entry of the nerve fibres into the optic disc is correspondingly displaced. This pattern means that lesions in or near the optic disc produce defects in the

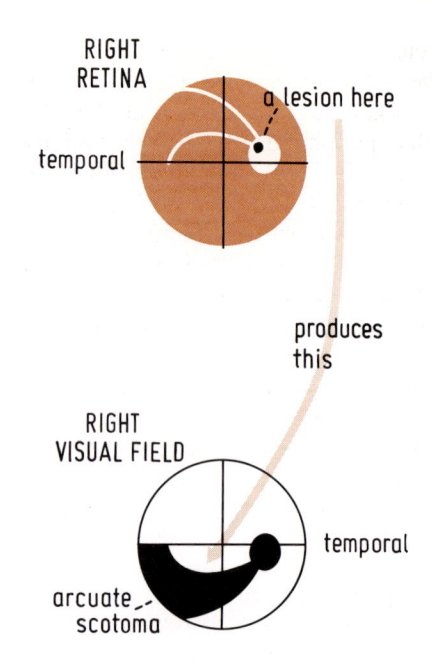

Fig 1-12 Anatomical basis of a nerve fibre bundle defect.

visual field which are quite distinctive. An example of this is the so called *nerve fibre bundle defect or arcuate scotoma* which occurs with glaucoma (Fig 1-12). The inevitable defect in the visual field caused by the optic disc itself is called the *blind spot*. From the optic disc the nerve fibres proceed by way of the optic nerve, optic chiasma, and optic tract to the lateral geniculate body.

The *visual receptors* are long, slender, highly specialized cells (Fig 1-13). Each is composed of an outer photoreceptor part united by a narrow cilium-like stalk to an inner cell body from which extends an axon with a terminal teledendron. They are of two types, the *rods* and the *cones*, which differ in detailed structure and in function. Foveal cones look superficially like rods but elsewhere in the retina cones are slightly tapered towards their tips.

The *photoreceptor segment* is composed of a stack of double membrane discs which are formed by infolding of the outer membrane (Fig 1-13). These discs contain the visual pigment molecules. In both the rods and cones the discs are continually being renewed; they are formed at the cell body end and discarded at the outer end of the receptor where the fragments are scavenged by the pigment epithelium.

The fine bridge between receptor and cell body is analogous to a cilium; it contains the ring of nine peripheral filaments or microtubules although it lacks the central two filaments of the characteristic 9 + 2 pattern. This suggests that the photoreceptors have perhaps evolved from cilia. In the *cell body* adjacent to the connecting cilium mitochondria are massed. Nearer the nucleus are ribosomes and a Golgi complex. The use of radioactively labelled aminoacids has shown that in rods protein formed here moves through the cilium to the base of the photoreceptor where it forms a transverse band which then slowly moves distally until eventually the labelled particles appear in the pigment epithelium.

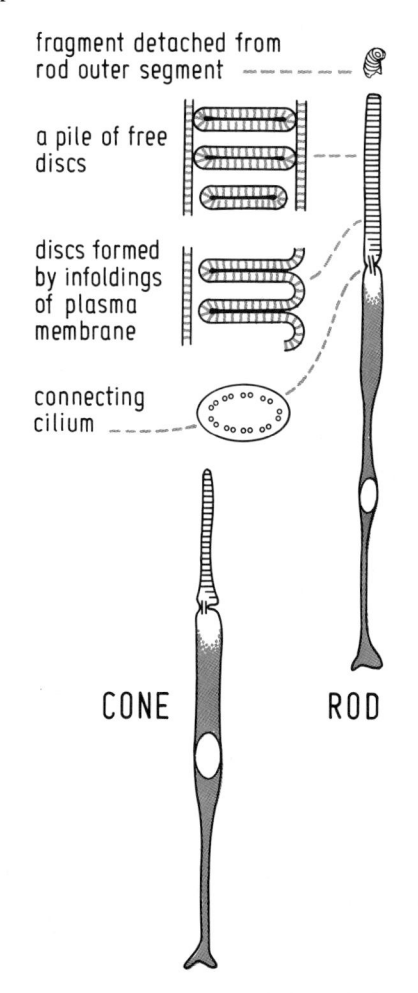

Fig 1-13 Human visual receptors.

Müller's cells are complex, elongated, giant glial cells which extend vertically through the full thickness of the neural retina from its internal surface outwards to the level of the photoreceptors. In addition to the structural framework which they provide they perform essential nutritional functions for the retinal neurones. The innermost surface of the retina, the *internal limiting membrane,* is a thick basement membrane formed by Müller's cells which has a remarkably smooth internal surface. Reflections from this glass-like membrane produce the glinting sheen which is commonly seen with an ophthalmoscope, especially in younger people.

The Optic Disc

The disc is a relatively pale, almost circular area (vertically ovoid) 1.5 to 2.0mm in diameter, 3mm nasal to the posterior pole of the globe, where the retinal nerve fibres leave and the retinal vessels enter and leave the interior of the eye (Fig 5-17).

In ophthalmoscopy the optic disc is found 15° nasal to the posterior pole, and the diameter of the disc (a *disc diameter* or dd) is used as a measuring unit. Sometimes the pigment epithelium and chorio-capillaris does not extend right up to the nerve, thus exposing a ring or crescent of white sclera (a scleral ring or crescent) (Fig 6-4). Another common normal variation is that called a pigment or choroidal crescent (Fig 6-1). This appears as a dark margin to part of the disc and is due to an accumulation of pigment epithelium (the term choroidal crescent is therefore wrong).

Most discs have a central depression, the *optic cup,* the diameter and depth of which vary from individual to individual. This physiological cupping can take the form of a small dimple, a slender funnel, a shallow hollow, a deep cup at the bottom of which the lamina cribrosa is visible, or a large excavation with overhanging edges which occupies up to 70% of the area of the optic disc (Fig 6-4). Pathological cupping, in which there is abnormal enlargement of the physiological cup, is the most important evidence of a serious type of glaucoma (Fig 6-5; Plates 1, 2, p. 121).

The periphery of the disc, especially on the nasal side, is commonly a little above the level of the surrounding retina. In some eyes this heaping up of the nerve fibres before they bend into the scleral formamen causes an appreciable elevation of the optic disc. This variation of normal anatomy is called *pseudopapilloedema* (Fig 6-7; Plate 5, p. 123). Papilloedema, with which it may be confused, is a pathological swelling or oedema of the disc (Fig 6-9; Plate 3, p. 122). This is always significant since it is caused by conditions such as increased intracranial pressure, dangerously high blood pressure, and inflammation of the optic nerve. The word papilloedema is derived from the old anatomical name for the optic disc of 'optic papilla', which also appears in the term papillo-macular bundle.

As seen with an ophthalmoscope the optic disc is a yellowish-red colour, often described as pink. The *colour* is due to a network of capilliaries among the translucent nerve fibres overlying the white lamina cribrosa. In contrast to the retina there is no layer of pigment to impart a dusky shade to the red colour. There are few nerve fibres and consequently few capillaries covering the lamina cribrosa in the region of the optic cup, which therefore looks whiter than the rest of the optic disc. The temporal part of the optic disc commonly looks paler than the nasal part.

The capillaries of the disc come mainly from the posterior ciliary arteries which pass through the adjacent sclera to the choroid (Fig 1-14). The small branches from these arteries may form an arterial circle in the sclera around the scleral foramen (the circle of Zinn) before supplying the disc and optic nerve. Contrary to expectation the disc receives little blood from the central retinal artery. On the other hand, venous drainage from the disc is mainly into the central retinal vein.

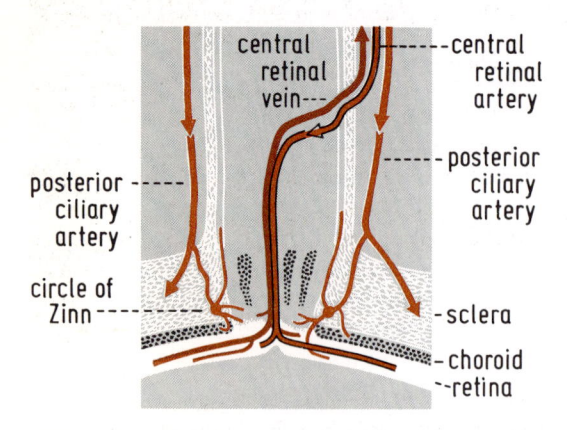

Fig 1-14 Posterior ciliary arteries and central retinal artery and vein.

The Central Area of the Retina

This region, 5 to 6mm in diameter, differs structurally and functionally from the rest of the retina. This is the part with a high concentration of cones which subserves clear form vision and colour vision (i.e. central vision), the peripheral retina being more concerned with vision in dim light and the detection of movement (peripheral vision).

The innermost part of the area centralis is called the *macula* (Fig 5-17). This is an area about the diameter of the optic disc which looks slightly darker than the surrounding retina because of heavier pigmentation of the underlying pigment epithelium. Within its periphery there are fine branches of the retinal blood vessels, but towards the centre these become more sparse until at the centre there are no blood vessels at all (Fig 1-19d). This local retinal avascularity enhances optical performance.

The *fovea* is a depression at the centre of the macula where the retina is thinned to a layer of cones only. The light of an ophthalmoscope is reflected from this concavity as from a tiny concave mirror so that its image is seen as a minute speck of light just anterior to the fovea (the foveal reflex).

The photoreceptor (outer) segments of the foveal cones are more slender (2.0 to 2.5 μm diameter) and longer than those of cones elsewhere and they are closely packed to form a fine-grained imaging surface (Fig 1-15). Since their cell bodies are more bulky (5 μm diameter) these have to be stacked in several layers. The related retinal cells with which they connect (bipolar, horizontal, amacrine and ganglion) take up even more room. They are accommodated by being displaced radially away from their cones, and the thickness of the retina gradually increases from the centre. As a consequence the foveal cones have long axons (up to 500 μm) and sweep horizontally in the retina. The centrifugal displacement of inner retinal cells continues outwards from the fovea to a gradually diminishing extent for about 3mm, that is nearly to the optic disc on its nasal side. Within this area the axons of the photoreceptors, both those of the fovea and those of their neighbours surrounding the fovea, form a layer more or less parallel to the surface of the retina, *Henle's layer*. In some retinal disorders hard exudates (p. 143) are radially orientated by the fibres of Henle's layer and can be seen with an ophthalmoscope as a 'macular fan' or 'macular star'.

The Retinal Blood Vessels

These arise from the *central retinal artery* which in turn is a branch of the ophthalmic artery. It enters the optic nerve about 1cm behind the globe and appears internally in the optic disc on the nasal side of the optic cup (Fig 1-14). It divides variably into branches which supply four quadrants of the retina (the superior temporal, inferior temporal, inferior nasal, and superior nasal quadrants) (Fig 5-17). The retinal veins from each of the four quadrants converge to form the *central retinal vein* on or in the optic disc and this vein leaves the eye in contact with and on the temporal side of the central retinal artery.

There is slight expansile pulsation of the retinal *arteries* on or near the optic disc but this is only seen with greater than usual ophthalmoscopic magnification. Pulsation is increased and becomes visible when the diastolic blood pressure approximates the intraocular pressure. This can occur either when diastolic pressure drops, as in aortic incompetence, or when intraocular pressure is raised above about 50mm Hg as in severe glaucoma.

A collapsing pulsation of one or more *veins* on the optic disc occurs spontaneously or can be induced by slightly increasing the intraocular pressure by gentle finger pressure on the globe through the lower lid. The intravascular pressure in the retinal veins is normally just greater than the intraocular pressure, otherwise the veins would collapse, and, because of the direction of blood flow, it must be lowest in the veins on the optic disc just before they leave the eye (Fig 1-16). With each systolic influx of blood into the intraocular uveal blood vessels there is a transient increase of intraocular pressure to above the level of the lowest venous pressure with consequent collapse of this part of the vein.

The central retinal vein crosses the subarachnoid space as it leaves the optic nerve about 1cm behind the globe (Fig 1-14). Here it is exposed to the CSF pressure and the intravenous pressure must be higher than the CSF pressure (110mm water = 8mm Hg) for blood to flow. If the CSF pressure rises the extraocular venous pressure will rise correspondingly. When the CSF pressure is higher than the intraocular pressure (15mm Hg = 200mm water) the intraocular venous pressure also rises to be higher than the intraocular pressure. The latter does not then control the intraocular venous pressure and pulsation of the retinal veins does not occur (Fig 1-16).

Retinal arteries and veins branch irregularly and between branchings a vessel does not taper but retains the same width. The terminal arterioles

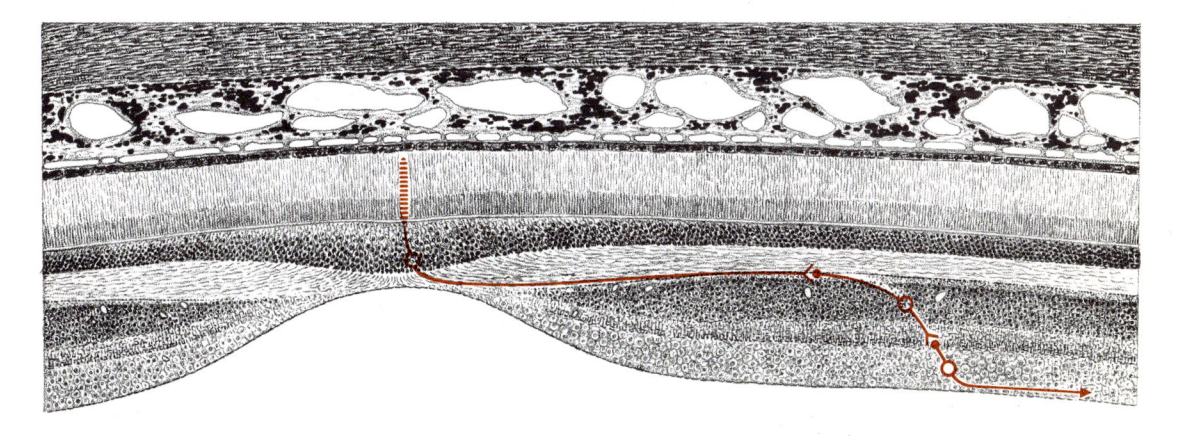

Fig 1-15 Transverse section through the fovea. In the centre there are only slender closely packed cone outer segments and several layers of cone cell bodies. Their indirect blood supply from the choriocapillaris is mediated by the pigment epithelium. Long cone axons run obliquely as Henle's layer to the centrifugally displaced cells of the inner retina. Where there are no inner retinal layers there are no retinal capillaries.

come off at almost right angles as side arm branches from the parent vessel.

The branches of the retinal artery and vein lie in the nerve fibre layer. The capillary network between them is found only in the portion of retina internal to the bipolar cells, the visual cells being nourished by the choriocapillaris (Fig 1-17). There are no large vessels in the central area of the retina and not even capillaries in the foveal retina where there are no internal retinal layers. In about one-quarter of all eyes a small artery appears over the temporal edge of the optic disc and this may be a *cilio-retinal artery* derived from a posterior ciliary artery (Plate 9, p. 125). The branches of the retinal arteries do not anastomose so that occlusion of one branch cannot be compensated for by neighbouring branches and loss of function in the territory supplied ensues.

The walls of the retinal vessels are normally transparent and therefore what one sees with an ophthalmoscope is the contained blood and not the blood vessels. Compared with their companion veins the arteries look narrower, are a brighter (arterial) red in colour and reflect the ophthalmoscope light more brightly from their convex surfaces. This linear reflection is called the vessel *light reflex*; it obscures about the middle third of the width of an artery, which at first sight may be mistakenly interpreted as a double blood column, whereas the venous light reflex occupies about one-fifth of the width of the vein. Arteries commonly cross veins *(AV crossings)* and less commonly veins cross arteries. At these crossings the two vessels are uniquely intimate with merging of their adventitial sheaths. As a consequence pathological changes in the arteries can modify the appearance of AV crossings.

The endothelial cells of the retinal capillaries and the 'tight' junctions between them are impermeable even to small molecules such as fluorescein (molecular weight 376). The choroidal capillaries are freely permeable to large molecules but these are prevented from diffusing from the choroid into the retina by the retinal pigment epithelium. Together the retinal endothelium and epithelium form a barrier to diffusion, the *blood-retina barrier,* which screens the retina from unwanted molecules and, by maintaining a tissue fluid with few large light-scattering molecules, enhances the transparency of the retina (Fig 1-18).

The blood-retina barrier enables the details of the retinal blood vessels to be examined clinically by *fluorescein angiography* (Fig 1-19). In this technique the fluorescent dye fluorescein is injected intravenously and the retina photographed while the blood containing the fluorescein is passing through the eye. Photographic filters are used so that only fluorescent light emitted from within the vessels reaches the film and a detailed image of the vessels is thus obtained. However if the vessels are damaged fluorescein leaks from them and the altered permeability is thus detected as a diffuse and persisting fluorescence (Figs 7-6; 8-5).

Mean ocular arterial pressure (60),
venous pressure (15.5),
tissue pressure (IOP)(15),
extraocular venous pressure (8).

Pressures at systolic IOP; increased venous collapse

Pressures at diastolic IOP; decreased venous collapse

Pressures when extraocular venous pressure higher than IOP; venous distension

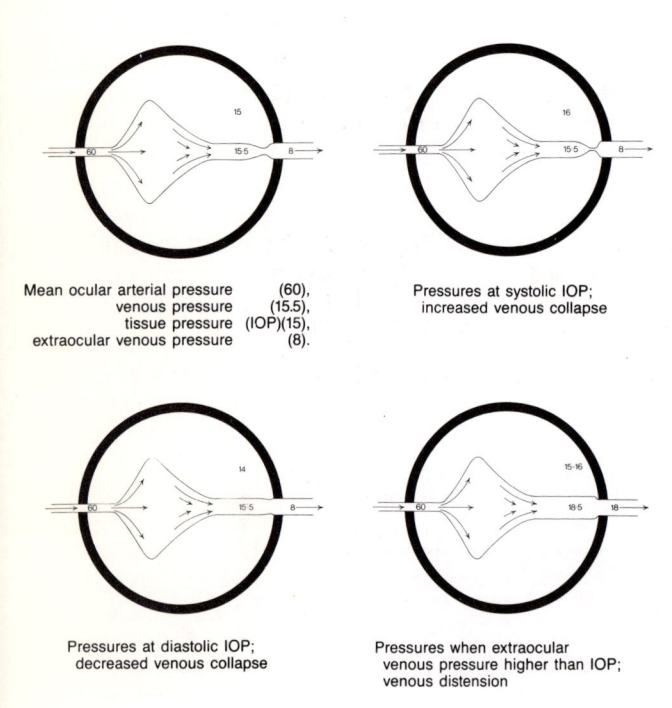

Fig 1-16 The haemodynamic consequences of blood flow into, through and out of a pressurized chamber. The IOP governs venous pressures within the eye. Therefore the ocular perfusion pressure (arterial inflow pressure minus venous outflow pressure) is arterial pressure minus IOP. Normally, venous pressure outside the eye has no effect on venous pressures within the eye. But if extraocular venous pressure is abnormally high and exceeds IOP, it is then the pressure which governs venous pressures within the eye. Pressures in mm Hg.

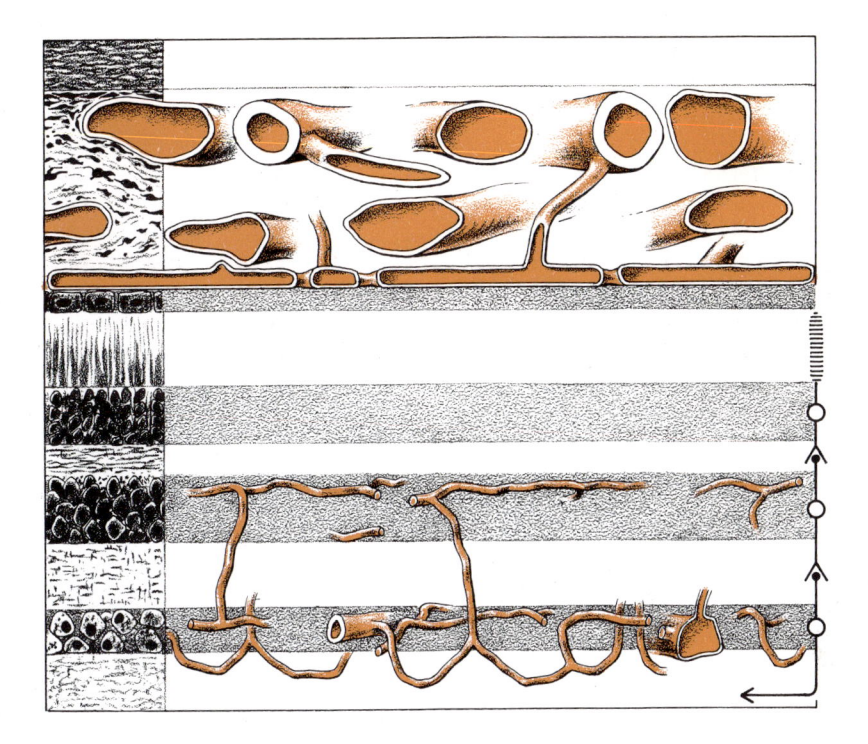

Fig 1-17 The two separate systems of retinal blood supply. The choroid, with a blood flow that is twenty times more than that in the retinal vessels, supplies from without the pigment epithelium and through it the outer half of the retina, while the retinal vessels penetrate the inner half of the retina which they supply. Superficial capillaries in the nerve fibre layer as shown here occur only where the retina is thicker in the neighbourhood of the optic disc and macula.

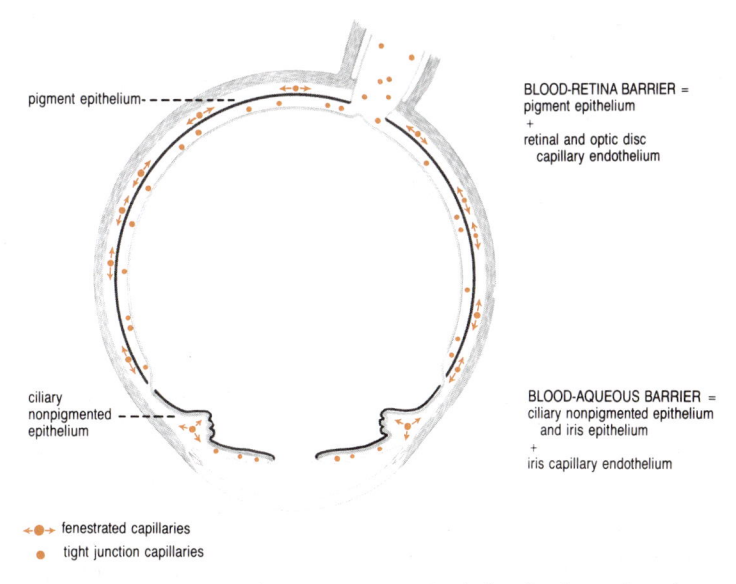

Fig 1-18 Blood-ocular barriers. Like the blood-brain barrier these obstacles to diffusion exclude from the retina unwanted molecules circulating in the blood.

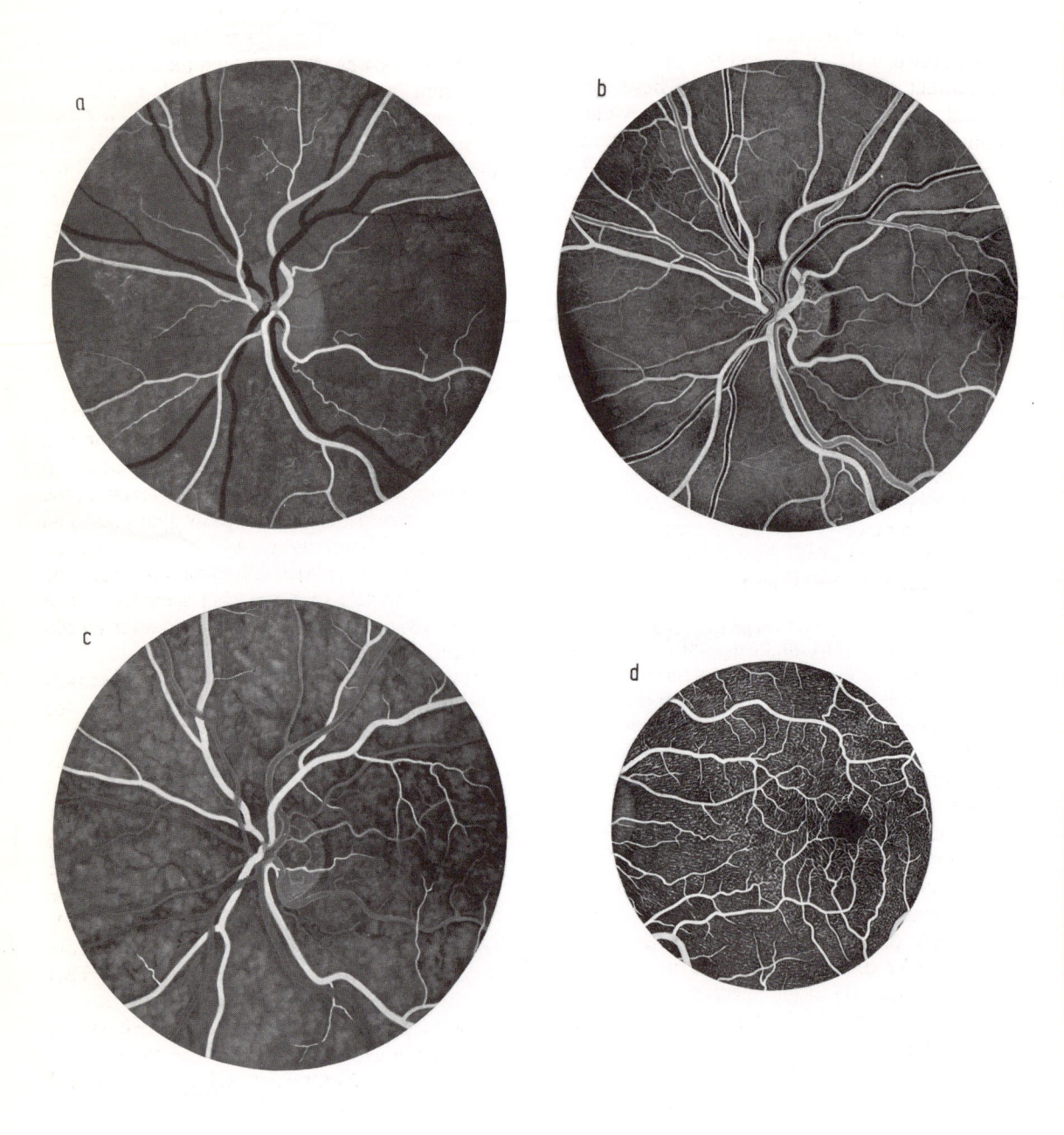

Fig 1-19 Normal sequence of fluorescein angiograms at different times after intra-venous injection of fluorescein, (a) at 10 sec (arterial phase), (b) at 12 sec (arterio-venous phase) and (c) at 20 sec (venous phase). Until all the venous blood contains fluorescein the laminar nature of flow in veins is apparent. (d) taken in the arterio-venous phase, shows the normal retinal capillary net in the peripheral part and the avascularity of the central part of the macula.

ANATOMY

The Optic Nerve

The optic nerve, being the axons of the ganglion cells between the globe and the optic chiasma, is a direct extension of the brain. These afferent visual and pupillary nerve fibres essentially constitute a tract of white matter; the myelinated axons run in a neuroglial framework and are enclosed in a meningeal sheath, the *optic nerve sheath*. The dural sheath is continuous at one end with the sclera and at the other with the dura of the optic canal of the skull. Between the arachnoid and pia sheathing the optic nerve there is a continuation of the sub-arachnoid space containing cerebrospinal fluid.

The nerve is conventionally considered in four parts:

1. The *intraocular* part, about 1mm long, occupies the scleral foramen. The optic disc is its ophthalmoscopically visible internal end. The diameter of this portion increases from 1.5mm internally to 3.0mm externally due to the acquisition of myelin sheaths by the nerve fibres.

2. The *orbital* portion runs backwards within the cone formed by the four rectus muscles of the eye. This part is tortuous and the nerve is therefore not stretched when the eye moves. The central retinal artery and central retinal vein pass through the meninges, cross the sub-arachnoid space, and enter the nerve about 1cm behind the globe. The pin-head sized *ciliary ganglion*, through which pass sensory fibres from the cornea and iris and sympathetic fibres to the iris dilator and in which parasympathetic fibres to the iris sphincter and ciliary muscle synapse, lies on the lateral side of the nerve near the apex of the orbit. An injection of local anaesthetic in this region, as well as paralysing the extra-ocular muscles, will therefore anaesthetize the eye and paralyse the intraocular muscles.

3. The *intracanalicular* part lies with the ophthalmic artery in the optic canal between the apex of the orbit and its intracranial opening anterolateral to the pituitary fossa.

4. The *intracranial* part is the short length before the nerve joins with the optic nerve of the other side to form the optic chiasma.

The Lens

The lens provides the adjustable part of the eye's refractive power. It lies behind the aqueous and in front of the vitreous; together with its *suspensory zonule* and the ciliary body it forms a second sort of diaphragm behind the iris diaphragm. Between the lens and the iris is the slit-like posterior chamber, while in the pupillary aperture the anterior lens surface is a boundary of the anterior chamber.

It is biconvex with the curvature of the posterior surface being greater than that of the anterior. It is about 9mm in diameter, about 5mm thick and the size increases slowly with age. Any opacity of the lens is called a *cataract*.

In youth the lens is transparent and colourless but with age it becomes less transparent and develops a yellowish colouration. This reduction in transparency can reduce the light reaching the retina to one-third of the amount that passed in youth and it can, by giving the pupil a grey appearance in oblique illumination, trap the unwary into falsely diagnosing a cataract. The yellow change can act as a filter to alter an old person's perception of colour.

Because it is transparent it has no blood vessels and it therefore depends on the aqueous for metabolic exchanges.

Externally there is an elastic *capsule* which is much thicker anteriorly than posteriorly and which is thicker towards the periphery than it is over the centre of the lens. The lens capsule is the unusually thick basement membrane of the underlying lens epithelium (the anterior capsule is the thickest basement membrane in the body). The suspensory zonule is attached to the capsule anterior and posterior to the lens equator. This attachment is quickly weakened by the enzyme alpha chymotrypsin, a solution of which can be used in the eye during the operation of intra-capsular cataract extraction to facilitate removal of the lens.

Beneath the capsule of the anterior surface only is a single layer of *lens epithelium*. At the equator these cells elongate markedly to become the *lens fibres*.

The *lens substance* is made up of lens fibres. They continue to be formed throughout life, later ones on the surface progressively enclosing the older central ones which lose their nuclei and are compressed to form a lens *nucleus*. This explains the layered onion-skin-like appearance of the lens so obvious when seen in an optical section with the slit-lamp microscope (Fig 5-5). After about the age of thirty years the nucleus of the lens becomes hard and insoluble so that if removal is necessary this cannot be done piecemeal as is possible at a younger age. The newer, still soft and soluble, living lens fibres surrounding the nucleus constitute the *cortex*.

The lens fibres run from the region of the equator towards the anterior and posterior poles, enclosing the earlier formed fibres. They are not long enough to reach from one pole to the other and those that end nearest the centre on one face terminate furthest from the centre on the opposite face. The ends of the fibres abut on each other along lines called *lens sutures* (Fig 1-20). The simplest pattern of sutures in the human lens is a triradiate branched one and these are the Y sutures seen with the slit-lamp microscope in front of and behind the central nucleus (Fig 5-3). (The anterior Y is erect, the posterior Y is inverted.)

When the zonule is relaxed in *accommodation* the anterior surface and to a lesser degree the posterior surface of the lens become more curved, especially centrally so that their shape becomes aspheric, the anterior surface and the equator of the lens are moved forwards, the lens diameter is reduced and the lens nucleus is thickened.

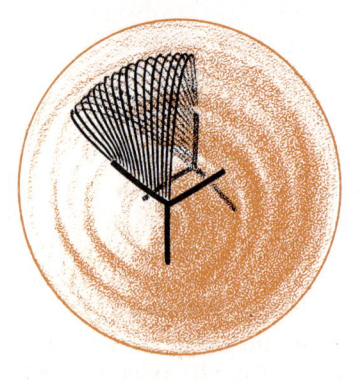

Fig 1-20 Terminations of the lens fibres form the Y sutures of the lens.

The Vitreous

The vitreous body is a transparent avascular jelly which fills the posterior segment (not the posterior chamber) of the globe behind the lens. Aqueous diffuses through it and it can be thought of as aqueous which is converted into a gel by the presence of micellae composed of very fine delicate collagen fibrils and an acid mucopolysaccharide, hyaluronic acid. These are most effective in creating a gel since the vitreous is 98% water. As with most gels there is a surface condensation (the hyaloid membrane).

The vitreous is normally attached to its surrounds at two sites, these being the limits of the retina anteriorly at the ora serrata and posteriorly around the margin of the optic disc. Abnormal attachments to the overlying retina can develop and these are a cause of holes forming in the retina with consequent retinal detachment if, as commonly happens with the passing years, the vitreous shrinks and separates posteriorly from the retina (Fig 1-21). When there are no vitreo-retinal adhesions this shrinkage is of no significance, the space between the gel surface and retina being filled with aqueous-like sol.

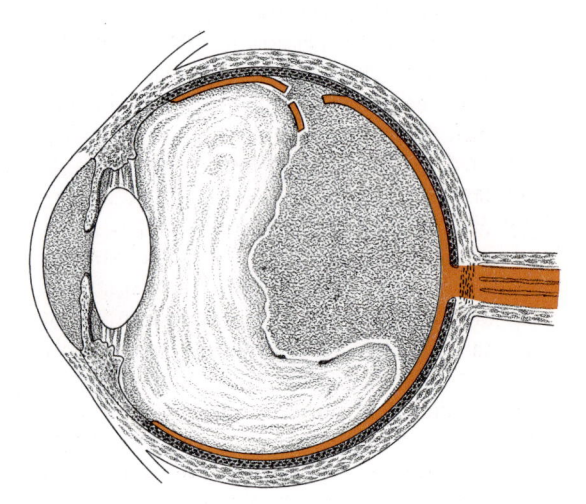

Fig 1-21 Senile shrinkage and posterior detachment of the vitreous. In this case in which there had been an abnormal vitreo-retinal adhesion a hole has been torn in the retina which is starting to detach. The normal attachment of the vitreous to the margin of the optic disc has also separated and would be seen with an ophthalmoscope as an opaque distorted ring. The space between the collapsed vitreous and the retina is filled with fluid similar to aqueous.

ANATOMY

The Aqueous Humour

This clear liquid, similar in composition to protein-free plasma, fills the anterior and posterior chambers. It is secreted by the ciliary processes into the posterior chamber from which it flows through the pupil into the anterior chamber. It seeps from the anterior chamber through the trabeculae into the canal of Schlemm. It is the nutritive medium for the lens and to a large extent for the cornea.

The Anterior Chamber (AC)

This aqueous-filled space is bounded anteriorly by the posterior corneal surface, posteriorly by the anterior surface of the iris and the lens, and peripherally by the angle of the anterior chamber where the corneo-sclera with the canal of Schlemm meets the ciliary body and iris.

The angle of the anterior chamber is of great clinical interest because it is the region where aqueous leaves the eye. If it becomes blocked, e.g. by the periphery of the iris coming into contact with the periphery of the cornea, the aqueous cannot escape and therefore the intra-ocular pressure rises. This increase in intraocular pressure is called glaucoma.

In antero-posterior section the AC is shaped like a plano-convex lens; it is 2.5 to 3.0mm deep centrally and narrows to a blunt angle peripherally (Fig 9-3a). The depth of the AC is genetically determined and some eyes have a *shallow AC* (depth less than 2mm) with a slit-like periphery (Fig 9-3b). In these eyes the AC is shaped more like a concavo-convex lens and the *angle* is said to be *narrow* (in contrast to the more common open angle). As a result of this anatomical variation it is these eyes which are susceptible to angle-closure glaucoma.

The angle is invisible to unaided clinical inspection because light reflected from it undergoes total internal reflection at the cornea-air surface and is therefore unable to leave the eye. This difficulty is overcome and the angle inspected by placing a contact lens on the cornea, a technique known as *gonioscopy*. The contact lens used is either one with an anterior surface more steeply curved than that of the cornea or one with a flat anterior surface and an internal mirror in which the chamber angle can be seen (Fig 1-22).

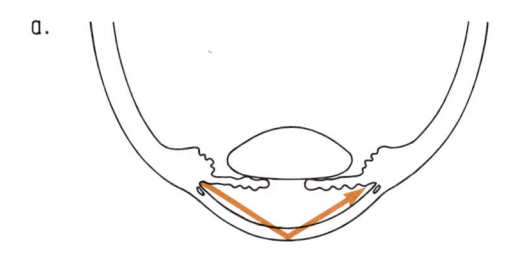

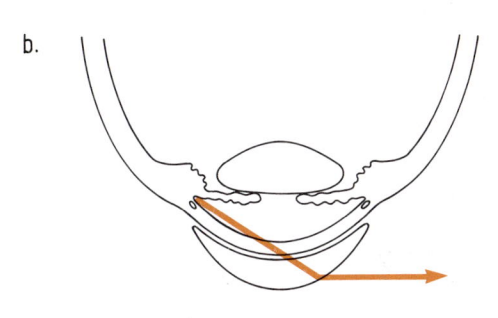

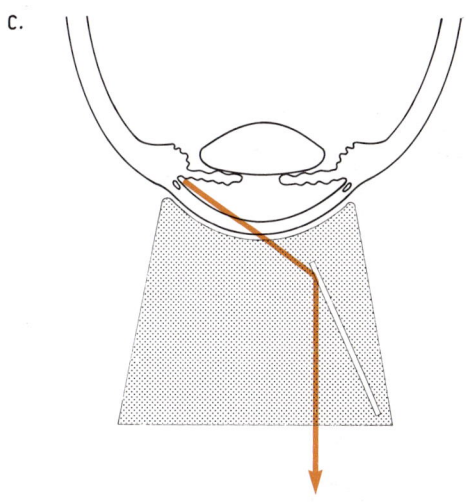

Fig 1-22 The optics of gonioscopy.

a Light reflected from the angle of the anterior chamber cannot emerge from the cornea because of total internal reflection.

b Light can emerge through a contact lens with an anterior surface more convex than that of the cornea.

c Light emerges from the anterior surface of a Goldmann contact lens after being reflected by the mirror within the solid plastic lens. It can be conveniently seen with a slit-lamp microscope.

THE ORBITS AND THE OCULAR APPENDAGES

The Orbits

The bony orbits are the sockets which contain the eyeballs and their muscles, nerves and blood vessels, the levator muscle of the upper lid, the lacrimal gland, the lacrimal sac, much fluid fat as packing, and a few nerves and vessels which pass through. The anterior opening of the orbit, the orbital *margin,* is not continuous; medially the upper margin spirals behind the inferior margin thereby creating the *lacrimal fossa* in which the lacrimal sac lies (Fig 1-23). Each orbit is approximately pyramidial in shape with *apex* posteriorly and four *walls*—medial, roof, lateral and floor. The medial walls of the two orbits are parallel while the two lateral walls are at an angle of 90° (Fig 1-24). The axes of the two orbits are at an angle of 45°; this perhaps explains why a sightless eye diverges.

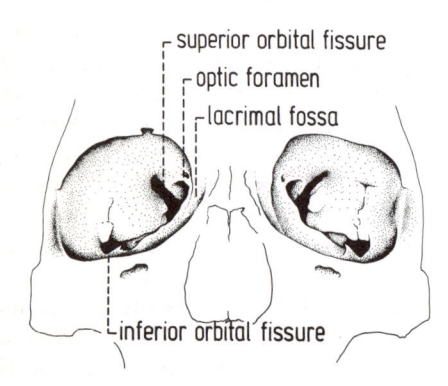

Fig 1-23 Orbital margins and apical openings from in front.

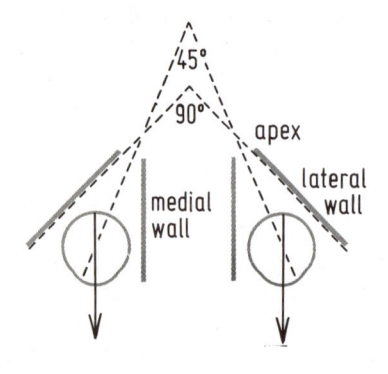

Fig 1-24 Orbital walls from above.

At the apex there are openings through which pass the optic nerve (the optic canal), the motor and sensory nerves to the eye, and the blood vessels. The four rectus muscles arise from the apex of the orbit. The inferior oblique muscle arises anteriorly from the infero-medial angle of the orbit and the effective or physiological origin of the superior oblique muscle, the trochlea, is directly above this on the supero-medial angle of the orbit. The anatomical origin of the superior oblique muscle is at the apex of the orbit. The levator palpebrae muscle also arises at the orbital apex.

The eyeball occupies only about one-fifth of the volume of the orbit and is situated anteriorly in the orbit just within the protective orbital margin.

The lacrimal gland lies in a shallow depression superolaterally just posterior to the orbital margin.

The orbits are related to the frontal sinus superiorly, the maxillary sinus inferiorly, and the ethmoidal and sphenoidal sinuses medially.

The Eyelids, Conjunctiva, Tenon's Capsule

The *lids*, upper and lower, are mobile folds which are essential for the wellbeing of the eye. Covered with skin on the outside and conjunctiva on the inside, each is stiffened by an internal plate of dense connective tissue (the *tarsus*) and contains the muscles and muscular insertions which move it. The free edges, the lid margins, which meet medially at the rounded *medial canthus* and laterally at the angular *lateral canthus,* form the boundaries of an adjustable opening in front of the eye, the *palpebral opening* (Fig 1-25). When the lids are normally open and the eye is directed straight ahead, the upper lid margin usually covers the uppermost 2 or 3mm of the cornea and the lower lid margin is at or just below the lower corneal margin. In infants, however, the upper lid margin is usually at or just above the upper corneal margin. The upper lid moves more than the lower lid and when it rises it moves backwards as well as upwards.

In addition to the cornea and conjunctiva-covered sclera, the following features are readily seen around and within the palpebral opening.

On the lid margins, which are about 2mm deep, are two or three irregular rows of eyelashes and

ANATOMY

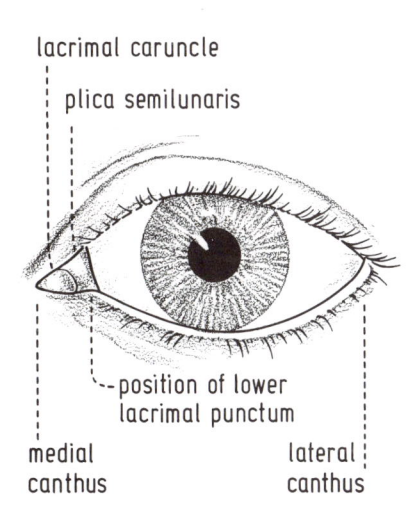

Fig 1-25 Palpebral fissure landmarks.

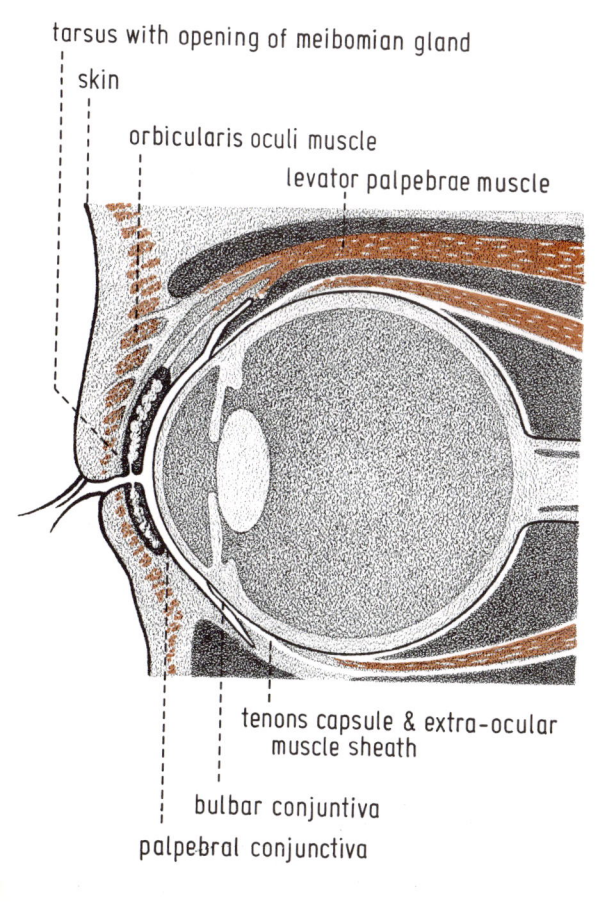

Fig 1-26 Saggital section of the lids and globe.

the openings of the *tarsal* (Meibomian) *glands*. These modified sebaceous glands are within the tarsus and if the lid is everted they show up as a series of cream streaks, perpendicular to the lid margin, beneath the conjunctiva. The secretion of the tarsal glands prevents tears from flowing over the lid margins and, as a very thin possibly monomolecular layer on its surface, retards evaporation of the corneal tear film.

Near the medial end of the lid margin is the *lacrimal punctum* which is the entrance into the lacrimal passages by way of which tears drain from the surface of the eye into the nose. The lower lacrimal punctum is directed posteriorly and it cannot be seen without slightly everting the lower lid.

A short horizontal ridging of the skin medial to the medial canthus is due to the underlying *medial palpebral ligament*, a stout fibrous tissue band which anchors the medial ends of the upper and lower tarsi to the bone in front of the upper part of the lacrimal fossa.

Deep to the medial canthus is a small pink nodule, the *caruncle*, which is a developmentally displaced piece of lower lid. It has hairs and contains sebaceous glands which produce the small blob of white secretion often found at the inner canthus. Immediately temporal to the caruncle is a small crescentic fold of conjunctiva, the *plica semilunaris*, which is a vestigial structure homologous with a nictitating membrane.

Two sets of antagonistic *muscles* close and open the lids. The *orbicularis oculi muscle* is an oval, subcutaneous sheet of sphincter-like muscle surrounding the palpebral opening from the eyebrows above to the cheek below (Fig 1-26). It is innervated by the seventh cranial nerve. Inability to close the lids or to blink fully in facial palsy is the most serious consequence of paralysis of this nerve. A reflex upward rotation of the eye (Bell's phenomenon) occurs with lid closure; this may mitigate the effects of a seventh nerve lesion (Bell's palsy). The orbicularis muscle aids the drainage of tears by virtue of a pumping action it exerts on the lacrimal sac; this explains the almost involuntary increase in blinking which occurs when an overflow of tears threatens.

The *levator palpebrae superioris muscle* arises at the apex of the orbit and runs forward to a wide insertion in the upper lid. It is innervated, along with four of the extraocular muscles, by the third cranial nerve. Inability to raise the upper lid is an obvious feature of a total lesion of the third nerve. Paralytic drooping of the upper lid, partial or total, is called ptosis and may be congenital due to maldevelopment of the muscle or its nerve supply. A small non-striated muscle, the *superior palpebral muscle of Müller,* is associated with the levator of the upper lid. This is supplied by the cervical sympathetic, a lesion of which results in a slight ptosis and miosis of the pupil (Horner's syndrome).

The **conjunctiva** is the transparent mucous membrane which covers the deep surface of the lids (the *palpebral* conjunctiva) and the anterior surface of the eyeball except for the cornea (the *bulbar* conjunctiva). The cul-de-sac where the one becomes continuous with the other is known as the *conjunctival fornix* and the potential space enclosed is called the *conjunctival sac.*

The conjunctiva is quite vascular but the vessels are usually constricted and not apparent. They rapidly dilate with irritation or inflammation of the conjunctiva (or of the anterior part of the eyeball) to cause a red eye (conjunctival injection or hyperaemia).

There are numerous mucus-secreting goblet cells in the conjunctiva. The mucus is obviously a lubricant and also by wetting the corneal epithelium it aids in the formation of a covering film of tears. Small accessory lacrimal glands in the conjunctiva are a secondary source of tears. Lymphoid tissue lies immediately under the conjunctival epithelium (the adenoid layer) and visible lymphoid follicles develop in this layer in some types of conjunctivitis. Hypertrophy of the conjunctival follicles commonly occurs in children concurrently with hypertrophy of the similar lymphoid tissue in the tonsils and the adenoids.

Tenon's capsule is a name given to the condensation of fibrous tissue which, like a capsule, encloses the sclera. It is loosely attached to the underlying sclera and to the overlying conjunctiva or orbital fat except anteriorly where, about 3mm from the limbus, it fuses with the conjunctiva and sclera. Because of this layer the bulbar conjunctiva can move freely on the sclera except adjacent to the limbus. At the insertions of the extraocular muscles it becomes continuous with the muscle sheaths.

The Lacrimal Apparatus

The *lacrimal gland* lies just behind the upper and outer orbital margin (Fig 1-27). The tears it secretes enter the conjunctival sac through about a dozen short ducts. Its parasympathetic nerve supply from the lacrimal nucleus runs by way of the facial nerve, greater superficial petrosal nerve, and vidian nerve to a synapse in the spheno-palatine ganglion and thence by branches of the maxillary division of the fifth cranial nerve.

The *lacrimal passages* consist of the upper and lower lacrimal puncta and canaliculi, the lacrimal sac, and the naso-lacrimal duct. The *punctum and canaliculus* of the upper lid are quite inefficient and unable to drain the normal tear production if the lower lid punctum and canaliculus cease to function. The *lacrimal sac* is merely that upper part of the naso-lacrimal duct which lies in the

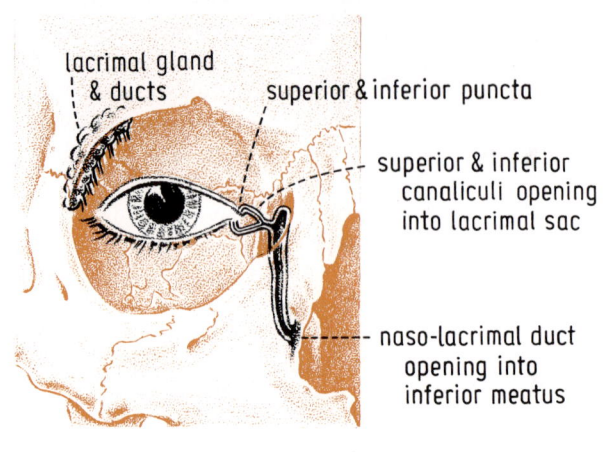

Fig 1-27 Lacrimal apparatus.

orbit in the lacrimal fossa. This hollow can be felt with a finger tip immediately below and behind the medial palpebral ligament.

The *naso-lacrimal duct* is the continuation of the lacrimal sac downwards into the nose, where it opens into the inferior meatus. Folds of the lining mucosa near this opening have a valve-like action and prevent reverse flow. The naso-lacrimal duct develops as a solid chord of cells which is later canalized. Often this is not complete at birth with resulting 'congenital obstruction of the naso-lacrimal duct'. This usually resolves spontaneously, especially if encouraged by regular gentle fingertip pressure on the lacrimal sac.

Opening and closing the lids as in normal blinking has a pumping effect on the lacrimal sac; with closure tears are drawn into the sac and with opening they are expressed into the nose.

Watering of the eyes can be caused by overproduction of tears (lacrimation) or by faulty drainage (epiphora). The former is caused by local irritation, emotional stimuli, or, rarely, following a facial nerve lesion when salivary gland secretory fibres find their way to the lacrimal gland (crocodile tears). Epiphora can result from displacement of the lower lid or from congenital, traumatic, inflammatory, or degenerative obstruction of any part of the lacrimal passages.

Although man's evolutionary emergence from an aquatic environment is very distant, our eyes are still under water. The essential covering of fluid is very thin, only 7 or 8 μm thick over the cornea, but without it the surface soon degenerates. The secretion of the lacrimal glands is the main component of the *tear film* which covers conjunctiva and cornea; the other constituents are mucus from the conjunctival glands and lipids from the tarsal glands. The pre-corneal tear film is a true film in that it resists gravity. It is renewed with each blink when the upper lid draws fluid up over the cornea from the meniscus of tears which lies along the lower lid margin. It is readily seen with the slit-lamp microscope especially if stained with the dye fluorescein.

Normal tears contain several antimicrobial substances which along with their mechanical flushing and mucus trapping help rid the conjunctival sac of pathogenic bacteria and fungi. Lysozyme, an ancient antibacterial enzyme found in plants as well as animals, was discovered in tears by Fleming in 1922 before his discovery of penicillin. Betalysin, lactoferrin, ceruloplasmin, IgA and IgC in tears also help in the defence of the ocular surface.

The Extraocular Muscles

There are four *rectus muscles* (superior, lateral, inferior, and medial) and two *oblique muscles* (superior and inferior) attached to each eye. The recti are inserted (at sites corresponding to their names) anterior to the centre of rotation of the globe; the obliques are inserted (at sites corresponding to their names) posterior to the centre of rotation (Fig 1-28). The vertical recti (i.e. superior and inferior) run forwards and outwards (in the line of the orbital axis) from their origin at the apex of the orbit; the obliques run backwards and outwards from their effective origins at the front of the medial wall of the orbit. With this information the actions of each muscle in all directions of gaze of the eye can be derived from elementary mechanics. (This is what should be memorized, not the tables which follow.) Fig 1-29 may help in the visualisation of the vertical rectus and oblique muscles of a patient who is facing you.

The lateral rectus is innervated by the sixth cranial nerve, the superior oblique by the fourth cranial nerve and the other four muscles by the third cranial nerve.

Movements of the Globe

Monocular Movements

All movements of each eye can be analysed into rotations about three axes — vertical, horizontal, and anteroposterior.

The rotations are named as follows:

Axis of rotation	Direction in which front of eye moves	Name of movement
vertical	medially	adduction
vertical	laterally	abduction
horizontal	up	elevation
horizontal	down	depression
anteroposterior	upper pole medially (inward twist)	intorsion
anteroposterior	upper pole laterally (outward twist)	extorsion

The *primary position* of the eye is the term given to the position of the globe when it is directed straight ahead with the head held vertically erect. The *visual axis* is the line from the fovea to the point of fixation.

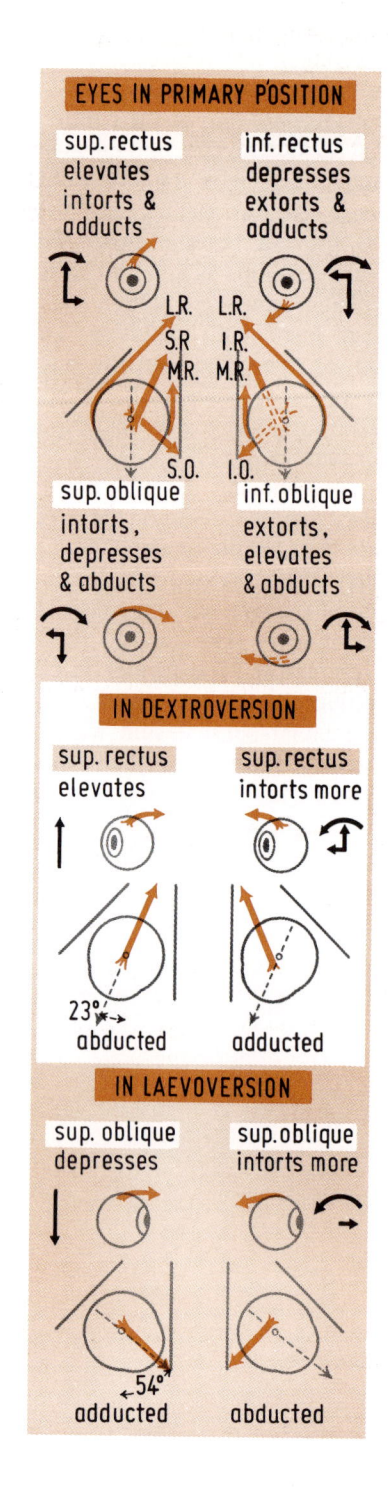

Fig 1-28 Actions of the extraocular muscles. Schematic representations of the orbits from above and of the globes from in front.

ANATOMY

The actions of the individual muscles from the primary position are:

lateral rectus — abduction
medial rectus — adduction

superior rectus — elevation, intorsion, adduction
inferior rectus — depression, extorsion, adduction

superior oblique — depression, intorsion, abduction
inferior oblique — elevation, extorsion, abduction

The major action of the vertical recti and of the obliques differs with the position of the globe. For example, when the globe is abducted 23° its axis coincides with that of the vertical recti and these then have only elevating or depressing actions respectively; when the globe is adducted the superior rectus becomes a more effective intorter and is less effective as an elevator, while the inferior rectus becomes a more effective extorter and a less effective depressor; the superior oblique is most effective as a depressor when the globe is fully adducted and has no depressing action when the globe is fully abducted.

This difference in action in different positions of gaze is made much use of clinically in determining which of the extraocular muscles is affected when eye movements are not normal. For example, if there is impairment of elevation of the right eye and this is greater in adduction than it is in abduction, the right inferior oblique and not the right superior rectus is at fault.

In an eye movement all six muscles work together, but for each rotation the principal muscles are as follows:

adduction — medial rectus; also superior and inferior recti
abduction — lateral rectus; also superior and inferior obliques

elevation — superior rectus, inferior oblique
depression — inferior rectus, superior oblique
intorsion — superior rectus, superior oblique
extorsion — inferior rectus, inferior oblique

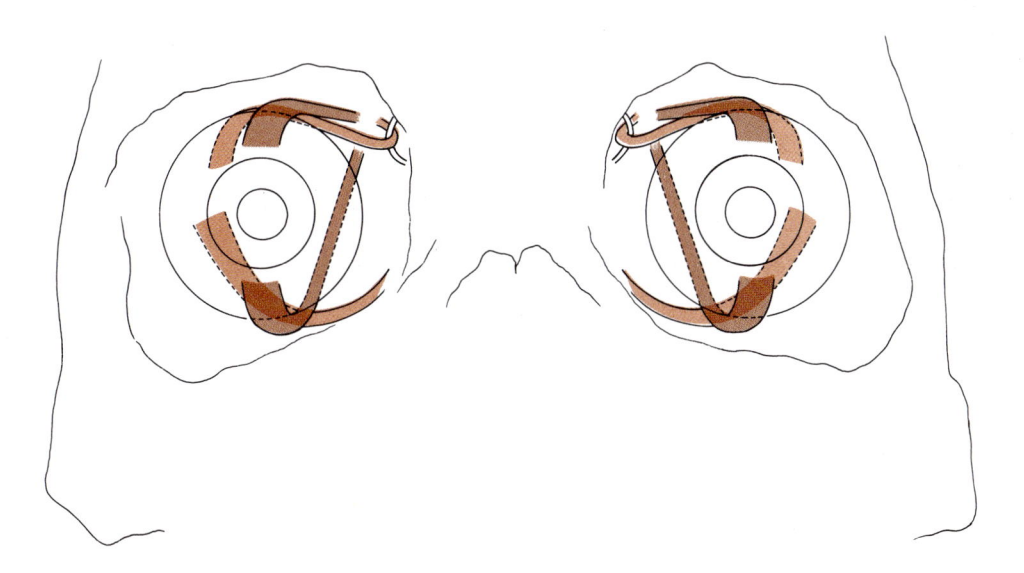

Fig 1-29 Vertically acting extraocular muscles: superior rectus, inferior rectus; superior oblique, inferior oblique.

Binocular Movements

Movements of the two eyes may be in the same direction (conjugate movements or versions) or in opposite directions (disjunctive movements or vergences).

Versions

The two eyes move together in a precisely co-ordinated way and corresponding muscles in the two eyes work together in pairs, sometimes called *yoke muscles*. For example, the right lateral rectus and the left medial rectus work together in dextroversion.

The names given to the versions in the so-called six cardinal directions (Fig 1-30) and the yoke muscles primarily involved in keeping the eyes looking in each of these directions are as follows:

Version	*Yoke Muscles*
dextroversion (to the right)	right lateral rectus left medial rectus
dextroelevation (up and to the right)	right superior rectus left inferior oblique
dextrodepression (down and to the right)	right inferior rectus left superior oblique
laevoversion (to the left)	right medial rectus left lateral rectus
laevoelevation (up and to the left)	right inferior oblique left superior rectus
laevodepression (down and to the left)	right superior oblique left inferior rectus

In any version the intensity of innervation is the same to each of a pair of yoke muscles (Hering's law). This happens even when one of the pair is not functioning normally. As a consequence, when there is a paresis of one muscle the resulting angle of deviation between the visual axes of the two eyes differs according to which eye is fixing, the deviation being greater when the eye with the affected muscle is fixing than when the other eye is fixing (Fig 1-31). For example, when there is a paresis of the right lateral rectus muscle and the right eye is fixing in a slightly dextroverted position an increased, perhaps maximal, innervation to the right lateral rectus is necessary to achieve this fixation. The same increased innervation goes to the unaffected left medial rectus and the left eye is therefore rotated far to the right. On the other hand, when the left eye is fixing, the normal innervation goes to both muscles and the right eye fails to reach the required slightly dextroverted position.

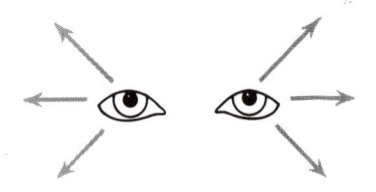

Fig 1-30 Six cardinal directions of eye movement.

A *squint* is that condition in which the visual axis of one eye (the squinting eye) is not directed to the object being looked at by the other eye (the fixing eye). A paralysis or paresis of an extra-ocular muscle will cause a squint and this is of the type called an *incomitant* squint, in that the angle of squint (the angle through which the visual axis of the squinting eye is deviated from what it should be if the eye was correctly directed to the point of fixation) will differ according to the direction of gaze (Fig 1-32). For example, when there is a paralysis of the right lateral rectus there will be no squint in laevoversion because the right lateral rectus is not required to contract in this direction of gaze. On dextroversion, however, there will be a squint and this will increase with increasing dextroversion (of the left eye).

The following common clinical situation is an example of the use made of the functional anatomy of the eye muscles (Fig 1-33). A person has a vertical squint in which the axis of the right eye is directed to a point higher than that of the left eye (in clinical jargon, 'a right over left' or R/L). This could be due to a weakness of one of four muscles, namely the two depressors of the right eye and the two elevators of the left eye. When the patient looks to the left the R/L increases. This reduces the possibly affected muscles to two, the right superior oblique or the left superior rectus. Finally, the R/L is greatest on laevodepression and therefore the faulty muscle must be the right superior oblique.

ANATOMY

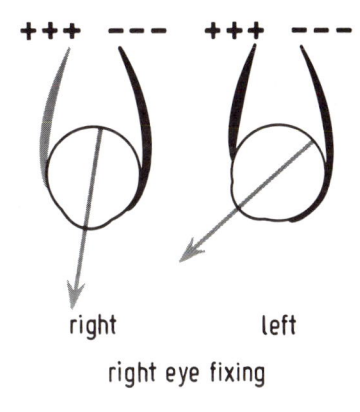

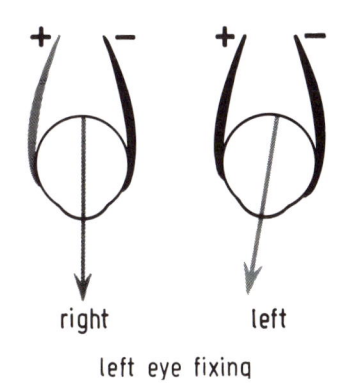

Fig 1-31 Paresis of the right lateral rectus muscle. The angle of squint is greater when the right eye fixes than when the left eye fixes.

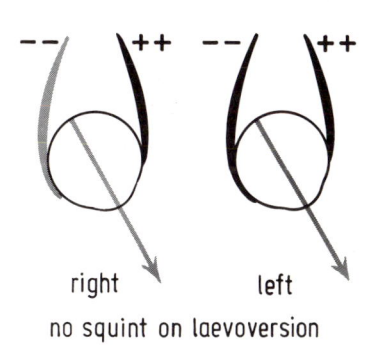

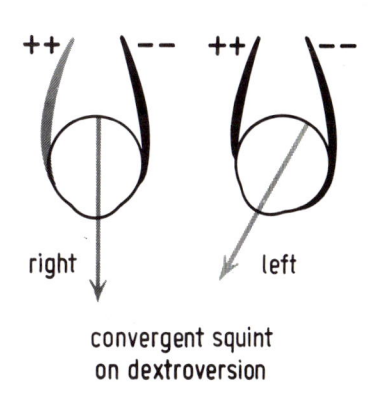

Fig 1-32 Paresis of the right lateral rectus muscle. The angle of squint differs in different directions of gaze.

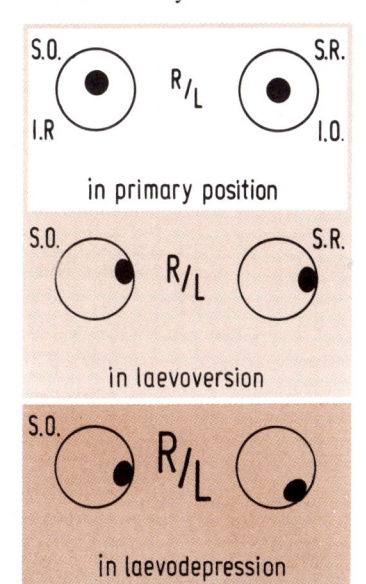

Fig 1-33 Analysis of a vertical diplopia due to paresis of the right superior oblique muscle.

Vergences

There are two disjunctive ocular movements, *convergence* when the visual axes converge and *divergence* when the visual axes diverge from a convergent position.

Convergence is linked with accommodation so that with near vision the two occur together and normally it is impossible to accommodate without converging and conversely to converge without accommodating. This linkage explains why a hypermetropic refractive error in a child may cause a convergent squint and why wearing glasses which correct the refractive error corrects the squint (p. 182).

NERVOUS PATHWAYS

The Intracranial Visual Pathway

The afferent visual pathway runs posteriorly in a horizontal plane from the nerve fibre layers of the two retinae by way of the optic nerves, optic chiasma, optic tracts, lateral geniculate bodies (LGB), and optic radiations to the visual cortex on the medial aspect and at the posterior pole of each occipital lobe (Fig 1-34). Throughout this pathway the visual fibres corresponding to each topographical region of the retina are mutually arranged in consistent anatomical patterns; a point-to-point correspondence of any area in the retina, and hence in the visual field, can be determined for any position along the pathway and in the visual cortex (Fig 1-35). Lesions at various sites therefore produce characteristic defects in the visual fields and these can be of clinical help in localizing the lesions (Fig 1-36). (The uniocular *visual field* is the portion of external space visible to one stationary eye. Points in the field are defined by polar co-ordinates from the *point of fixation*. A *hemianopia* is a defect in the visual fields of both eyes caused by a lesion in one region of the visual pathway. A *scotoma* is a non-seeing area within a seeing area.)

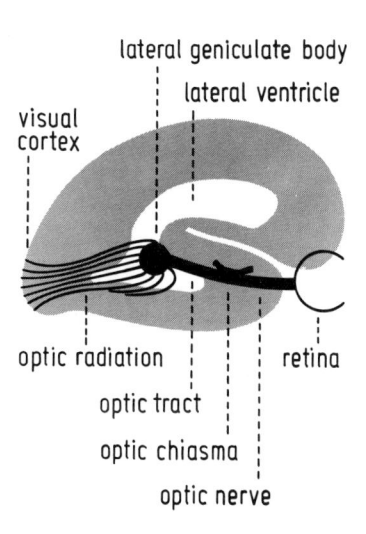

Fig 1-34 Visual pathway.

The simplest as well as the most fundamental subdivision of the visual fibres is into those which originate in the temporal part of the retina and those which originate in the nasal part, the division between the two groups being a vertical line through the fovea. (Note that this division of the retina into two physiological halves differs from the anatomical and ophthalmoscopic division by a vertical line passing through the optic disc.) This is a fundamental subdivision because at the chiasma the fibres from each nasal hemiretina cross the midline to the optic tract of the other side; the temporal hemi-retinal fibres do not cross. As a result of this partial decussation in the chiasma, stimuli from the homonymous (= the same side) halves of the two visual *fields,* e.g. temporal of right eye and nasal of left eye, reach the visual cortex of the opposite side, e.g. left. In other words, just as each hemisphere dominates the general sensory and motor activities of the opposite half of the body, we 'see' with the cortex on the opposite side.

The next basic subdivision of the visual fibres is into upper and lower parts according to whether they originate above or below a horizontal line through the fovea. The corresponding lower and upper halves of the visual fields are separated by a horizontal line through the fixation point. The upper/lower relationship of the fibres is retained throughout the pathway, e.g. an upper retinal localization corresponds to an upper cortical one.

Combining these two subdivisions gives the standard division of the fibres into four groups originating from the upper temporal, lower temporal, upper nasal, and lower nasal quadrants of the retina. (Again note that these quadrants centred on the fovea are different from the ophthalmoscopic and anatomical quadrants centred on the optic disc.) A further useful division in each of these quadrants is into those fibres subserving central vision from the macular region and those subserving peripheral vision from the rest of the retina.

The **optic chiasma** is the central bridge of the X formed by the two optic nerves anteriorly and the two optic tracts posteriorly. Its posterior border forms the lowermost part of the anterior wall of the third ventricle and is close to the hypothalamic nuclei. Immediately posterior the pituitary stalk passes downwards and forwards to pierce the diaphragm of the sella turcica which, with the underlying pituitary gland, is a few millimetres inferior to the chiasma. On either side is the internal carotid artery which here divides into middle and anterior cerebral arteries.

Expanding lesions of these neighbouring structures, e.g. pituitary tumour, arterial aneurysm, may damage the visual fibres in the chiasma. The function of the crossing fibres is commonly destroyed first and therefore the characteristic manifestation of chiasmal compression, e.g. from a pituitary tumour, is an initial *bitemporal hemianopia*.

Each **optic tract** runs posteriorly around the cerebral peduncle, deep to the temporal lobe, to enter the lateral geniculate body (except for the afferent pupillary fibres which go to the nearby pretectal nucleus). It is the first part of the retro-chiasmal pathway, the part in which lesions cause homonymous defects in the visual fields. Because the fibres from corresponding areas of the retinae of the two eyes are at first not together in the tracts these homonymous defects may be incongruous, i.e. dissimilar in the two fields.

Each **lateral geniculate body** (LGB) forms a slight bump on the postero-lateral aspect of the pulvinar of the thalamus but most of it is deep to the optic tract. Internally it is composed of six layers of grey matter alternating with white matter and in these the ganglion cell axons synapse with cells whose fibres constitute the optic radiation. Crossed fibres synapse in layers 1, 4, and 6, uncrossed fibres in layers 2, 3, and 5, and fibres from corresponding areas of the two retinae synapse in adjacent sites in the layers.

Because the ganglion cell axons end in the LGB, lesions of the visual fibres central to the LGB (supragenicular lesions) do not cause an atrophic pallor of the optic disc (optic atrophy) as is commonly the case with infrageniculate lesions.

Each **optic radiation** passes compactly through the most posterior part of the internal capsule and then spreads to form a broad band which runs posteriorly over the outer surface of the lateral ventricle through the parietal lobe to the occipital lobe. Because the radiation is part of the internal capsule, vascular lesions of this area can cause a hemianopia at the same time as a hemiplegia. The lower fibres are diverted forwards to form a loop (Meyer's) in the temporal lobe before passing posteriorly and therefore a lesion here can cause an upper quadrantanopia. Fibres from corresponding areas of the two retinae run together in the radiation so that lesions here usually produce field defects which are congruous, i.e. of the same shape in the two fields.

Each **visual cortex** is an area (area 17) of cortex on the medial aspect and posterior pole of the occipital lobe. Because on section it has a conspicuous white line in the grey matter it is also known by the old name of *striate area*. Much of the area is buried within a deep antero-posterior fissure, the calcarine fissure; yet another name derives from this, the *calcarine cortex*.

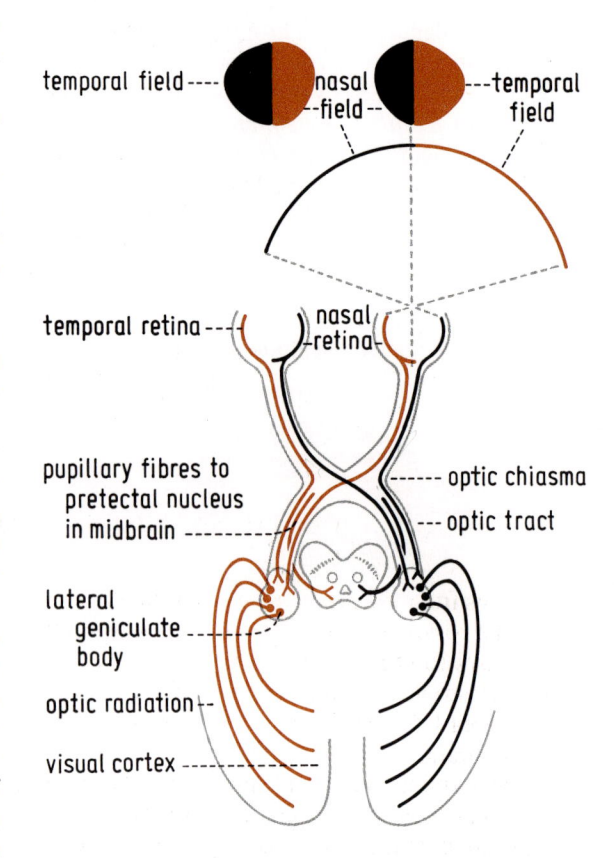

Fig 1-35 Visual pathway (and afferent pupillary fibres) with corresponding visual fields. (Visual fields are conventionally represented as seen by the subject).

ANATOMY

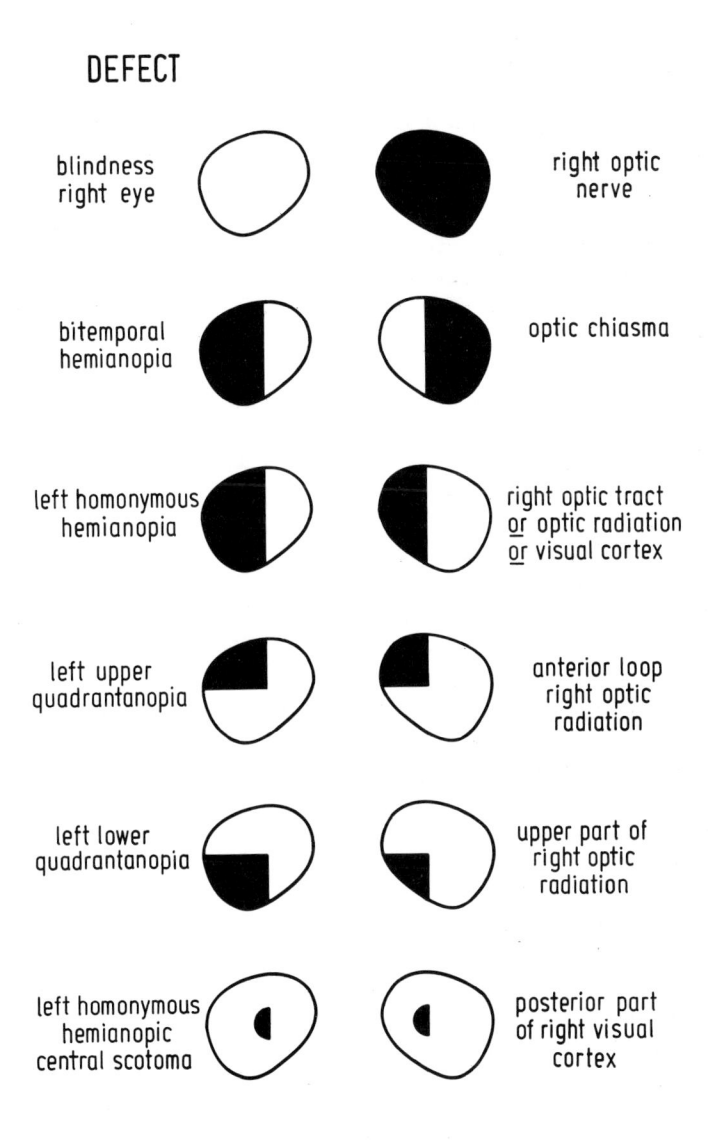

DEFECT

Defect			Location
blindness right eye	○ ●		right optic nerve
bitemporal hemianopia	◐ ◑		optic chiasma
left homonymous hemianopia	◐ ◐		right optic tract or optic radiation or visual cortex
left upper quadrantanopia			anterior loop right optic radiation
left lower quadrantanopia			upper part of right optic radiation
left homonymous hemianopic central scotoma			posterior part of right visual cortex

Fig 1-36 Schematic examples of visual defects.

Axons from the LGB synapse with cells in layer 4 of the cortex and from these there are countless pathways to other cells in the visual cortex, to the parastriate area (area 18) and the peristriate area (area 19), and indirectly to most other parts of the brain.

The terminations of fibres in the cortex are such that those corresponding to upper retinal areas are dorsal to those corresponding to lower retinal areas and those corresponding to central retinal areas are posterior to those corresponding to more peripheral areas. The area representing the macula is disproportionately large; it is as large as that representing the rest of the retina. This magnification is greatest for foveal representation; the width of two foveal cones (5 μm) corresponds with a cortical area 100 times as wide. This anatomical disproportion based on functional importance and precision is similar to that occurring throughout the general sensory and motor nervous system.

Central vision is commonly retained (macular sparing) when a lesion of the visual cortex causes a homonymous hemianopia. This is possibly because the temporal and nasal halves of the retina overlap in a narrow band running vertically through the fovea; from this zone some axons project to the visual cortex on one side and some to that on the other.

The Pupillary Pathways

The function of the pupil is to control the amount of light which reaches the retina. The size of the pupil is mainly determined by the parasympathetic nervous system causing contraction or relaxation of the sphincter muscle. The sympathetic system has a secondary role only; it maintains a constant tone in the dilator muscle which aids relaxation of the sphincter. The two most important *pupillary reflexes* which control pupil size are the light reflex and the near reflex in which constriction of the pupil results respectively from light and from looking at near objects.

The pathway for the *light reflex* is subcortical and therefore this reflex can be retained when there is total blindness due to bilateral cortical

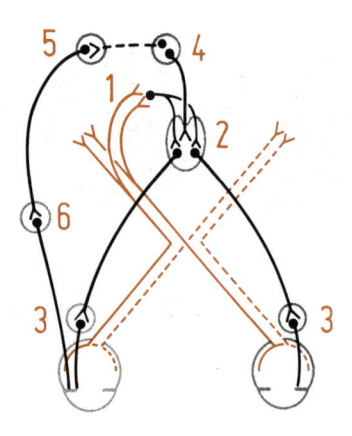

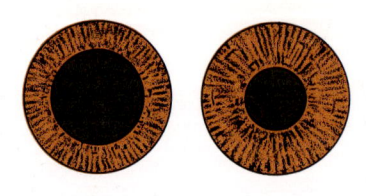

Fig 1-38 Fixed dilated pupil in oculomotor nerve paralysis.

lesions (cortical blindness) (Fig 1-37). The afferent fibres from both rods and cones run with the visual fibres until just before the LGB where the pupillary fibres leave the optic tracts to synapse in the pretectal nuclei in the region of the superior colliculi. Since fibres from each eye go to the nuclei on both sides, a light stimulus to one eye causes constriction of both the pupil of that eye (the *direct reaction* to light) and the pupil of the other eye (the *consensual reaction* to light). From each pretectal nucleus impulses go to the parasympathetic portion of the oculomotor nuclei (the nucleus of Edinger-Westphal) on both sides. The efferent pathway is via the third nerve to a synapse in the ciliary ganglion from which postganglionic fibres go by the short ciliary nerves to the sphincter muscle of the iris. A total lesion of the third nerve thus produces a fixed dilated pupil on the same side (Fig 1-38).

Normally both the accommodation and the convergence which occur when a near object is looked at initiate the pupillary constriction of the *near reflex*. But either can do this alone when the other is eliminated, accommodation with convex lenses or convergence with prisms. The precise afferent pathways are not known but they involve the visual cortex (Fig 1-39). From there the outflow via the peristriate area passes to the nucleus of Edinger-Westphal. The efferent pathway from this nucleus is similar to that of the light reflex.

Lesions in the pretectal region, e.g. neurosyphilis, may abolish the pupillary light reflex, both direct and consensual, while leaving the near reflex intact. This is called the *Argyll Robertson pupil* (Fig 1-40). A somewhat similar dissociation of the pupillary reactions to light and to near occurs in what is called the *myotonic* or *Adie's pupil* (Fig 1-41). Whereas Argyll Robertson pupils are miotic and often irregular, are usually bilateral, and signify neurological disease, an Adie's pupil

1 pretectal nucleus
2 Edinger-Westphal nucleus
3 ciliary ganglion
4 hypothalamic centre
5 cilio-spinal centre
6 superior cervical ganglion

Fig 1-37 Pupillary pathway, light reflex.

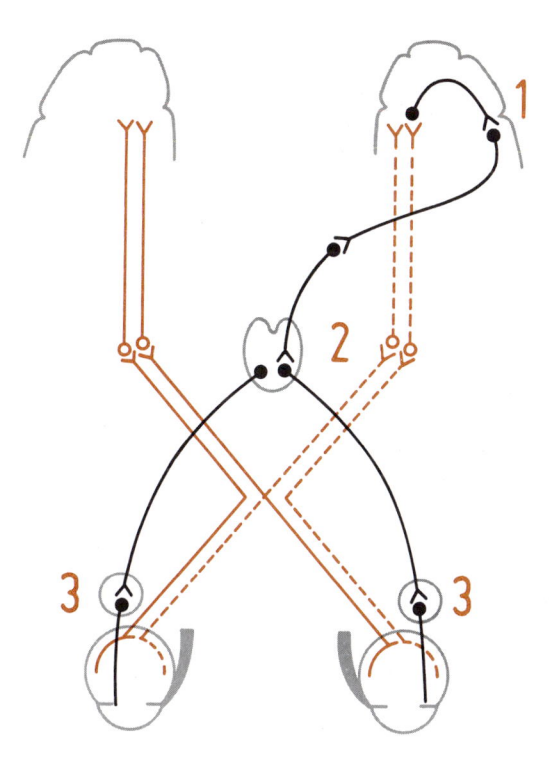

ANATOMY

of Edinger-Westphal, e.g. when the pupils dilate as a result of emotional stimuli, and conversely when the pupils constrict in sleep because of lowered sympathetic activity. In accordance with the subsidiary role of the dilator muscle, lesions of the sympathetic pathway cause only slight miosis (Horner's syndrome) and do not greatly interfere with pupillary reaction (Fig 1-42).

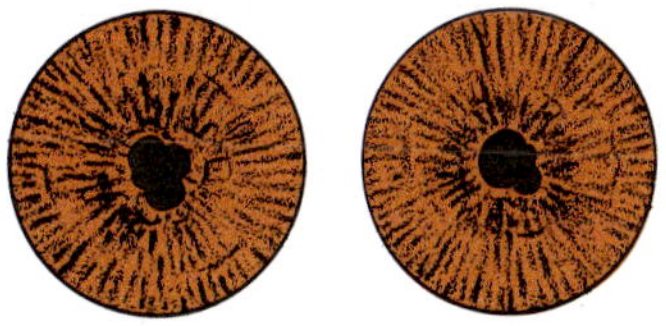

Fig 1-40 Miotic irregular Argyll Robertson pupils.

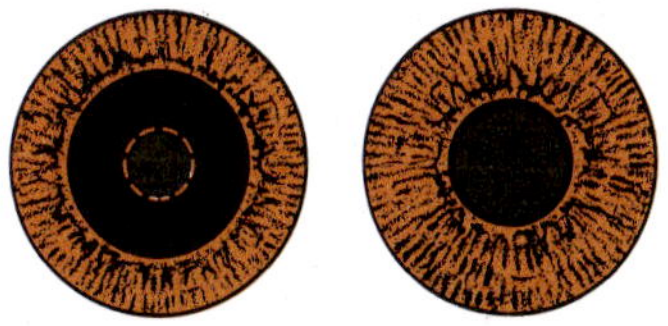

1 peristriate area
2 Edinger-Westphal nucleus
3 ciliary ganglion

Fig 1-39 Pupillary pathway, near reflex.

is usually larger than its fellow (occasionally it is smaller), is usually unilateral, and is an entirely benign change often associated with reduced tendon reflexes. The myotonic pupil reacts very little, if at all, to light. It constricts fully but in a slow and delayed fashion to near stimuli and after cessation of the stimulus redilatation is noticeably slow.

The *sympathetic innervation* of the dilator muscle of the iris originates in the hypothalamus, passes to the cilio-spinal centre in the upper part of the spinal cord, and from this region preganglionic fibres pass in the cervical sympathetic trunk to the superior cervical ganglion. Postganglionic fibres reach the eye by way of the internal carotid plexus, a branch of the fifth nerve and the ciliary nerves. The hypothalamic centre also influences pupil size by inhibiting the nuclei

Fig 1-41 Larger (or smaller) myotonic pupil.

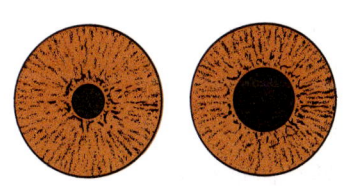

Fig 1-42 Miotic pupil in Horner's syndrome.

The Accommodation Pathway

The accommodation reflex is initiated by blurring of the retinal image and the afferent pathway is with the visual fibres to the visual cortex (Fig 1-43). From here a connection is made with the peristriate area of the occipital cortex. The efferent pathway is by way of a corticotectal tract to the parasympathetic nuclei of Edinger-Westphal and thence to the ciliary ganglion and on to the ciliary muscle which is caused to contract. The role of the sympathetic system is doubtful but it may induce some relaxation of the ciliary muscle.

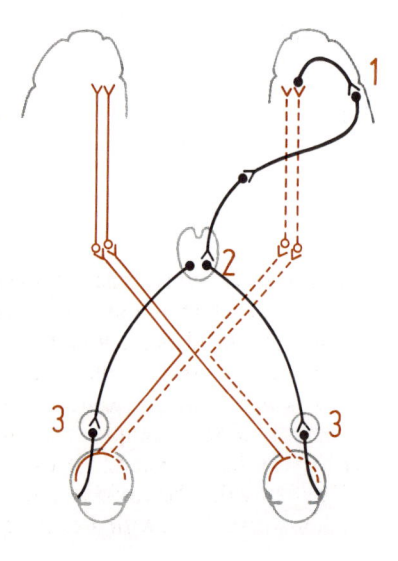

1 peristriate area
2 Edinger-Westphal nucleus
3 ciliary ganglion

Fig 1-43 Accommodation pathway.

The Motor Pathways

An outline of the functional systems of eye movements and the purpose they fulfil will be given first because this makes it easier to understand the anatomy of the ocular motor pathways. It is also true that more is known of the physiology than of the detailed anatomy of the motor pathways.

Functional Systems of Eye Movements

In animals whose eyes are directed sideways and who have no fovea the main purpose of eye movements is to stabilize the retinal images in spite of movement of the animal and of movement of its visual target. This is achieved by the *vestibular system,* which compensates for head and body movements, and a *smooth pursuit* (or *reflex following*) *system,* which enables the eyes to track a moving target. A third component, a fast *resetting system,* is needed to return the eyes to the neutral position after each excursion. If either of the primary movements continues beyond the mechanical limits of eye rotation, the resetting system returns the eyes rapidly to a central position from which the primary movement again moves them. In this way an oscillatory movement of the eyes, called *nystagmus,* arises and allows perception to occur during the brief phases when the image is not moving on the retina. Without this, visual perception would be blurred out during any movement of the animal or its target. Think of a rabbit fleeing through undergrowth; instead of a clueless streaking past of the environment the physiological nystagmus allows flashes of useful vision.

In animals with a fovea and with forward-directed eyes and therefore overlapping fields of vision, two additional eye movement systems are required. These are a *saccadic system* (probably evolved from the more primitive resetting system), which enables the eyes to move so that the visual target is quickly imaged on the fovea, and a *vergence and fusion system,* which controls the degree of convergence of the visual axes so that the target is imaged on the fovea of each eye for all distances.

Fundamentally these systems of eye movement constitute a *tracking system.* Any tracking system which is on a moveable base and which records distance must fulfil four functions. Consider a gunnery tracking system on a ship. The four requirements are: a stabilizing system to compensate for movements of the ship, a system to rapidly fix a given target, a system to follow movements of the target, and a range-finding system. In man the analagous four systems of eye movement are: vestibular to compensate for movements of the head in the environment, saccadic to acquire a target, smooth pursuit to track the target if it moves in the environment,

ANATOMY

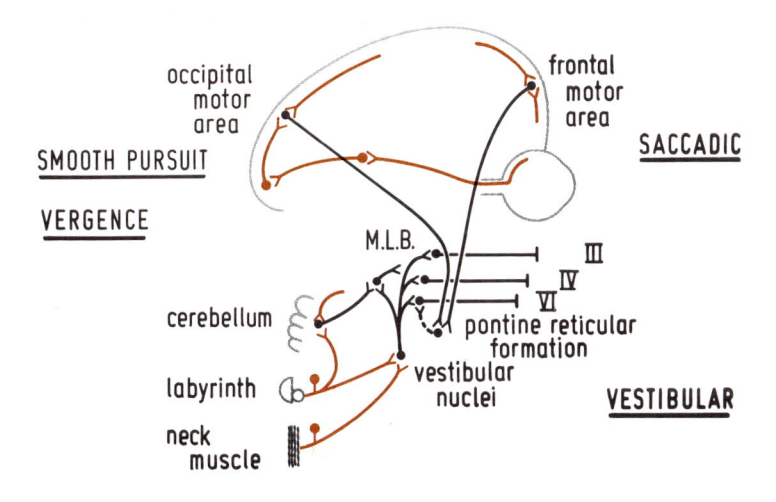

Fig 1-44 Four eye movement systems for tracking visual targets.

and vergence for tracking in depth (Fig 1-44).

Almost all eye movements are combinations of movements produced by these four systems. Although they combine smoothly together the central pathways for each of these tasks are separate.

The vestibular system derives information about head and body movement from the labyrinths, the muscles of the neck, and the ocular muscles themselves. The afferent stimuli for the other three systems are visual from the retina to the occipital cortex. (Saccadic movements can also be initiated voluntarily without visual stimuli.) The final common path for all four systems is the ocular motor nuclei, their nerves, and the twelve extraocular muscles.

Vestibular movements occur with very brief latency, occur reflexly as a result of changes in the static position of the head or of changes in the velocity of the head, can be neutralized by pursuit or saccadic movements (e.g. when head and eyes turn in the same direction), and, if rotation of the head continues in the same direction, alternate with resetting reflex saccades to produce vestibular nystagmus (for a period of about 10 seconds). The effectiveness of compensatory vestibular eye movements compared with pursuit movements is demonstrated by our greater ability to continue reading a text while shaking our head than if the text is similarly moved while our head is stationary.

Saccadic movements are very fast, are the movements which change fixation and can be reflexly caused, as for example by a movement in the periphery of the visual field, or can be voluntarily initiated. The rapid eye movements (REM) that are associated with dreaming are also saccades.

Smooth pursuit or *following movements* match eye velocity to target velocity (up to a maximum of about 45°/sec), are reflex but require visual 'attention', and in situations where most of the visual environment is continuously moving, alternate with reflex saccades to produce optokinetic nystagmus.

Vergence and fusional movements are slow and occur reflexly as a result of the difference between the off-target errors of each eye.

Ocular Motor Nerves, Nuclei and Internuclear Connections

The extraocular muscles are innervated by the third, fourth, and sixth cranial nerves. The nuclei of these nerves lie close to the midline on each side of the mid-brain (third and fourth nerve nuclei) and the pons (sixth nerve nucleus). They are linked together and to the vestibular nuclei by the *medial longitudinal bundle* (MLB), a fasciculus of nerve fibres which runs through the brain-stem close to the midline, and they are connected to multisynaptic circuits in the brain-stem (reticular formations) and the cerebellum (Fig 1-45).

A lesion of the MLB results in *internuclear ophthalmoplegia*. In this condition there is weakness of adduction of the eye when this is part of a lateral version movement, but not when it is part of convergence; there is also usually nystagmus of the abducting eye on horizontal versions and vertical nystagmus on elevation of the eye.

In the brain-stem adjacent to the nuclei there are regions where fibres subserving common functions come close together. Clinically these are called *gaze centres* because localized lesions in these areas can selectively interfere with particular binocular movements. The *pontine paramedial reticular formation* ventral to the MLB at the level of the sixth nerve nucleus may be called the 'centre' of lateral versions, and nuclei in the *pretectal region* near the superior colliculi constitute a 'centre' for vertical movement.

Central Organization

Vestibular system. Afferent fibres from the labyrinths and from muscle proprioceptors synapse in the vestibular nuclei and from there fibres run in the medial longitudinal bundle to synapse directly with the ocular motor nuclei and indirectly through neuronal pathways in the pontine reticular formation and the cerebellum. Occasionally, when a supra-nuclear lesion destroys other eye movements, the reflex which attempts to maintain an unchanging direction of gaze of the eyes in spite of movements of the body and head may be unmasked clinically as the doll's head phenomenon. Lesions of the labyrinths or of the brain-stem in the region of the vestibular nuclei commonly cause a pathological vestibular nystagmus.

Saccadic system (fronto-pontine system). The efferent pathway for voluntary saccadic movements begins in the frontal ocular motor centre (the premotor cortex). Fibres from this area travel with other fibres from the motor cortex through the anterior part of the internal capsule, and decussate below the level of the fourth nerve

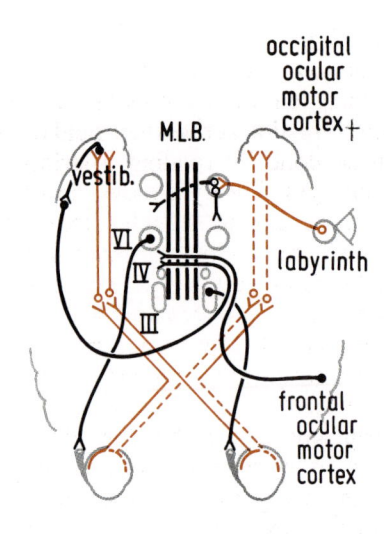

Fig 1-45 Motor pathways for eye movements.

nuclei to reach the pontine paramedian reticular formation. From here fibres go to all the ocular motor nuclei by way of the MLB. Impulses from the frontal centre of one side cause the eyes to move to the opposite side.

Irritative lesions of a frontal motor centre may cause involuntary deviation of the eyes to the opposite side. Destructive lesions cause a temporary volitional gaze palsy to the opposite side with retention of reflex following movement of the eyes in this direction, i.e. the patient may be unable to voluntarily look towards one side, but can follow a moving object with his or her eyes to that side.

Smooth pursuit or following system (occipito-pontine system). The efferent pathway for reflex pursuit movements begins in the occipital ocular motor centre (peristriate cortex). Fibres from this area pass on the medial aspect of the optic radiation to eventually reach the region of the superior colliculus. From here the pathway crosses the midline to join the fronto-pontine fibres and then recrosses the midline with them to terminate in the pontine paramedian reticular formation. This double decussation is postulated to explain the clinical observation that impulses from the occipital centre on one side cause the eyes to move to the *same* side. This must be one of the very few examples of apparent ipsilateral cortical control.

Optokinetic nystagmus is induced in people with a normal oculomotor mechanism by exposing them to recurrent visual stimuli passing in the same direction across their field of vision. This can be done by rotating a striped drum before their eyes. The eyes move slowly in the same direction as the stimulus (slow phase) alternately with rapid refixation movements in the opposite direction (fast phase). Because frontal oculomotor control is contralateral and occipital oculomotor control is ipsilateral, both phases of optokinetic nystagmus are mediated through the same hemisphere. Interruption of the occipito-pontine pathway impairs the slow phase, while involvement of the fronto-pontine pathway leads to loss of the fast phase and consequent steady deviation of the eyes in the direction of movement of the stimulus.

The smooth pursuit system is readily disturbed by fatigue, sedatives, anticonvulsants, excess alcohol, and general central nervous system disease. In such conditions smooth pursuit movements are abolished and tracking can only be carried out by saccadic pursuit movements (cogwheel movements).

Vergence and fusion system. The efferent pathway for vergence and fusional movements from the occipital peristriate area is probably similar to that for following movements.

Involvement of the pretectal region, e.g. by pressure from a tumour of the pineal gland in young adults, results in absent voluntary, following, and reflex elevation of the eyes above the primary position with retention of depression of the eyes. This is called the Sylvian aqueduct syndrome or Parinaud's syndrome.

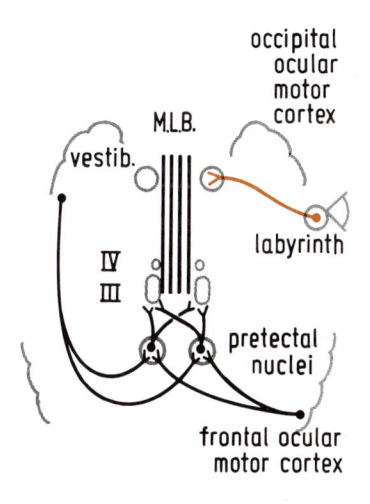

Fig 1-46 Supranuclear pathways for vertical eye movements.

Vertical Eye Movements

There are similar saccadic, following, and vestibular systems for vertical movements. Fronto-mesencephalic, occipito-mesencephalic, and vestibular pathways all proceed to the pretectal region on both sides (vertical gaze 'centre') where synapses occur and impulses to the third and fourth nerve nuclei for vertical eye movements are co-ordinated (Fig 1-46).

Closing the eyelids is usually accompanied by an upward rotation of the eyes (Bell's phenomenon) and can be demonstrated by holding the lids open while the patient attempts to close them. Elevation of the eyes as a result of this reflex may be preserved when voluntary and following elevation is absent due to a lesion of the cortico-mesencephalic pathways. A similar retention of reflex elevation of the eyes in the presence of supra-nuclear lesions is seen in the doll's head phenomenon.

Chapter 2

OPHTHALMIC OPTICS

THE EYE AS AN OPTICAL INSTRUMENT

Image formation
   Image formation by the eye

Accommodation
   Presbyopia

Refractive errors
   Myopia
   Hypermetropia
   Astigmatism
   Correction with spectacles
   Measurement of refractive errors
   Pin-hole test
   Contact lenses
   Intraocular lenses
   Indications for spectacles
   Surgical correction of refractive errors

PHYSICAL AND GEOMETRICAL OPTICS

Diffraction and interference

Polarized light

Spherical aberration

Chromatic aberration

Image formation by a lens with opacities

Reflecting surfaces of the eye

Visualization of intraocular opacities

THE EYE AS AN OPTICAL INSTRUMENT

Image Formation

Because light travels in straight lines and because every luminous or illuminated object scatters light in all directions, an optical image can only be formed by selection of rays (Fig 2-1). A pin-hole camera (originally, camera obscura = dark chamber) is one of the simplest image-forming devices (Fig 2-2). From each point on the object only a few rays can pass through the pin-hole aperture and these strike a corresponding point on the surface opposite the hole. Further, light from all other points on the object is prevented from falling on this particular point. In this way a point image of each point of the object is formed. Because only a small portion of the light emanating from the object can enter a pin-hole camera the image is dim. A convex lens in place of the pin-hole refracts the light and thus, also acting as a ray selector, it also forms an image (Fig 2-3). It does however pass much more light and therefore gives a brighter image. The eye is an image-forming camera obscura (Fig 2-4).

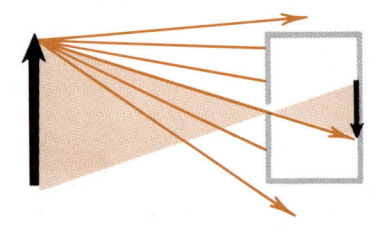

Fig 2-2 Image formation by a pin-hole camera.

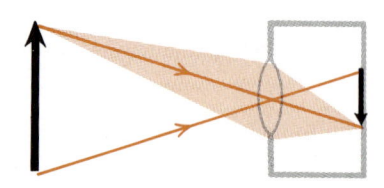

Fig 2-3 Image formation by a convex lens.

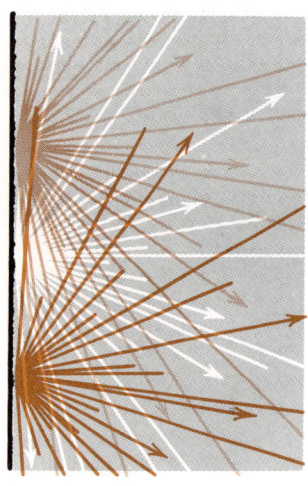

Fig 2-1 Light emitted from a point source or light reflected from each point of a surface travels in all possible directions.

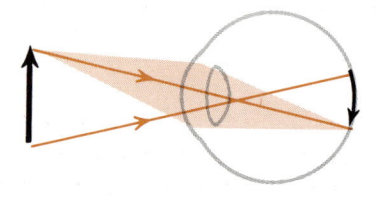

Fig-2-4 Image formation by the eye.

OPTICS

Image Formation by the Eye

Refraction of light entering the eye is complex because it encounters several changes in refractive index in its path through the transparent ocular media (air 1, cornea 1.376, aqueous 1.336, lens cortex 1.386, lens nucleus 1.406, vitreous 1.336).

This complexity is overcome by approximations of various types, the simplest of which is the *reduced eye* or equivalent eye (Fig 2-5). In the model described by Listing a single spherical refracting surface is assumed to be situated 1.5mm behind the anterior surface of the cornea. The surface is assumed to have a radius of curvature of 5.7mm and to separate a medium with the refractive index of water (1.336) from air. The posterior focus of the surface is 24.4mm posterior to the cornea, and this is where the retina is located in an eye of average length.

The refractive power in doptres of a lens in air is the reciprocal of its focal length measured in metres. The diopric power of a single spherical refracting surface in air, such as that of the reduced eye, is the reciprocal of its (second) focal length multiplied by the refractive index of the medium. The total power of this reduced eye is therefore 1.336/0.0229 = 58 dioptres (D).

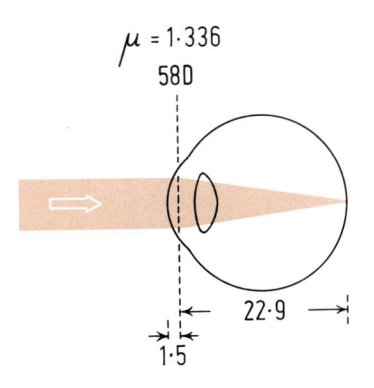

Fig 2-5 Reduced eye.

Parallel rays of light from an object at infinity come to a focus on the retina (Fig 2-6). Rays from an object nearer than infinity will come to a focus behind the retina (Fig 2-7). For these to be focused on the retina an increase in the refractive power is required, e.g. an increase of 3D when the object is at a distance of ⅓ metre from the eye. This increase in refractive power is called accommodation.

Accommodation

The appropriate changes in the total refraction of light entering the eye come from alterations in the curvature of the lens which contributes the smaller but adjustable part of the eye's refractive power. The ciliary muscle provides the motive power for accommodation. On contraction it causes the ciliary body to move forward and to thicken and thereby relaxes the tension of the suspensory zonule of the lens. This in turn permits elastic contraction of the lens capsule which moulds the lens to a more spherical shape (p. 20).

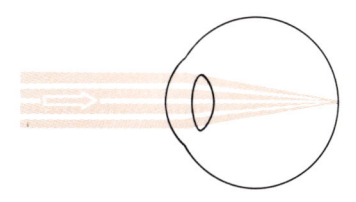

Fig 2-6 Parallel rays of light from infinity are refracted by the cornea and lens to come to a focus on the retina of an emmetropic eye.

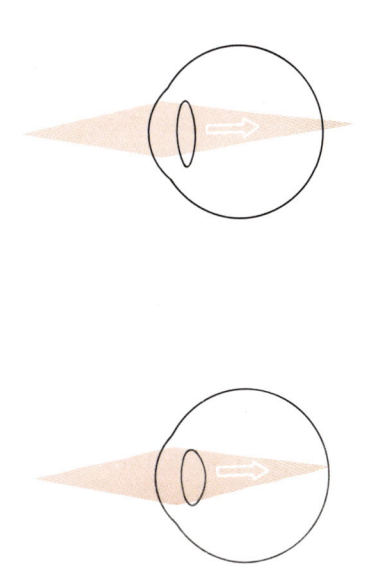

Fig 2-7 Upper Rays from a near object come to a focus behind the retina of the unaccommodated eye.

  Lower The accommodated eye focuses rays from a near object on the retina.

The ciliary muscle is controlled by parasympathetic fibres originating in the Edinger-Westphal nucleus in the mid-brain which travel via the third nerve with a synapse in the ciliary ganglion. Parasympatholytic drops in the eye will therefore paralyse accommodation and this is used in determining refractive errors, especially in children, to temporarily inhibit all accommodation so that the refraction of the unfocused eye can be determined.

The stimulus for accommodation is a blurred retinal image. When the eye is accommodated there are fluctuations of about two cycles per second in the refractive power. This is a form of 'hunting' and suggests that this servo-mechanism determines by trial and error which action diminishes blur.

In childhood the power of accommodation is about 10D, that is a child can see clearly an object 10cm from the eye. From childhood onwards the power of accommodation steadily diminishes so that at 45 years it is 3.5D and at 65 years it is only 1.0D. This steady loss of accommodative power is called **presbyopia**. It is due not to any loss of power of the ciliary muscle, but to a progressive hardening of the lens and also to the steady increase in size of the lens with age.

Usually about the age of 45 or 50 years the universal presbyopic reduction in accommodation makes near visual tasks difficult and 'reading glasses' are required (Fig 2-8). The convex lenses of the spectacles used for this purpose supply the increased power for near vision which the individual is no longer able to produce. Inevitably distant vision through reading glasses is blurred because of the artificial myopia which they create. *Bifocal spectacles* are used to provide clear vision for both far and near; they obviate the need to remove the near spectacles for distant vision or, if distance glasses are also required, to use two pairs of glasses. Every few years the strength of an individual's near correction has to be increased until about the age of sixty-five when all accommodation has to come from spectacles and the strength of these is at the maximum required.

Refractive Errors

The normal condition of the eye in which, with no accommodation, parallel light is focused on the retina is called *emmetropia*. Any optical departure from this condition is called a *refractive error* or *ametropia*. There are three kinds of refractive error, namely myopia, hypermetropia, and astigmatism.

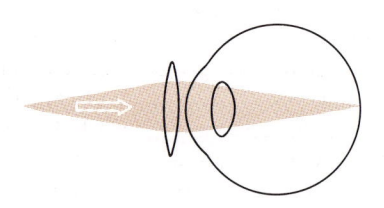

Fig 2-8 Correction of presbyopia with a convex spectacle lens.

In **myopia**, the eye is too long for its refracting system or the refracting system is too powerful for its length (Fig 2-9). Consequently parallel rays of light from a distant object are focused in front of the retina and accommodation only increases the error. On the other hand near vision is possible with less than normal or, if the error is large enough, no accommodation.

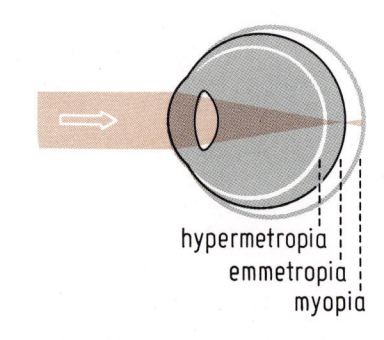

Fig 2-9 Hypermetropia, emmetropia and myopia.

In **hypermetropia** the eye is too short or the refraction is too weak (Fig 2-9). *Aphakia,* that is when the lens has been removed from the eye as in a cataract operation, is a special case of hypermetropia.

Astigmatism results when the curvature of some component of the optical system of the eye, for example the cornea, is not spherical but is *toric.* That is, the refracting surface is more curved in one meridian than in the meridian at 90° to it (as occurs in a dessert spoon, whereas the bowl of a soup spoon is more or less

OPTICS

spherical). Therefore a point image of a point object is not possible (Fig 2-10). Astigmatism can be myopic, hypermetropic, or mixed. Accommodation cannot completely correct astigmatism, but sometimes the continuing search for clear vision by the accommodation mechanism causes ocular discomfort due to afferent impulses from the overworked ciliary muscles.

There is no one normal length or normal power for an emmetropic eye, these two variables being correlated in individual eyes to achieve emmetropia.

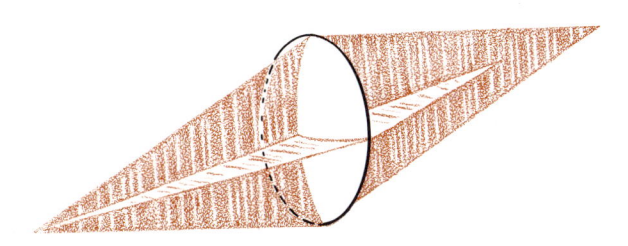

Fig 2-10 Astigmatic refraction by a toric surface.

Correction with Spectacles

For a *myopic* eye there is a point nearer than infinity from which rays of light come to a focus on the retina when the eye is not accommodating. Therefore if a concave lens is provided so that it diverges parallel rays of light as if they came from this near point, these will be focused on the retina (Fig 2-11). This is the basis of using concave lenses to correct myopic refractive errors. Because the myope does not need to accommodate to see near objects he or she can read without glasses after the onset of presbyopia. Sometimes in old people the lens becomes stronger due to an increase in its refractive index, myopia occurs and with it the ability to read without spectacles. This is the basis for 'second sight' of old people.

Hypermetropia can be corrected by a convex lens (Fig 2-12) or, provided the hypermetropia is not too great, accommodation can be used to achieve clear distant vision. However, accommodation for distant vision is interfered with by presbyopia and therefore spectacles become necessary for distant vision at, for example, 30 years of age. For the same reason a hypermetrope requires reading glasses at a younger age than an emmetrope. Further, if glasses are not worn the need for prolonged excessive accommodation may give rise to ocular discomfort, especially if much close work is done.

For *aphakia* a convex lens of approximately +12.0D is required for distant vision and about +15.0D for near vision. For optical reasons the retinal image in corrected aphakia is one-third larger than that of a normal eye. This is why spectacles cannot be used to correct unilateral aphakia if the phakic eye is also to be used because the different sized images of the two eyes cannot be fused and a form of double vision would occur.

Cylindrical lenses are used in the correction of *astigmatism*. A *cylindrical lens* is one in which the surface is curved (convex or concave) in one meridian and flat (plane) in the other (Fig 2-13). For example, a slab from the side of a solid glass cylinder is a convex (or positive, or plus) cylindrical lens. The meridian in which there is no curvature is the *axis* of the cylinder. A cylindrical curvature can be combined with a spherical curvature in a lens which is then called a toric surfaced lens. In astigmatism the surface of the cornea is toric instead of spherical. The appropriate axis as well as the strength of the correcting cylindrical lens must be determined and incorporated in spectacles if these are required.

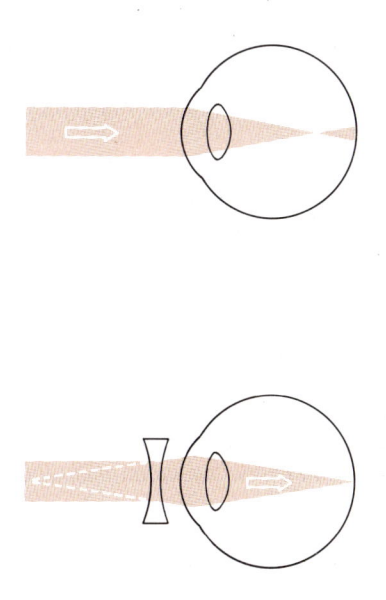

Fig 2-11 Myopia and its correction with a concave lens.

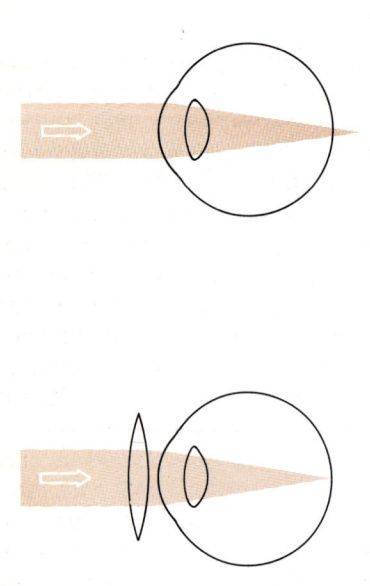

Fig 2-12 Hypermetropia and its correction with a convex lens.

Measurement of Refractive Errors

It has been claimed that, 'Of all aspects of medicine the prescription of spectacles or contact lenses gives to more people more comfort and increased efficiency than any other medical technique'.

Determination of the refraction of a patient, or, as it is commonly called, refracting a patient, can be done objectively, when no response is required from the subject, or subjectively, when the subject helps in finding the precise lens with which his or her vision is clearest and most comfortable.

The method most commonly used in *objective refraction* is called retinoscopy. In this procedure a beam of light from a retinoscope, which is an instrument somewhat like an ophthalmoscope, is directed through *trial lenses* into the patient's eye and moved within his or her pupil. By looking through the retinoscope and comparing the movement of light seen reflected from the subject's fundus with the movement of light from the retinoscope the refractionist can select the trial lens which corrects any refractive error which may be present. Because accommodation by the subject's eye would alter refraction by an unknown amount it is necessary that this does not occur during retinoscopy. In most adult subjects this can be achieved by having them look fixedly at a distant object. With babies and children accommodation is temporarily paralysed by instilling parasympatholytic drops in the eyes prior to refraction.

There are numerous techniques of *subjective refraction*. Essentially the subject looks critically at a distant object, e.g. the lowest line which he or she can read on a Snellen test-type (Fig 3-14) 6m from him or her, while combinations of trial lenses are placed in front of the eye being tested and he or she is asked which of a pair of alternative lens combinations gives clearest definition of the test object. The lenses are placed in a *trial frame* worn like spectacles by the subject or they are contained in a mechanised optical refracting unit which can be moved into position in front of the patient's face. Subjective measurement of refraction will be misleading or impossible unless the patient is co-operative, has understanding, and is a reasonable observer. For this reason, and also to reduce

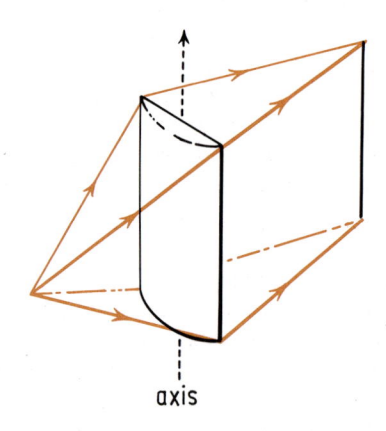

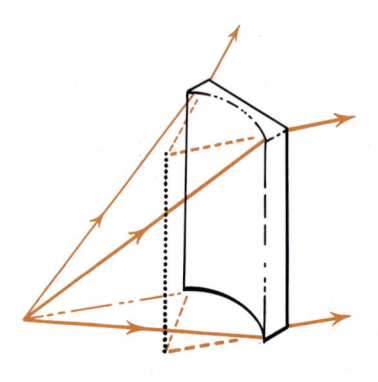

Fig 2-13 Image formation by cylindrical lenses.

OPTICS

the time spent in trial-and-error testing, subjective refraction is usually preceded by retinoscopy and the subjective test is then used to verify and to increase the accuracy of the objective findings.

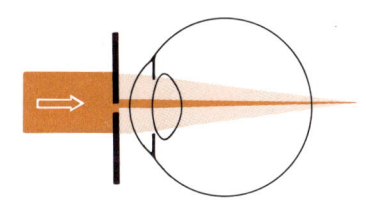

Fig 2-14 A pin-hole aperture reduces the size of the blur circle on the retina in an ametropic eye.

Pin-hole Test
When visual acuity is reduced because of an uncorrected refractive error a pin-hole aperture of about 1mm diameter held in front of the eye will improve acuity appreciably by reducing the size of the blur circles which comprise the retinal image (Fig 2-14). In similar fashion poor vision due to partial corneal or lenticular opacities is improved with a pin-hole. On the other hand lowered vision due to lesions of the retina or optic nerve is worsened by a pin-hole because it reduces the light reaching the retina. Clinical use of a pin-hole is therefore a very useful simple test for determining whether or not a patient's reduced acuity is due to disease of the retina or its nerve.

A small size of the pupil, such as occurs in a bright light, similarly diminishes the effect of a refractive error and of the spherical and chromatic aberrations of the eye. Too small a pupil, however, worsens image formation because of the increased effect of diffraction at the pupil margin. The optimum pupil size is about 2mm.

Some myopes who do not wear glasses, perhaps because they think them disfiguring, habitually screw up their eyelids to make a narrow, slit-like palpebral aperture and thereby reduce the blurring of their distant vision.

Contact Lenses
Plastic lenses worn in contact with the eye under the lids are used as an alternative to spectacles for cosmetic reasons and for some occupations and sporting activities. In some cases of corneal scarring and irregularity, e.g. keratoconus (conical cornea) in which the central cornea becomes thinned and cone shaped, and in high degrees of myopia, contact lenses give much better vision than is possible with spectacles. This occurs because when a contact lens is worn refraction of the light entering the eye takes place mainly at the air-lens interface and the cornea itself is largely eliminated as a refracting surface. This overcomes corneal astigmatism as well as irregularities. Any refractive power needed is provided by appropriately curving the front surface of the lens. Contact lenses may also permit binocular vision by patients with unilateral aphakia because the disparity in the retinal image sizes of the phakic and aphakic eyes is much less than with spectacles. Further, the defects and distortions of aphakic vision are much less with contact lenses than with spectacles (p. 191).

Corneal contact lenses are made of either hard (polymethylmethacrylate) or soft, water-absorbing (hydroxyethylmethacrylate) plastic. Hard lenses are smaller in diameter than the cornea on which they move with blinking and eye movements. The tears beneath them are thus kept fresh enough to supply the corneal epithelium with oxygen. Soft lenses are slightly larger than the corneal diameter and are relatively stationary on the eye but their high content of water permits some oxygen to diffuse through the lens. Hard lenses have to be removed (and disinfected) each night, but some soft lenses can be worn continuously by those patients who need but cannot handle contact lenses, e.g. aged aphakics, provided they can be regularly supervised. Compared with hard lenses, soft lenses are more comfortable but they give less clear vision, last for a shorter time, cost more, and cannot correct more than modest amounts of astigmatism or keratoconus. In a few corneal diseases and degenerations they are useful as 'bandage lenses'.

Intraocular Lenses
Another way of correcting the refractive error of aphakia is to insert a plastic lens into the eye when the cataract is surgically removed.

The intraocular lens (IOL) is fixed in position either in front of or, more frequently and better, behind the pupil. This 'pseudophakia' is the best optical solution for aphakia and, unless there are contra-indications, a posterior chamber IOL is

Indications for Spectacles

There is a widespread fallacious folk-lore of sight and it includes wrong reasons for wearing glasses. Many assume, and some are persuaded by a few of those who profit from the use of spectacles, that wearing glasses will preserve their eyes or strengthen their sight. In a sense this can be true for some children, but for adults it is without foundation. There are only three reasons why an adult should wear glasses and the individual him or herself is the one to judge whether any of these apply to him or her. The indications are (1) to see more clearly, (2) to see more comfortably, and (3) to protect the eyes from injury—mechanical, actinic, thermal, or chemical. It is entirely reasonable for a patient to prefer blurred vision or ocular discomfort to the nuisance of wearing glasses or contact lenses. No harm to the eyes can result from this choice.

On the other hand it can be critically important for the development of normal seeing that some infants and children consistently wear an optical correction during their growing years. Examples of conditions which demand this are some types of squint, and amblyopia due to markedly unequal refractive errors in a pair of eyes (p. 185). Children who are myopic when young should also wear glasses most of the time, not only to relieve such obvious handicaps as not seeing blackboard work, but to forestall the narrowed range of interests and restricted personality which can result from a child growing up in a world in which only near things are clearly seen.

Surgical Correction of Refractive Errors

The curvature and hence the refractive power of the cornea can be altered by grafting a precisely lathe-shaped 7 to 9mm diameter button of donor cornea on to the centre of the recipient cornea. This type of onlay lamellar keratoplasty, in which only the recipient corneal epithelium is removed, is called *epikeratophakia,* and it will probably be increasingly used to treat selected patients with aphakia or keratoconus. The corneal curvature can be flattened by making eight peripheral radial incisions in the cornea down to the level of Descemet's membrane. This procedure, called *radial keratotomy,* is being done with increasing frequency in some countries to correct moderate degrees ($-3D$ to $-6D$) of myopia.

RELEVANT PHYSICAL AND GEOMETRICAL OPTICS

Diffraction and Interference

The phenomenon of *diffraction* refers to the bending of rays of light which occurs when they pass the edge of an opaque object. As a result the rays are spread out beyond the edge and therefore a shadow of even a point source of light is never truly sharp. When light passes through a small aperture this deviation of light rays at all points of the aperture margin results in the light splaying out behind the aperture so that if the light is intercepted on a screen the image of the aperture is surrounded by a less bright zone of light (Fig 2-15).

This is in conflict with the assumption that light can be represented as rays which travel in straight lines, the rectilinear propagation of light, which is the basis of geometrical optics. In practice, however, the methods of geometrical optics are satisfactory so long as apertures and distances are large compared with the wavelength of light.

The effects of diffraction can occasionally be seen without special apparatus: for example, at sunrise in the mountains when, just before the sun appears over the skyline, the dark outline of the tops in the direction of the sun is surrounded by a brilliant rim of light; the light from the sun is bent over the hill.

Interference is the term used for the interaction which occurs when two or more wave motions meet. When lights from two mutually coherent sources meet, interference occurs so that at some points there is reinforcement and at other points there is cancellation of the wave motion. *Coherence* of lights means that their phase relationship is constant, for example when light from a single source is divided into two separate parts which are then able to overlap. Laser light is coherent.

When light passes an opacity which has a straight edge and is then intercepted by a screen, a fine pattern of lines is formed parallel to the edge of the shadow. This is a *diffraction pattern* and it is the result of interference of the diffracted

OPTICS

rays. The diffraction pattern caused by a circular aperture takes the form of a bright central disc surrounded by concentric dark and light rings (Airy's disc) (Fig 2-15).

A regular pattern of very fine slits, holes, etc., which alternately let light through and stop it is called a *diffraction grating* and this produces diffraction patterns of greater intensity than does a single aperture. With white light the pattern is composed of spectral colours, a diffraction spectrum. Any structure within the eye which acts as a diffraction grating will produce a diffraction spectrum when a bright point of light is viewed and this is seen as a rainbow-coloured *halo* (red outermost) surrounding the light. When the intraocular pressure is acutely raised (acute angle-closure glaucoma) oedema of the corneal epithelium occurs and this, acting as a diffraction grating, gives rise to haloes around lights, a most significant symptom. A halo can be readily experienced by looking at a distant light through a clean glass microscope slide on which you have created a film of droplets of moisture by breathing on it.

Diffraction limits the resolving power of any optical system. In the eye, blurring of the retinal image as a result of diffraction at the pupil increases with decreasing pupil size and becomes significant with pupils less than 2mm in diameter. On the other hand, decreasing the aperture of the eye reduces the effects of aberrations (p. 50) and of ametropia and it is found that with pupil sizes larger than 3mm, visual acuity is independent of pupil size because a decrease in diffraction is counter-balanced by an increase in aberration. The optimum pupil size for best acuity (in good illumination) is between 2 and 3mm.

Scattering of light by very fine particles is a diffraction effect and the colour of a blue iris, like the blue colour of the sky, is due to this. A blue iris is one in which there is little pigment in the stroma. The microscopic cell structures of the stroma scatter blue light more than the longer wavelengths; some of the blue therefore escapes absorption by the pigment of the posterior epithelial layers whereas most of the relatively unscattered green and red is absorbed (p. 9).

Polarized Light

The wave vibrations of light are transverse, i.e. the vibrations take place in a plane perpendicular to the direction of propagation of the wave. In ordinary light transverse vibrations take place in all the possible directions. When light does not vibrate symmetrically in all directions it is said to be *polarized*. In plane-polarized light the vibrations tend to be restricted to one direction (Fig 2-16).

Polarization can result from reflection from a smooth non-metallic surface, e.g. the surface of water or snow; from scattering by dust particles or gas molecules, e.g. light from a blue sky; from passage through crystals which split light into two beams with opposite polarizations (birefringent

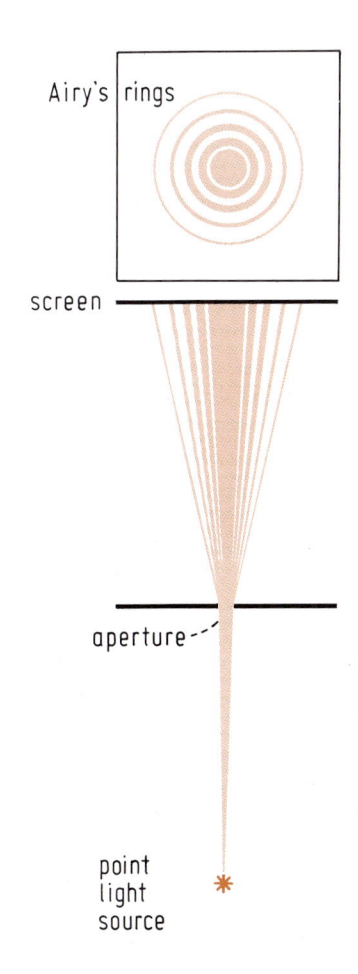

Fig 2-15 Diffraction by a circular aperture and the diffraction pattern resulting from interference of the diffracted rays.

crystals); and from passage through filters which are birefringent and also absorb one of the polarized beams (dichroic polarizers), e.g. 'Polaroid' filters.

In ophthalmology, polarizing filters are used to present different images to the two eyes, e.g. in a stereoscopic slide projector; to eliminate unwanted reflections, e.g. in some ophthalmoscopes; to act as 'light rheostats' or 'light valves' in varying the intensity of a light; and to reduce glare by blocking or preventing reflected glare light, e.g. in sun glasses in which the (transmission) axis is vertical (useful in dry fly fishing), and in desk lights.

Spherical Aberration

Rays of light which pass through the peripheral portion of a lens with spherical surfaces are brought to a focus nearer to the lens than are rays which pass through the centre of the lens (paraxial rays). As a consequence, a point image of a point on the object is not formed and this is known as spherical aberration (Fig 2-17). To eliminate this aberration the lens surfaces must be aspheric. These are not often used because they are difficult to make, but aspheric lenses of plastic are used when strong spectacles are needed, e.g. after cataract extraction, for subnormal vision.

Spherical aberration can be reduced by using an aperture in front of a lens so that only paraxial rays can pass, but this reduces the brightness of the image. Selection of the best shapes of lenses (e.g. biconvex, planoconvex, etc.) and combinations of lenses are used to reduce spherical aberration in optical instruments (aplanatic lenses).

The spherical aberration of the human eye is small because of the peripheral flattening of the cornea and because the core of the lens is more refractive than the periphery.

Chromatic Aberration

Because the refractive index of any material varies with the wavelength of light, being smaller for longer wavelengths and larger for shorter wavelengths, the component wavelengths of white light are refracted to different degrees by a given material (dispersion). In a simple lens this causes chromatic aberration; for example, with a convex lens the blue rays, being refracted more strongly, come to a focus nearer to the lens than the red rays. As a consequence, instead of points an image is composed of blur circles. The diameter of these depends on the diameter of the lens and they can therefore be reduced in size and the image sharpened by reducing the aperture of a lens.

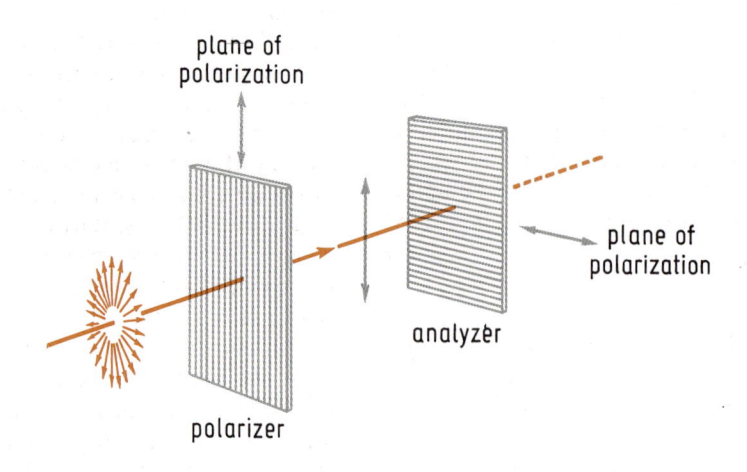

Fig 2-16 Plane polarization of light by one dichroic filter (polarizer) and its subsequent absorption by a second crossed filter (analyzer).

OPTICS

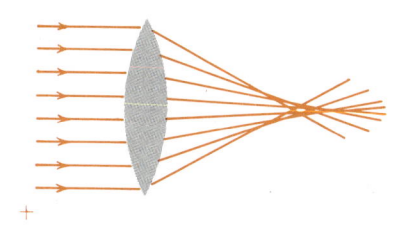

Fig 2-17 Spherical aberration of a biconvex lens.

Dispersion and refractive index for different materials do not run strictly parallel and it is therefore possible to make an achromatic lens by combining glasses with different dispersions and refractive indices.

Red neon signs are seen more clearly than blue or green ones because for red the eye is relatively hypermetropic and this can be compensated for by accommodation; no such correction is possible with the shorter wavelengths to which the eye is relatively myopic.

Chromatic aberration is one of the more serious defects of the human eye but, except under laboratory conditions, its effects are rarely seen; this may be because there is a neural mechanism which suppresses the chromatic fringes on the retina. It can be demonstrated by looking at a small distant light through a cobalt glass which transmits light only from the blue and red ends of the spectrum. What is seen will depend on any refractive error; with hypermetropia there is a blue spot surrounded by a red ring; with myopia there is a red spot surrounded by a blue ring (Fig 2-18). This test could be used in determining refractive errors, but a more refined test is the *duochrome* test in which black letters on green and on red retro-illuminated backgrounds are viewed. When the green and red are equally clear the refractive error is precisely corrected.

Image Formation by a Lens with Opacities

When an image of an object point is formed by a lens, all parts of the lens contribute to the formation of the image. This means that a localized opacity of part of the lens does not prevent an image being formed although it will reduce its brightness. It follows that localized cataract changes may interfere only slightly with vision. It also follows that ophthalmoscopy is

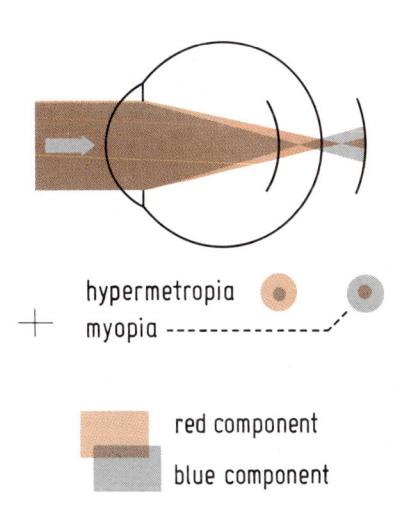

Fig 2-18 Chromatic aberration in the eye.

possible in an eye in which the lens is partly opaque provided a clear part of the lens is chosen to look through; this is usually very much easier when the patient's pupil is dilated with drops.

An opacity centrally in the lens may obstruct vision when the pupil is small and with this type of cataract patients often see less well in bright light. They can be helped by regularly using eye drops to dilate their pupil.

Reflecting Surfaces of the Eye

At any surface where refraction occurs, that is where a surface separates media of different refractive indices, there is also reflection. Much use is made of these mirror surfaces of the eye. And they can also be a nuisance; for example, reflection from the cornea, the corneal light reflex, is a difficulty in ophthalmoscopy. By measuring the sizes of the reflected (catoptric) images of known objects from the anterior and posterior corneal surfaces and from the anterior and posterior lens surfaces (the Purkinje-Sanson images) the curvature of these surfaces can be determined, as can also the changes which occur in the lens surfaces on accommodation.

Keratoscopy is a method of examining the reflected image formed by the cornea of concentric circles and thereby assessing its curvature and especially any irregularities of its surface or loss of surface lustre (Fig-19). This is a more elaborate way of performing a very simple but basic clinical test. In practice the light of a focusing pocket torch or an ophthalmoscope is shone obliquely from several directions in turn on to the cornea and imperfections of its mirror surface looked for. With this technique minute irregularities, e.g. abrasions, ulcers, which are invisible with direct illumination can be easily detected.

Keratometry is a method of precisely measuring the radius of curvature of the central portion of the cornea, again by measuring the size of the reflected image of an object of known size. The information it gives is necessary for fitting contact lenses.

The positions of the corneal light reflexes when a light is looked at are regularly used to check whether there is a squint (p. 102).

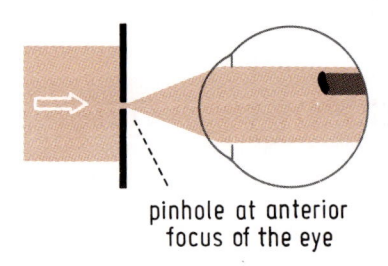

Fig 2-20 Optical arrangement which increases the visibility to an observer of an opacity in his or her vitreous.

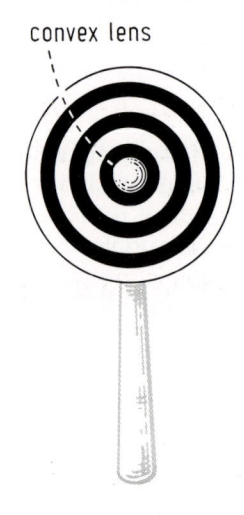

Fig 2-19 Placido's disc for keratoscopy.

Visualization of Intraocular Opacities

Fine opacities in the vitreous are almost universal and most people will have at some time noticed these muscae volitantes (flying flies) when looking towards a bright surface, e.g. the sky. Their shadows on the retina are made more distinct if the optical conditions are so arranged that the rays of light within the vitreous are more or less parallel. This requires a small source of light at the anterior focus of the eye. The simplest way to achieve this is to make a small hole (e.g. 0.2mm) in a card, hold this 15mm in front of the cornea and look through the hole at a bright light (Fig 2-20).

Chapter 3

PHYSIOLOGY OF VISION

VISUAL SENSATION
Stimulus and sensation
Dual visual systems
Methods of investigation

PHOTOCHEMICAL TRANSDUCTION
Psychophysical studies

THE SENSATION OF LIGHT
Brightness
Threshold
   Spatial summation
   Temporal summation
Visual field
Adaptation
   Apparent brightness
   Local retinal adaptation
Spectral sensitivity
Differential light threshold, contrast
   Simultaneous contrast
   Relation between intensity and brightness
Time relationship between stimulus and sensation
   Latency
   Duration of sensation

FORM VISION
Visual acuity
Regional differences of the retina
Relation between intensity and acuity
The optical and anatomical basis
Visibility of a single line
Contrast sensitivity

COLOUR VISION
Attributes of colour
   Hue
   Brightness
   Saturation
Stimuli for colour
Colour mixtures
Mechanism of colour vision
   Trichromatic receptors
   Opponent-pairs process
Colour matching
Clinical testing
Defective colour vision

ELECTRO-PHYSIOLOGY OF VISION
Methods applicable to human subjects
   Electro-oculography
   Electroretinography
   Visually evoked response
Methods applicable to animal subjects
   Retinal cells
   Receptive fields
   Visual cortex
   Colour coding
   Columnar organization
   Higher cortical areas
   Interference with normal development

BINOCULAR VISION
Visual direction
   Oculocentric direction
   Egocentric direction
Binocular vision
   Corresponding retinal points
   Horopter
Stereopsis
Suppression, retinal rivalry, stereoscopic lustre
Diplopia
The synoptophore
   Simultaneous perception
   Fusion
   Stereopsis
Binocular motor co-ordination
Heterophoria

THE PHYSIOLOGY OF VISION

VISUAL SENSATION

Sensation and Perception

In the analysis of sensory experience it is customary to distinguish between sensations, the elemental sensory impressions, and perceptions, the final products in consciousness which are syntheses of sensations, experience, and expectations, which require attention and which give the sensations some meaning. In some degree this distinction corresponds with those aspects which can be studied by the methods of physiology and those which require the methods of psychology. However, these distinctions, while of some use, are largely arbitrary and artificial. In fact it is impossible to experience a pure and isolated sensation. It would be silly in an introduction to the physiology of vision to discuss only physiology and omit the psychological culmination of the process. The following largely descriptive account is therefore a mixture of physiology and psychology.

Stimulus and Sensation

In considering sensation it is important to differentiate between the physical stimulus and the subjective sensation. Confusion of stimulus and sensation is encouraged by the ordinary use of words. For example, 'a red light', which can really only describe a sensation, is commonly used to describe a stimulus which for pedantic accuracy should be described as 'radiation of such and such wavelengths' or 'light which generally gives rise to a sensation described as red'.

The table summarizing visual sensation illustrates this distinction and will also serve as a guide to what is initially a confusing topic. Like any analysis this is artificial and over simplified. For example, brightness and form discrimination vary with colour, and the colour of a sensation is influenced by other variables than the wavelength.

Dual Visual Systems

The visual process is based on a double mechanism and the results of this are apparent in the study of almost every aspect of seeing. There is a *scotopic* mechanism, more active in dim light, mediated by the rods, which is especially concerned with the appreciation of low intensities of light and of movement and is achromatic. And there is a *photopic* mechanism, more active in bright light, mediated by the cones, which is especially concerned with the appreciation of form and colour. The two receptors have different structures and photopigments, have a different topographical distribution in the retina and have differing patterns of neural connections in that many rods converge on to a single pathway while each cone has a more individual pathway to the central nervous system.

Methods of Investigation

Information about the physiology of vision comes from three main sources, *psychophysical* studies of visual sensation and perception, *photochemical* studies of the peripheral mechanism, and *electrophysiological* studies of the visual pathways from receptors to cortex. In psychophysics the sensations aroused by precisely known stimuli are systematically studied to establish the quantitative relationships which exist between stimulus and response. The physiological events which occur between stimulus and sensation are ignored, the nervous system being treated more or less as a 'black box'. In photochemistry and electrophysiology the contents of the black box are studied and, although the results are beginning to explain some of the mechanisms which link stimulus and sensation, it is not possible to unify all the information obtained by these different approaches.

In this survey an outline of the photochemistry of vision is followed by a description based largely on the findings of psychophysical investigations. Some of the more noteworthy results of the electrophysiological approach follow the account of colour vision.

PHYSIOLOGY

SUMMARY OF VISUAL SENSATION

	Stimulus	**Sensation and Perception**
	Light 400-760 nm	Sight[1]
	Low Intensity	Scotopic vision
	High Intensity	Photopic vision
Quantity	Intensity (luminance)	Brightness[2]
		Threshold
		Differential threshold
Spatial distribution	Objective direction	Subjective direction (visual direction)[3]
	Constant stimulus	Autokinetic movement
	Temporal change	Movement[4]
	Multiple	
	Subthreshold	Spatial summation[5]
	Suprathreshold	
	Effect of adjacent stimuli	Inhibition (contrast)[6]
	Simultaneous stimuli	Form discrimination[4]
Temporal distribution	Objective timing	Subjective timing[7]
		Latency
		After image
	Constant stimulus	Adaptation[8]
	Spatial change	Phi movement
	Multiple	
	Subthreshold	Temporal summation[5]
	Suprathreshold	
	Effect of previous stimuli	Dark adaptation[8]
		Light adaptation
	Continuing stimuli	Flicker fusion
Quality	Wavelength	Colour[9]

1. The *adequate stimulus* is light between 400 and 706 nanometres (nm).
2. The *intensity* (quantity) of the stimulus is discriminated — *brightness*.
3. Each sensation is given a location in space — *visual direction*.
4. Because of (3), there is discrimination between spatially separated simultaneous stimuli — *form*, and there is discrimination of change in position of a stimulus — *movement*.
5. Summation of subthreshold stimuli separated in space or time may result in a sensation — *spatial and temporal summation*.
6. The sensation resulting from one stimulus may be *inhibited* by another stimulus — *contrast*.
7. Stimulus and sensation are not coterminous. There is an interval of time between the onset of the stimulus and the sensation — *latency*. Sensation may outlast the stimulus — *after image*.
8. *Adaptation* to a constant stimulus occurs so that brightness diminishes. A period of absence of stimulus results in lowered threshold — *dark adaptation*.
9. The *wavelength* (quality) of the stimulus is discriminated — *colour* (hue).

PHOTOCHEMICAL TRANSDUCTION

Electromagnetic radiation is without effect unless it is absorbed (Fig 3-1). The portion of the spectrum between about 400 and 700nm is light because this is the wave band which is absorbed by the photoreceptors of the eye, the rods and cones. The light-absorbing materials they contain are the *visual pigments* (not to be confused with the melanin pigment of the pigment epithelium which also absorbs light and converts it into heat). These pigments are the transducers which initiate the conversion of light-energy into neuro-electrical impulses. When they absorb quanta of light their molecules break down with release of energy. Resynthesis of the molecules is effected by an enzyme mechanism within the retina.

The pigment in rods is rhodopsin and it absorbs most readily light of wavelength 500nm (blue-green) (Fig 3-2). Each cone contains one of three different visual pigments. These have maximum absorptions respectively at 419nm (blue), 531nm (green), and 559nm (yellow) and provide the basis for wavelength discrimination which gives rise to the perception of colour (Fig 3-3). (Although the peak absorption of the 'red' pigment is of a 'yellow' wavelength it does absorb 'red' wavelengths as well.)

These visual pigments are conjugated proteins, a globular supporting protein, opsin, being combined with a chromophore carotenoid chain. The chromophore group, retinal, is the aldehyde of vitamin A, retinol, and a nutritional deficiency of vitamin A can cause night-blindness due to malfunctioning of the rods. The four human visual pigments contain the same chromophore, retinal, united with four different opsins. It is not known how differences in the opsins alter the absorption spectra of the same chromophore which is presumably the part which absorbs the light. Retinal can exist in a number of cis-trans stereoisomers and it is thought that the primary action of light is to isomerize the retinal from the bent (11-cis) to the straight (trans) shape. This slight alteration in form sets off a chain of reactions that result in a change in shape of the whole pigment molecule, bleaching of the molecule and finally separation of retinal from opsin. Regeneration of rhodopsin from retinal and opsin requires isomerization of trans retinal back to the 11-cis form and this is facilitated by an enzyme system contained in the pigment epithelium of the retina. This is one of the

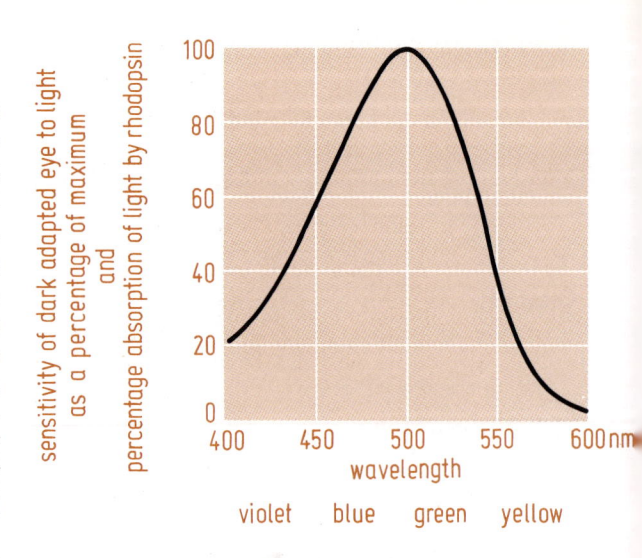

Fig 3-2 Scotopic spectral luminosity (or sensitivity) curve and spectral absorption curve of rhodopsin.

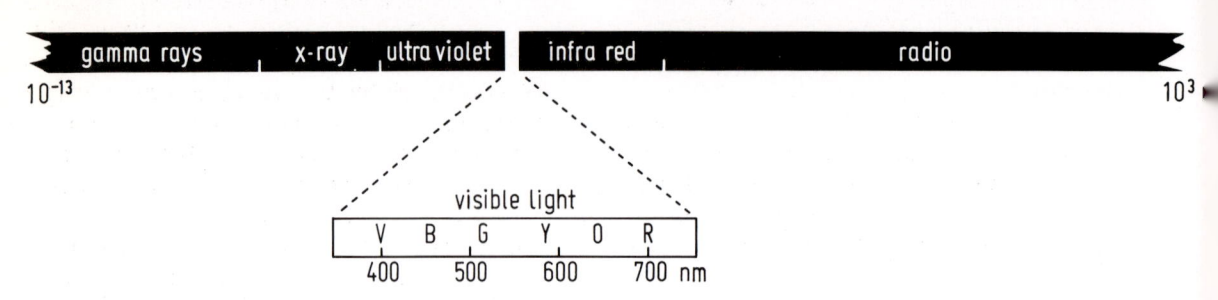

Fig 3-1 Wavelength spectrum of electromagnetic radiation.

reasons for the loss of vision in retinal detachment and explains why recovery of vision can occur when the detached retina is reapposed to the pigment epithelium.

Psychophysical Studies

Measurement of Sensation

Accurate quantification of subjective sensations is not possible. For example, we cannot say that one sensation is three times brighter than another sensation. The three features of a sensation which can be determined are:

1. The threshold of the sensation.
2. The equality of two sensations, e.g. matching for equal brightness; matching of their colours.
3. The minimum detectable difference between two sensations, e.g. differential light threshold; discrimination of hues.

In each case it is the stimulus which is measured and it is assumed that equal sensations are evoked by equal stimuli under identical conditions.

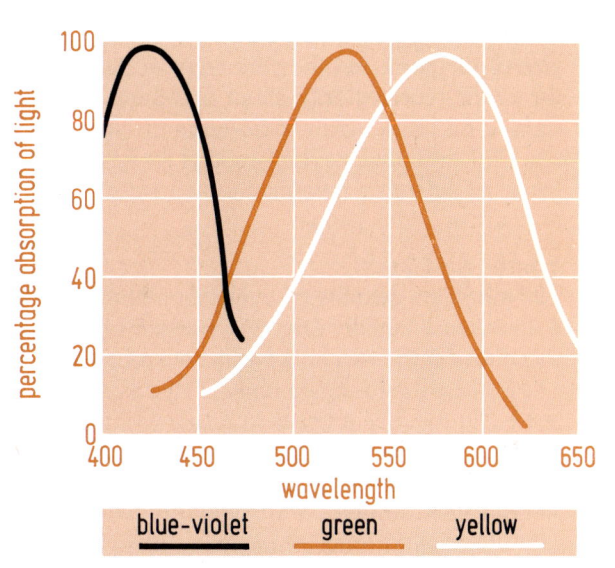

Fig 3-3 Spectral absorption curves of the three cone pigments.

THE SENSATION OF LIGHT

Brightness

This is the simplest visual sensation, the sensation of light itself. The nearest approach to the pure sensation can be experienced when the whole visual field is uniformly filled with diffused light. The absence of light gives rise to a sensation of blackness. That this also is a sensation will be realized by thinking of the space behind your head. From here there is no sensation, there is nothing. This is probably the nearest we can come to experiencing what it is like to be blind.

Assessment of the perception of light as such involves measurement of the *threshold*, the intensity of light which can just be detected, and the *differential light threshold*, the smallest difference in intensity which can be appreciated. The reciprocal of the threshold, *sensitivity*, is often used because of its greater convenience.

Threshold

At best the eye is very sensitive to light; when dark-adapted it is more sensitive than most artificial light detectors. Light as faint as that from a candle about 17 miles away in a non-absorbing atmosphere can be seen. The energy involved in this is unimaginably small, 10^{-10} erg/sec.

Because of the uncertainty underlying quantum fluctuations at low intensities and biological variations, absolute threshold is not a sharply defined intensity of stimulus. It is an arbitrarily defined probability of seeing and a 50% frequency of seeing is usually chosen as indicating the threshold level.

The minimum number of quanta of light absorbed by the retinal photoreceptors which can elicit a sensation of light is probably about 4. Note that this is the light which reaches and is absorbed by the retinal photoreceptors; 40 to 100 quanta have to enter the eye for 4 quanta to arrive at the retina. It is thought that a retinal rod can be stimulated by the absorption of a single quantum. But this does not give rise to a sensation because it cannot be distinguished as a signal from the spontaneous random discharges from the retina ('dark noise').

In practice, threshold is affected by many factors, e.g. refraction of the eye, the size of the pupil, direction of entry of light into the eye, wavelength, duration and area of the stimulus, the region of the retina stimulated, age, and the attention of the subject. The importance of age is shown by the fact that, owing to the smaller size of the pupil and the yellowing of the lens, the retina receives only about one-third of the light at 60 years that it received at 20 years of age. This has obvious implications for selecting levels of desirable illumination and for driving at night by older people.

Spatial Summation

The minimum quantity of light required to elicit a sensation is equally effective whether concentrated on a small area of the retina or spread over a larger area (up to certain limits). That is, a large test patch requires a lower luminance (intensity per unit area) than does a smaller area for it to be seen. This means that spatial summation of sub-threshold stimuli occurs, and it is due to the convergence of groups of receptors on to single ganglion cells. This explains why summation occurs over much larger areas in the periphery of the retina than at the centre where cones converge much less and may even have a one-to-one relation to individual ganglion cells.

Temporal Summation

Within a certain range of times temporal summation of sub-threshold stimuli occurs. The time-span required by the eye to integrate energy is about 0.1 second. Again, it is the total number of quanta reaching the receptors which determines the emergence of sensation.

Visual Field

The visual field is the portion of external space visible to one stationary eye. Put another way it is the locus of all points on a surface in front of and concentric with the stationary eye from which a visual sensation can be stimulated.

In testing the field of vision the *threshold* intensity of a stimulus required to evoke a sensation from various parts of the field is determined. The intensity of the stimulus is varied by using test objects of different sizes and luminances and peripheral vision is measured by determining the most peripheral position of the test object when it is just seen. This position is described by polar co-ordinates from the fixation point (so many degrees from fixation in such and

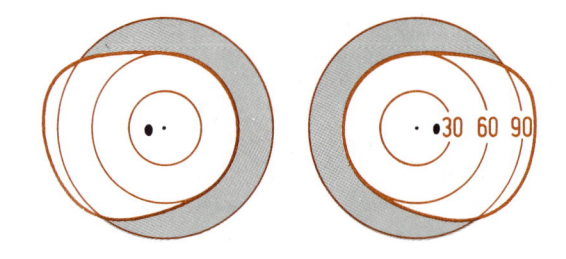

Fig 3-4 Boundaries and blind spots of normal visual fields conventionally charted as seen by the subject. The fixation points and the 30°, 60° and 90° distances from fixation are shown.

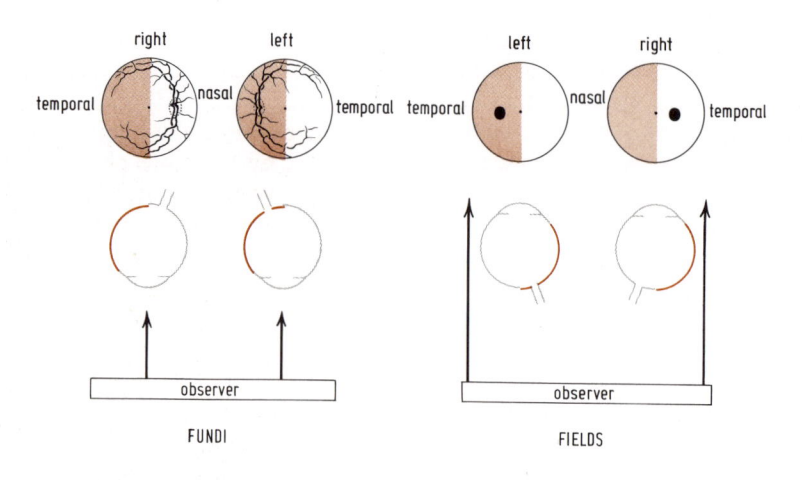

Fig 3-5 Corresponding areas of fundi and fields.

such a meridian). The line connecting the points where a given test-object is seen is called an isopter (Fig 3-4). By custom the field is drawn on a chart as it is seen from the subject's eye. Because a map of the visual field is charted in this way there may be confusion as to the corresponding points on the fundus as seen with an ophthalmoscope unless a careful mental transposition is made (Fig 3-5). A verbal transposition is an easy and safe way out (superior → inferior, temporal → nasal, etc)!

Two devices which are used clinically to examine visual fields are the arc- or bowl-shaped perimeter, in which the testing distance is one-third of a metre and with which the whole visual field can be examined, and the flat black tangent (Bjerrum's) screen, in which the testing distance is one or two metres and with which only the central field out to about 30° from fixation can be examined. In a commonly used perimeter, the Goldmann perimeter, spots of light of selected sizes and intensities are projected on to and moved over the inside surface of a hemispherical bowl which is diffusely illuminated to provide an appropriate background illumination (Fig 9-6). The subject's head is positioned so that the eye being tested is at the centre of the sphere and fixes a small light at the centre of the bowl. With the tangent screen a small white disc of a selected size at the end of a fine black wand is moved in front of the black screen. Compared with the perimeter the tangent screen magnifies any defects in the central visual field. The simplest way to test a patient's visual fields is by 'confrontation' (p. 101) but, although this can yield much useful information, quantitative studies with instruments are frequently required.

Adaptation
This refers to the common experience that the sensitivity of the eye adjusts to the general level of illumination. With low intensities vision is scotopic, with high intensities it is photopic and the transition between the two occurs at light intensities corresponding to about that of full moonlight. The threshold alters with the amount of light to which the eye has been exposed in the recent past.

Dark adaptation results in a 20-times increase in sensitivity of the central retina after about seven minutes in the dark and a 10,000-times increase in sensitivity of the peripheral retina after about one hour. Dilatation of the pupil which occurs in the dark gives an increase in sensitivity of only 16 times.

The course of dark adaptation can be followed by determining at regular intervals the threshold intensity of a stimulus for a subject kept in the dark. When an area of the retina containing both rods and cones is tested the adaptation curve (threshold intensity plotted against time) shows a shoulder at about 7 minutes corresponding to the limit of cone-adaptation and beyond which the slower but much greater rod-adaptation continues (Fig 3-6).

Because the sensitivity of cones increases much less than that of rods with dark adaptation, there is a relative central scotoma under conditions of dim illumination. It is well known that faint stars can be seen when viewed eccentrically but disappear when looked at directly. Deliberate use of eccentric vision may be important in such activities as night-flying.

Red light is relatively poorly absorbed by rods and it is therefore a relatively inefficient stimulus for them. Consequently it does not interfere with their dark adaptation as much as lights of shorter wavelength. For this reason useful levels of dark adaptation can be achieved by wearing dark red goggles (through which cone vision is possible) instead of by being in complete darkness.

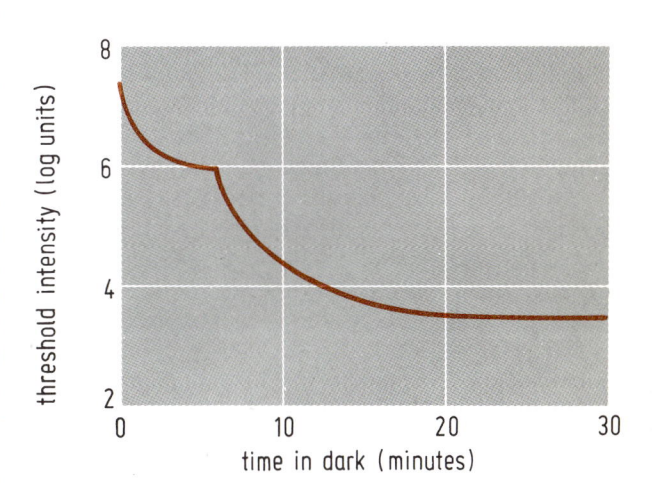

Fig 3-6 Dark adaptation curve.

Dark adaptation is due to both regeneration of the visual pigments and to neural mechanisms in the retina and central nervous system.

Light adaptation, the decreased sensitivity with increased intensity of illumination, is more rapid than dark adaptation. The time required is about two or three minutes and a very large increase in threshold occurs during the first few seconds.

Apparent Brightness

As well as its effect on threshold, adaptation affects the apparent brightness of above threshold stimuli. With increasing dark adaptation a low intensity stimulus looks brighter and brighter, while with increasing light adaptation a high intensity stimulus looks less and less bright. In fact, over a range of intensities of about 1,000 to 1, compensation is such that the final brightness is the same for stimuli of different intensity. For example, if the image is completely stabilized on the retina, a pattern of different shades of grey will within a few minutes become a uniform unpatterned grey.

Local Retinal Adaptation

In normal seeing the state of adaptation of the retina changes from place to place and from time to time as images of differing intensities fall on various parts of the retina. As a consequence the relative brightness of an array of objects does not change when the intensity of the illumination slowly changes with time, e.g. as a cloud passes across the sun (brightness constancy).

Troxler Effect

If the eye does not move, objects in the periphery of the visual field, and particularly in low levels of lighting, disappear from sight. This is a local adaptation effect which you can readily experience for yourself. It is not usually experienced for objects near fixation because the normal involuntary eye movements (physiological nystagmus) preclude steady fixation. However, if the retinal image is truly stabilized by the use of an optical system so that the image moves precisely with all eye movements, a simple pattern fails in about five seconds and a complex pattern fragments. Unsteady fixation is necessary for normal seeing; what might seem to be a defect of the tracking system of the eyes is made use of by the central nervous system. This is another indication that one of the major functions of the central nervous system is the detection of change in the environment.

This local adaptation partly explains why we are unaware of the *shadows cast by our retinal blood vessels* on the underlying receptors. If the retina is illuminated with light coming from an unusual angle, e.g. by shining the light through the sclera instead of through the pupil, the shadows of the vessels are displaced on to receptors which are not relatively dark-adapted and the pattern of retinal vessels is perceived in surprising detail. The simplest way to experience this is to gently rub your eyeball with the lit-up naked bulb of a torch through a closed lid just inside the lower or the upper orbital margin. The dark optic disc and the avascular area of the macula are readily appreciated.

Spectral Sensitivity

The colour of a stimulus affects its brightness. Lights of different wavelengths but each of the same intensity produce different brightnesses, those from the middle of the spectrum looking most bright. That is, the eye is maximally sensitive to yellow and this colour is therefore the best for distress signal lights and survival clothing.

The curve in which sensitivity to light is plotted against wavelength of light is called the spectral luminosity curve or spectral sensitivity curve. (Note that it is brightness which is measured without reference to colour, which may or may not occur.) This differs depending on whether the eye is dark-adapted or light-adapted. The two curves are similar in shape, but the light-adapted curve is nearer to the red end of the spectrum, the *Purkinje shift,* so that in scotopic vision the eye is most sensitive to green (500nm), while in photopic vision it is most sensitive to yellow (560nm) (Fig 3-7). Purkinje described this phenomenon (the Purkinje effect) in a form which is easily repeated at sunset or sunrise. As the sun sets and the general illumination diminishes, red flowers look progressively darker than blue flowers even though in daylight they looked more or less equally bright. Eventually the red flowers look black or are invisible while the blue flowers are seen as greyish patches and vision is colourless.

As intensity of illumination increases and vision changes from colourless scotopic to coloured photopic, or as a stimulus is moved from the periphery towards the centre of the retina, there is a *photochromatic interval* during which coloured stimuli all appear blue-grey before they excite a sensation of colour. Rods are relatively (e.g. 1,000 times) more sensitive than cones to the blue end of the spectrum, while foveal cones are slightly more sensitive than rods to the extreme red end of the spectrum. It is fortunate that if a red light is seen, e.g. a signal light, it is seen as red, i.e. for deep red there is almost no photochromatic interval. In examining the visual fields with coloured objects it is usually the recognition of the colour which is tested and the photochromatic interval has to be ignored.

The spectral absorption curve for rhodopsin corresponds so closely to the rod spectral sensitivity curve that this is strong evidence for rhodopsin being the pigment in rods which absorbs light and thereby initiates the visual process (Fig 3-2).

Differential Light Threshold. Contrast

This refers to the ability to discriminate between differences of intensity, either between two neighbouring stimuli (differential threshold) or between a stimulus and its background (incremental threshold). Contrast between an object and its background is the basis of seeing objects at all. When we look at the sky in daylight the quanta of light from the stars still reach our eyes but we do not see them because the stimulus they provide

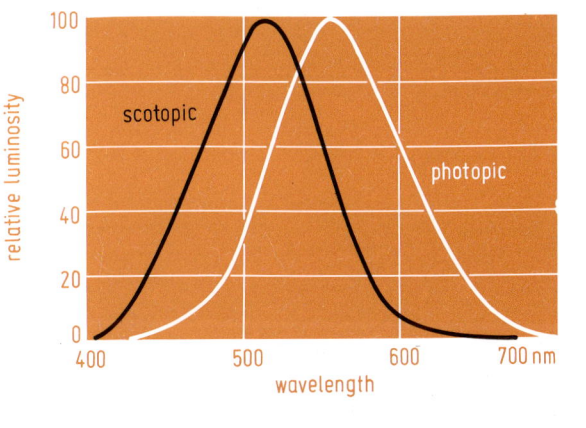

Fig 3-7 Purkinje shift. Relative scotopic and photopic spectral luminosity curves. Note that the actual sensitivity is much greater in scotopic than in photopic vision.

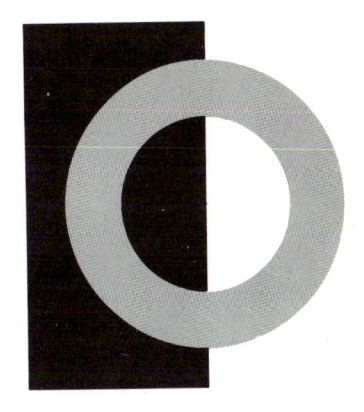

Fig 3-8 Simultaneous contrast. Grey on black seems lighter than the same grey on white.

in addition to that of the background stimulus is too small to be detected.

Simultaneous Contrast

The brightness of the area surrounding a stimulus greatly affects the apparent brightness of the stimulus. For example, the same grey patch appears dark if surrounded by white but light if surrounded by black (Fig 3-8). Similarly, a given colour looks more intense when it is surrounded by its complementary colour.

It is the local border contrast rather than the average contrast between a surface and its surroundings which influences the apparent brightness of the surface. If the change in luminance at the border between adjacent surfaces of *unequal luminance* is gradual the surfaces can appear to be *equally bright* (Fig 3-9). This occurs under natural conditions when, for example, the gradual change in the intensity of illumination along the wall of a room lit by a single light near one end may not be perceived. On the other hand abrupt changes of luminance enhance the brightness difference at sharp-edged borders of objects. Brightness depends so much on border contrast that when two adjacent surfaces of *equal luminance* are separated by a border in which there is a local difference in luminance, the surfaces appear to be *unequally bright* (the Craik-O'Brien-Cornsweet illusion) (Fig 3-10). Both retinal and central mechanisms are involved in this process of lateral inhibition (spatial induction). It plays an important role in form vision.

Fig 3-9 (a) The luminances of the two half fields are different (physical contrast 3.5%). As shown in the luminance profile there is an abrupt step transition between the two sides and as expected they appear to be unequally bright.

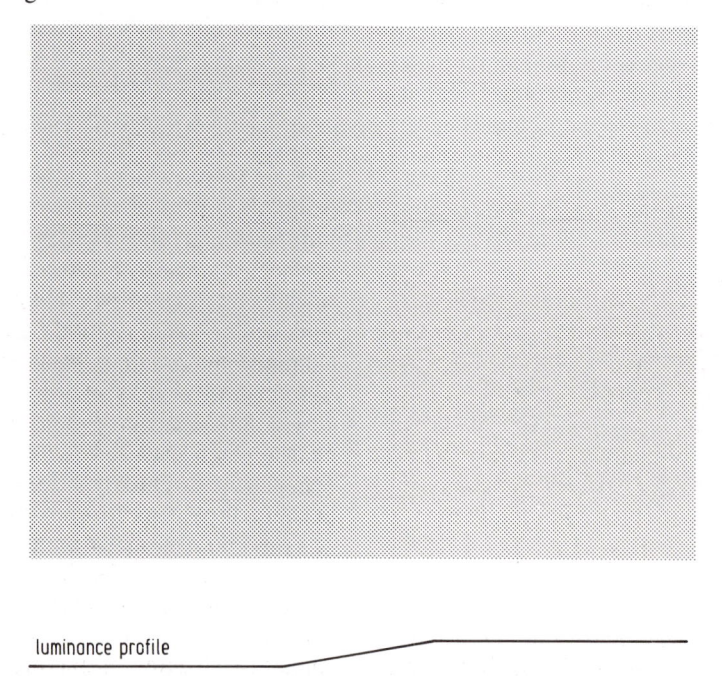

(b) The luminances of the half fields are the same as in Fig 3-9(a) but as shown by the ramp in the luminance profile the transition between them is gradual. It is difficult if not impossible to detect the expected difference in brightness between the two sides. In this figure and in Fig 3-10 the luminance of a surface depends on the size of the individual dots and these were regulated by computer control of a laser printer.

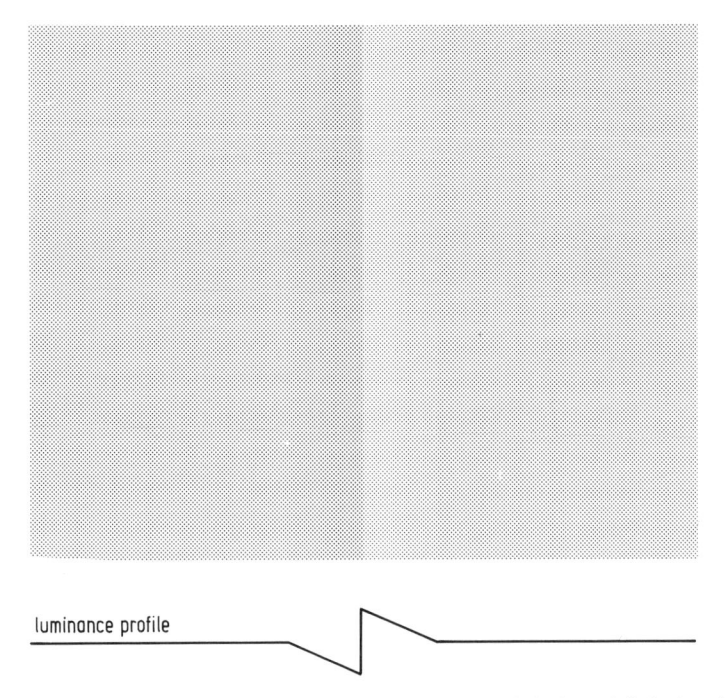

Fig 3-10 The luminance profile shows that apart from the central dark and light bands the luminance is uniform, but the two half fields appear to be unequally bright. Cover the border between the two halves with an opaque strip and the difference in brightness will disappear.

Quantitative Relation between Intensity and Brightness

The relation between a stimulus and the resulting sensation in general was thought to be such that the smallest difference in a stimulus which can be detected is proportional to the whole stimulus (Weber's Law; $\triangle I/I$ = constant). For light this is suggested by the observation that an extra candle makes an appreciable difference to the brightness of a room lit by one or two candles, but no difference to a room normally lit by electricity. Weber's Law is approximately true for vision over medium intensities where we can detect a change in intensity of about 1% of the background illumination.

Another attempt to relate intensity to brightness was 'Fechner's Law' which states that brightness increases in proportion to the logarithm of the intensity of the stimulus. In other words, for brightness to increase steadily (arithmetically) intensity has to be increased more and more (geometrically).

Time Relationship between Stimulus and Sensation

Latency

The latent period between stimulus and sensation varies between 0.05 and 0.5 second. It is such that if two pilots are flying at Mach 3 on a collision course and one emerges from cloud 200 metres from the other they would collide without ever seeing each other.

The latent period increases with decreasing intensity of the stimulus and it has been suggested that this is due to temporal summation, a process which increases retinal sensitivity by increasing the time during which the energy of a stimulus can be integrated. This increased latency in dim light means that the reaction time of drivers is lengthened and the increased integrating time makes localization of moving objects, as in ball games, less accurate.

This effect is indirectly demonstrated by the *Pulfrich pendulum effect* (Fig 3-11). If a pendulum is observed swinging across the line of sight with

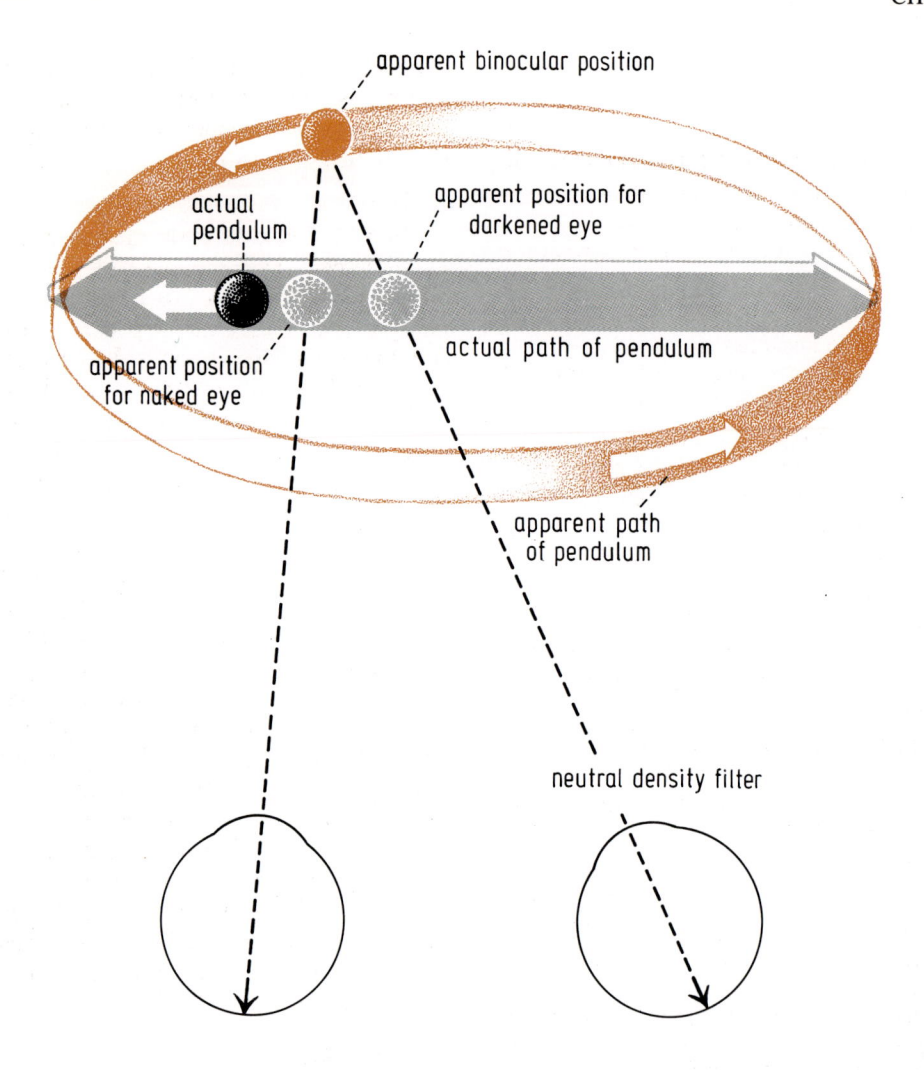

Fig 3-11 Pulfrich pendulum effect.

both eyes, one of which has a dark glass before it, the pendulum will appear to swing in an ellipse instead of in a straight line. The pendulum is seen by the eye with reduced illumination after it is seen by the other eye and therefore its position as seen with the darkened eye trails behind its position as seen with the other. This disparity gives rise to a stereoscopic displacement of the pendulum and this is greatest at the centre of swing where the movement is fastest. Hence the pendulum is seen to follow an elliptical path.

The Pulfrich effect can be elicited without using a dark filter when a patient has pathological changes, e.g. demyelination in multiple sclerosis, which delay conduction in one optic nerve more than the other. A simple clinical test with a swinging pendulum can thus detect asymmetry of the conduction times in the right and left visual pathways. Conduction times are more precisely assessed by measuring the latencies of the visually evoked response (p. 74).

Duration of Sensation

After the cessation of a stimulus sensation continues *(visual persistence)* for a time which varies with intensity, adaptation, etc. A *positive after-image* is an example of this and may be experienced by looking towards a light with one eye covered and the other screened by a card. If the card is rapidly jerked aside and immediately replaced as rapidly as possible the light will be briefly seen as if through the card, so clearly in fact that details not noticed while exposed to the light may be seen in the after-image.

A brief exposure is likely to produce a positive after-image, that is one which is bright against a darker background. It is as if retinal activity continues after the stimulus stops.

A more prolonged exposure (e.g. for 30 seconds) without movement of the eye to a visual field containing a localized stimulus of high intensity is likely to produce a *negative after-image,* that is one which is dark against a brighter background. (The words positive and negative are used by analogy with their use in photography.) This is readily experienced by fixing a naked light and then looking at a uniform surface when a black spot will be seen. If the light is coloured the negative after-image is tinged with the complementary colour.

Local light adaptation in the region of the retina subjected to the bright illumination obviously plays a part in the production of a negative after-image but there is evidence that central parts of the nervous system as well as the retina are concerned in after-image formation. In any case the one after-image can change from negative to positive and vice versa, e.g. with the opening and closing the eyes.

The mechanisms which give rise to after-images are sometimes called successive contrast or temporal induction. These terms emphasize that the effect of a retinal stimulus is not limited to the actual time of the stimulus, just as the terms simultaneous contrast or spatial induction (p. 61) emphasize that the effect of a stimulus is not limited to the actual area of the retina stimulated. A stimulus induces changes which are temporally and spatially different from its actual occurrence.

Cinema and television are only possible because of visual persistence which causes a discontinuous stimulus to produce a continuous sensation. The discontinuity of the cinema stimulus will be appreciated when it is realized that the screen is dark for about half the time. The movement seen in the movies and in moving illuminated signs is due to another effect, called the *phi phenomenon* or beta-movement. This is the sensation of continuous movement which results from successive stimulation of neighbouring retinal regions by brief stationary stimuli provided both the distance and the time interval between the stimuli are within a certain range.

Flicker

If a light flashes on and off the separate flashes will be perceived if the frequency is low, but when the frequency becomes faster than a certain rate the light is seen continuously as a steady light. This lowest rate for fusion is the *critical fusion frequency.* It is about 30 per second for moderate intensities and about 50 per second for bright lights.

The original rate of sixteen frames per second at which films were projected was chosen because, with the intensities of light used, the majority of people did not experience flicker, although many did and hence the old name, 'the flicks'. Modern projectors interrupt the light 72 times per second which is above the critical fusion frequency.

Similarly in television the frame rate must be fast enough (together with the decay time of the screen phosphor) to avoid flicker, although this may occur and in a very few susceptible people it has induced photogenic epilepsy. Flicker produced by the rotor blades of a helicopter near the ground or by driving past a row of trees with the sun on the far side can be a similar hazard. The 50 per second fluctuation of fluorescent light tubes may give rise to flicker in some people when seen in the peripheral field.

FORM VISION

Form vision or the form sense refers to the ability to discriminate spatially separated visual stimuli. *Visual acuity* is a measure of the accuracy of form vision and, in general usage, visual acuity means the ability to distinguish the details and the shape of objects. It is a measure of the resolving power of the eye.

In its more precise use visual acuity is the measure of visual resolution. It is conveniently defined as the visual angle (in minutes of arc) subtended at the eye by the smallest detail the presence of which the subject can detect in a test object. This is referred to as the threshold visual angle or as the minimum angle of resolution (MAR) of the test. For example, with Landolt rings (broken circles in which the gap is in one of eight positions) the MAR is the width of the gap in the ring (Fig 3-12). Detection is assumed when 50% (or 75%) of the answers are correct. In man the maximum visual acuity when tested with Landolt rings is about 24 seconds (equivalent to 6/2.4).

The following approximate relationships and dimensions are given as an aid to understanding:

A visual angle of 1° corresponds to twice the diameter of the sun or the full moon and to 300 μm on the retina, which is the diameter of the rod-free area.

A visual angle of 1 minute corresponds to about 3cm at 100m and to 5 μm on the retina.

A visual angle of 12 seconds corresponds to 1 μm on the retina.

The distance between foveal cones is 2 to 2.5 μm.

There are as many visual acuities as there are test objects, e.g. letters; black bars on a white background (a grating); faint binary stars; a golf ball at 300m.

Clinical Measurement of Visual Acuity

Unfortunately, for historical reasons, visual acuity is seldom expressed simply and straightforwardly as the MAR in minutes of arc. Experience in astronomy led to the opinion that for a pair of binary stars to be seen as two separate stars they must be separated by one minute of arc. This came to be accepted as the normal resolving power of the human eye and it is the basis on which the universally used *Snellen letter charts* are constructed. In this test, letters are arranged in lines and the size of the letters in each line is such that the details of the letters each subtend one minute of arc at defined distances from the eye (while the whole letter subtends five minutes

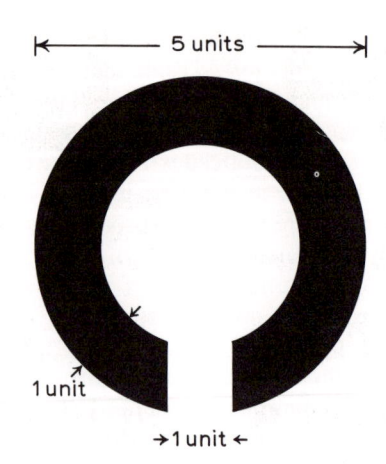

Fig 3-12 Landolt ring. The size of the gap is the critical detail which determines the threshold visual angle or the minimum angle of resolution (MAR).

of arc) (Fig 3-13). The distances at which this angle of one minute is subtended range from 60m down to 4m (Fig 3-14). The test is usually conducted at a distance of 6m (20 feet) (because at this distance the effects of accommodation [1/6D] can be ignored) and the line of smallest letters which the subject can correctly read is determined. The result is expressed as a pseudo-fraction in which the numerator is the testing distance (6m) and the denominator is the distance at which the letters of the correctly read line have a MAR of one minute of arc. For example, if the 6m line is read the vision is recorded as 6/6, the theoretical normal acuity. If only the 60m letter can be read the vision is 6/60, while if the 4m line is read the vision is 6/4. Many young people have this latter acuity, which only goes to show

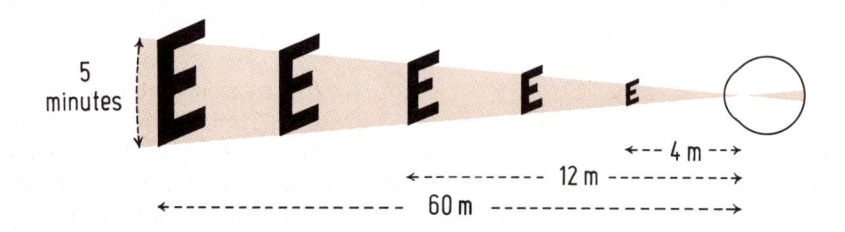

Fig 3-13 Basis of the Snellen chart. The sizes of the letters are such that at the defined distance from the eye the width of the strokes of the letters subtends an angle of 1 minute of arc and the whole letter subtends 5 minutes of arc, that is the letter has a MAR of 1 minute at the defined distance.

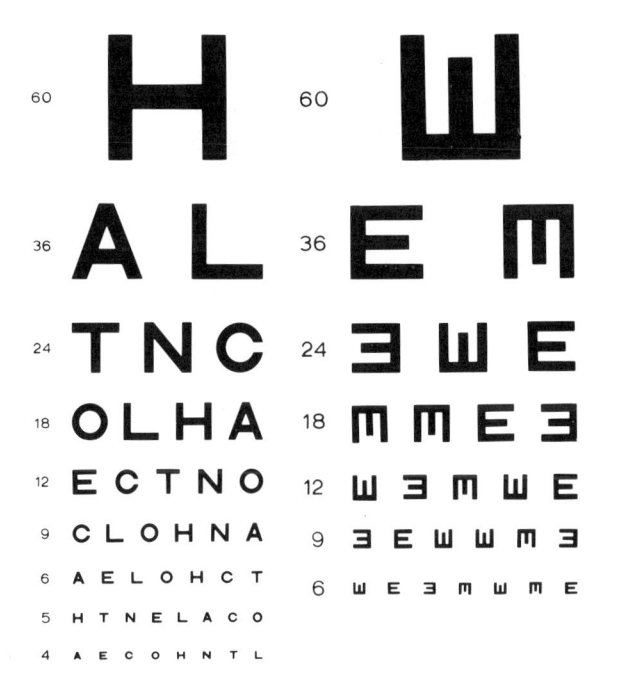

Fig 3-14 Snellen letter and illiterate E test-types.

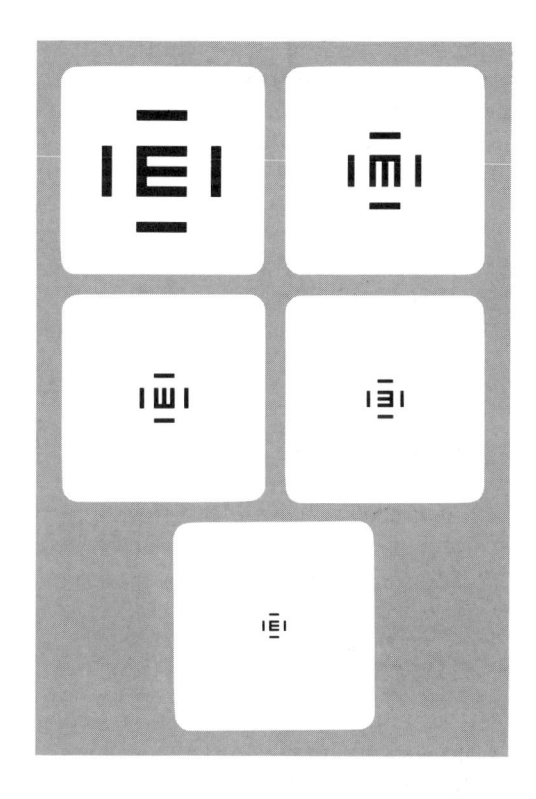

Fig 3-15 Set of single E test cards for use at 4m. With this version in which each E is surrounded by 'confusion bars', visual acuity is similar to that found with lines of Es on a chart. With single Es without the bars a patient's visual acuity can be misleadingly better than it is with Es in lines.

that while 6/6 may be 'normal' for this test it is less than the normal acuity often found.

The MAR of any size of letter is the reciprocal of the Snellen fraction, e.g. at 6m distance the MAR of a 60m letter is 10 minutes, and of a 12m letter it is 2 minutes.

Although 6m is the customary testing distance, tests designed for use at a distance of 4m (13ft) have the advantage of being more easily accommodated, e.g. in doctors' rooms, and they are preferable for young children. The shorter testing distance requires 0.25D of accommodation but correction for this small error is easy. With tests at this distance 4/4 is equivalent to 6/6 (MAR = 1'), 4/12 to 6/18 (MAR = 3'), 4/40 to 6/60 (MAR = 10') and so on.

The illiterate E test is commonly used to test young children (Fig 3-14). In this instead of letters the chart shows a series of letter Es randomly orientated in one of four directions, to the right, to the left, up, and down. The examiner points in turn to each E and the child is asked to point the fingers of his or her hand in the same direction as the 'fingers' of the E. More young children are able to do the test when a set of cards each with a single E of one of the required sizes is used instead of a chart with lines of Es (Fig 3-15).

Another useful test for infants is the letter-matching test (Fig 10-6). In this the child shows that it can recognise the shape of a letter shown individually on a card by pointing to the same letter on a key card bearing all the five or seven letters (O A X T H V U) used in the test.

Visual acuity is often better when tested with isolated symbols than when lines of symbols on a chart are used. This is due to contour interaction of adjacent stimuli (the crowding phenomenon). In some cases of amblyopia (p. 185) the difference between line acuity and single E or single letter acuity can be as much as seven or eight minutes in the MAR. This defect of isolated symbol tests is overcome by surrounding the symbol on all four sides with an adjacent black bar (Fig 3-15).

If a subject's visual acuity is less than 6/60 the distance from the test chart can be progressively reduced down to 1m to discover if his or her acuity is between 1/60 and 6/60, or the ability to 'count fingers' can be tested by holding up a hand with a varying number of separated outstretched fingers.

The recognition of letters involves more than the resolution of detail because the overall shapes of the letters and the subject's educational background also influence the result. For scientific studies the Landolt rings are therefore used.

Testing of *near vision* introduces additional variables, especially those related to accommodation. Clinically it is used most often as a test of the power of accommodation, but it is also useful when testing of distant vision is inconvenient or impossible. A chart based on Snellen principles is not usually used for near vision but an empirical one consisting of examples of print of different sizes is used (Fig 4-13). The British Faculty of Ophthalmologists Reading Type consists of a series of passages in 'Times Roman' print of different sizes from 5 to 48 point. The notation used is N (indicating 'near') followed by the point number of the print size, i.e. N5 to N48.

Regional Differences of the Retina

The centre of the fovea has a much higher acuity than the rest of the retina and the fall-off is very abrupt. At 3° from the centre acuity is about half of central acuity and at 5° it is about one-eighth. This is associated with the anatomical features of the fovea, at the centre of which there is an area with only cones, and these cones are distinctive in their shape and their central connections. As previously stated, this rod-free area has a diameter of about 300 μm which corresponds to a visual angle of 1° (twice that of the sun or full moon).

Variation of Acuity with Intensity of Light

With black test objects against a luminous background, the acuity increases with increasing luminance up to a maximum beyond which it does not increase. This conforms to the every-day experience that in dim light we cannot read fine print which can be read with higher illuminations and that no matter how bright the light there is a limit to the finest of detail which we can see. It should perhaps be mentioned here that in spite of the frequently heard admonishment, no harm can result from reading or attempting to read in a poor light. Discomfort may result but this does not signify damage to the eyes. At levels similar to full moonlight acuity is roughly one-eighth of that in daylight.

At very low levels of light many rods combine as a group to act as a light detector and these fewer groups of many rods form a coarser mosaic than the many groups of fewer rods which are the functional units above threshold levels. At higher levels of acuity there is a similar reduction in the number of cones in each functional unit as the illumination increases. The whole range of functional groups is from thousands of rods in the periphery to a single cone at the fovea.

The Optical and Anatomical Basis

The optical and anatomical factors which limit visual resolution are the sharpness of the image on the retina and the fineness of the 'grain' of the retinal mosaic of receptors. Because of diffraction and chromatic aberration the actual image on the retina is blurred and much larger than the geometrical image. Although it is thus attenuated there is still a pattern of different light intensities on the retina corresponding to the pattern of the geometrical image. For example, whereas the perfect image of a grating would have light intensities of 100% corresponding to the white bars and zero corresponding to the black bars with abrupt transitions between light and dark, the actual retinal image might have intensities of 60%, corresponding to the centres of the white bars, gradually falling to minima of 40%, corresponding to the centres of the black bars (Fig 3-16). However, differences in the illumination of neighbouring cones even less than this can be discriminated. In fact this difference of 60 to 40 is what occurs with the finest grating which can be resolved. It follows that the limit of resolution is ultimately determined by the fineness of the cone mosaic and not by the imperfections of the image. This is supported by the finding that the width of the bars in the finest grating which can be resolved corresponds to 2.3 μm on the retina and that the intercentre distance (= diameter) of foveal cones is 2.0 to 2.5 μm.

PHYSIOLOGY

GEOMETRIC IMAGE   RETINAL IMAGE

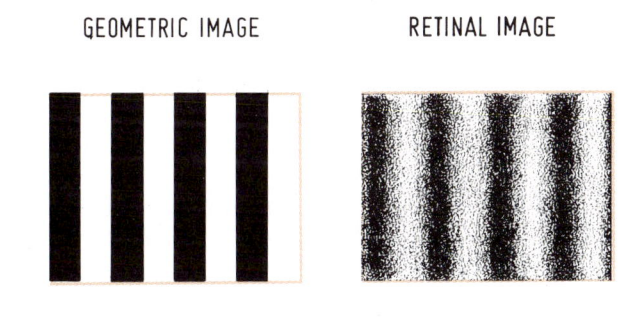

corresponding graphs of light intensity

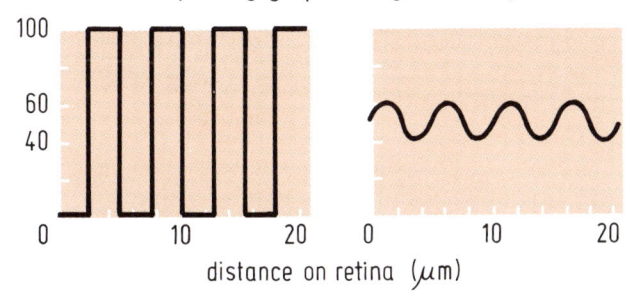

distance on retina (μm)

Fig 3-16 Light intensities in the image of a fine grating on the retina.

Visibility of a Single Line

We can detect a long black line subtending an angle of only 0.5 seconds of arc. This corresponds to a geometrical image of about 0.04 μm or 1/60 of the diameter of a cone, but the actual image is much wider due to diffraction. The row of cones covered by the centre of this long shadow receives only 1% less light than the adjacent cones but this is sufficient for the line to be detected.

An illuminated slit on a black background is always visible however thin it may be, provided it is sufficiently bright.

Vernier acuity, the ability to detect a break in an edge, is also high and is used in many precision measuring instruments. It is possible to detect a discontinuity of alignment of 10 seconds of arc (corresponding to a retinal image of 0.7 μm). It is one example of what has been called hyperacuity and depends on the relative localization of the suprathreshold features rather than the discrimination of threshold brightness differences.

Contrast Sensitivity

Seeing involves not only the detection of fine, high-contrast detail as is measured in the conventional tests of visual acuity, but also the ability to detect coarser features of low contrast, such as quite large objects seen murkily through a fog — or through an oedematous cornea or a cataract. A person's contrast sensitivity can be measured by using as test objects gratings of parallel, equal width, bright and dark bars in which the brightness changes in a sine-wave manner (sinusoidal gratings) (Fig 3-17). The width of the bars determines how coarse or fine the grating is and this is expressed as the spatial-frequency of the grating (number of cycles of one bright plus one dark bar per degree of visual angle; thirty cycles/degree is equivalent to 6/6). The contrast between maximum and minimum brightness is also varied. Test gratings are usually generated on an oscilloscope screen and the least contrast required for a grating of a given frequency to be seen is determined. The reciprocal of this threshold is the contrast sensitivity for this frequency. For most subjects contrast sensitivity is greatest for a frequency of about 5 cycles/degree (corresponds to 6/36) and is appreciably less for higher (and also lower) frequencies. Fine detail (high frequency) will be seen only when the contrast is high. The highest frequency detected when contrast is 100% (black on white) corresponds to visual acuity as usually tested.

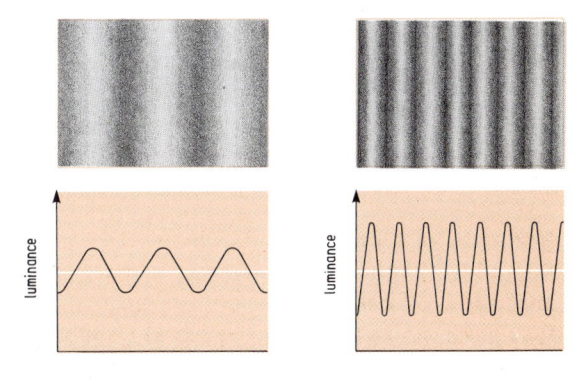

Fig 3-17 Examples of sinusoidal gratings. Both the spatial frequency and the contrast of the grating on the left are lower than those of the one on the right. At 55cm distance the frequencies are respectively about 1.0 and 2.5 cycles per degree.

Less precise but more simple tests of contrast sensitivity are used clinically. Some consist of sets of *printed gratings* of selected frequencies and contrasts, e.g. the Arden Gratings, the Ginsberg 'Vistec' Vision Contrast test and the Cambridge Low Contrast Gratings. An alternative is to test a patient's visual acuity with *low contrast letter charts* in which the letters are a faint grey instead of the customary black on a white background. For example, with a letter contrast of 1.5% the average acuity is 4/24 whereas a person with reduced contrast sensitivity may not see even the 4/40 letter at this reduced contrast although his or her acuity with maximum letter contrast is 4/4. Another simple test, the *border contrast test* is based on the detection of a difference in brightness between the two halves of a surface which have slightly different luminances when the transition between the two luminances is gradual (p. 61). The steepness of the slope of the ramp in the luminance profile is increased, that is, the transition from the lower luminance of one half to the higher luminance of the other half is made more abrupt, until a difference in brightness is detected (Fig 3-9). The better the contrast sensitivity the less steep the ramp in the luminance profile needs to be for detection.

Some patients who have normal Snellen acuity, including a few who are aware that in spite of this their vision is impaired, are found to have reduced contrast sensitivity. Some of the conditions which may cause this are multiple sclerosis, diabetic maculopathy and chronic open-angle glaucoma.

between stimulus and sensation is approximately

STIMULUS	SENSATION
Wavelength	*Hue*
380 - 450	Violet
450 - 490	Blue
490 - 550	Green
550 - 590	Yellow
590 - 630	Orange
630 - 760	Red

An average observer can distinguish between 150 and 200 hues and in the blue-green and yellow regions can detect a difference of 1nm in wavelength. At both ends of the visible spectrum the just-noticeable difference is 4 to 7nm.

Simultaneous or successive contrast from an adjoining or preceding chromatic stimulus, and the brightness and the saturation of a stimulus, also influence the hue perceived. A surround which is brighter than a coloured surface induces a 'blackness' in the surface (brightness contrast). This induced darkness alters the colour which is perceived. Most 'dark colours' are seen as darker versions of the same hue which is seen when there is no brightness contrast, e.g. dark red, navy blue, olive green, but brown is an exception. A surface that looks orange changes to brown when it is surrounded by a brighter surface (Fig 3-18).

COLOUR VISION

Attributes of Colour

Colour vision, like other sensations, is a private affair. However, it is common experience that there are three ways in which subjective colour sensations can differ and these psychological attributes of a colour, as they are called, are hue, brightness and saturation.

Hue is described by words such as red, yellow, green, and is dependent primarily on the wavelength of the stimulus. The correspondence

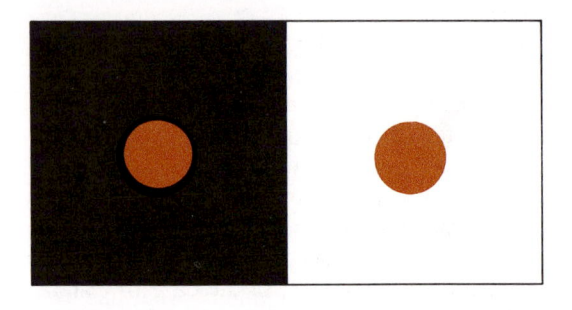

Fig 3-18 The discs are printed with the same colour but they look different. The one surrounded by black is seen as a dull orange, the other surrounded by white as a darker brown.

Simultaneous colour contrast, which is important to painters, is illustrated by the fact that when a yellow-green colour is surrounded by a red area it looks green and when surrounded by a white area it looks yellow. The effect of brightness on the subjective appearance of a colour (Bezold-Brücke phenomenon) is such that, with the exception of a blue, a green, and a yellow, the hue changes with luminance (within the photopic range). For example, an orange which looks a reddish orange at low luminances looks yellowish orange at high luminances. Desaturating (adding white to) a stimulus (except for a yellow) alters its hue; for example, a yellow-green becomes yellower.

Brightness is described by words such as very dim and dazzling, and is dependent on the luminance of the stimulus. Artists use the word shade to describe the reduced brightness of the colour of a pigment obtained by an admixture of black. The relative brightness of different wavelengths changes with the luminance; in dim light (scotopic conditions) blue-green colours are brightest, whereas in bright light (photopic conditions) yellow colours are brighter (Purkinje shift, p. 60).

Saturation refers to the paleness or whiteness of a colour and depends on the purity of the dominant wavelength in the stimulus. A saturated colour has little white while a less saturated or desaturated colour, a tint in artist's terminology, has more white. Pink is desaturated red.

Stimuli for Colour

'White light' is a mixture of wavelengths within the range of the visible spectrum (400-760nm). 'Coloured light' results from an alteration of this mixture. Such a change can be produced in the white light from a continuous source by optical methods such as dispersion, diffraction, interference, or absorption, which isolate specific wavelengths. Alternatively, specific wavelengths may be produced by a discontinuous source such as a gas discharge lamp or a laser. Objects appear coloured when their pigments selectively absorb certain wavelengths and, in the case of opaque objects, reflect others, or, in the case of transparent objects, e.g. filters, transmit others. (Interference filters transmit only a narrow band of wavelengths and reflect the rest of the incident light.)

Colour Mixtures

There are two different types of colour mixture, *additive* when lights are mixed and *subtractive* when pigments are mixed. This distinction explains the difference between spectral (lights) primary colours and artists' primary colours. *Primary colours* are a trio of selected wavelengths from which all spectral hues and white can be obtained by mixing (trichromatic colour mixing). Three spectral primary colours are a blue, a green, and a red. From these yellow can be produced by additively mixing red and green, for example by superimposing on a screen these two wavelengths, one from each of two projectors. Three artists' primary pigments are blue, yellow, and red, while three primaries for colour photography or lithography are cyan (blue-green), yellow, and magenta (blue-red). From these green can be produced by subtractively mixing blue or cyan and yellow. If green and red pigments are mixed the result is not yellow but a dirty black. Spectral blue and yellow can be subtractively mixed to produce green by placing a blue and yellow filter both in the light beam from the same projector. Additively mixed light from these same two filters would produce white. The pointillist school of painters mixed pigments additively by using small dots of colours adjacent to each other. Subtractive mixtures always reduce the luminosity.

There are numerous pairs of spectral colours which when mixed produce the sensation of grey or white. Such pairs are called *complementary colours*. Examples are blue and yellow, orange and greenish-blue, and red and a blue-green. Green does not have a spectral complement because it requires the addition of some red and blue to produce white.

Mechanism of Colour Vision

In man there are three colour receptors, one maximally sensitive to orange, one to green, and one to blue. These are the cone photoreceptors each of which contains one of three photopigments (p. 56). 'Red' and 'green cones' are at least five times more numerous than 'blue cones'. At this peripheral level in the visual pathway colour vision is *trichromatic* and the three cone pigments are the physiological basis for the trichromatic colour mixing described above whereby all of the 150 to 200 spectral hues can be matched by mixing in various proportions three properly chosen spectral primaries. Congenital colour vision defects are probably due to a deficiency or an absence of one or more of the cone pigments.

Centrally in the visual pathway, from ganglion cell level, the colour information is coded and transmitted by what is called the *opponent-pairs process*. This theory is based on both psychophysical and electrophysiological findings (p. 78). Briefly, there are two functional subdivisions of nerve cells and fibres, those which transmit information about green and red and those responding to blue and yellow. Further, each subdivision behaves in an opposite manner for its pair of colours. For example, in one class of spectrally opponent cells the discharge rate either increases when a red stimulus is turned on and decreases when a green stimulus is applied (R+ G−) or decreases with red and increases with green (G+ R−). The other class of cells behaves in opposite ways to blue and yellow. In effect, at some stage four unique types of sensations emerge from three types of receptors. This fits in with a number of psychological observations. By introspection there seem to be four distinct colour sensations, namely blue, green, yellow, red. These perceptually homogeneous sensations are called the four *primal* hues. It will be noted that it is yellow which has been added to the three *primary* hues of blue, green, and red. The opponent-pairs process also explains why mixtures of complementary colours can produce, not an intermediate hue, but by neutralization an achromatic white sensation and why the after-image of a coloured stimulus is coloured with its complementary colour.

Colour Matching

Subjective experiences cannot be measured (absolute pitch is perhaps an exception). It is therefore not possible to directly relate quantitatively the magnitude of sensations to the magnitude of stimuli which gives rise to them. But obviously there is some psychophysical relationship between a sensation and the cause of the stimulus; for colour vision the relationships are those between hue and wavelength, between brightness and luminance, and between saturation and purity.

Although sensation cannot be measured it is possible to say whether two sensations which are close together in space or time are the same or different, and matching of sensations is a useful tool in studying the physiological mechanism relating a stimulus to its corresponding sensation.

An *anomaloscope* is a device in which a variable mixture of two coloured lights can be compared with and matched to a light of another colour. Most commonly red and green lights are additively mixed in varying proportion to produce a match for a yellow light. Colour matches such as these are based on the fact that the same subjective colour sensation can result from stimuli with different spectral composition. This means that when colours look alike they do so either because they are physically identical (an *isomeric* match) or because, although they are physically different, they nevertheless stimulate the three types of cones in the same proportions (a *metameric* match). A common illustration of the phenomenon of metamerism is that colours which seem the same under one illuminant such as daylight do not match under another illuminant such as an artificial light. In anomaloscopes the colours to be matched are a metameric pair; the two fields seen side by side in the viewing aperture evoke the same sensation, but are spectrally different. Although testing with an anomaloscope and interpretation of the results is not simple this is the best method for fully identifying all defects and minor variations in colour vision. The *anomaloscope* detects and differentiates *anomalies* of colour vision.

Clinical Testing of Colour Vision

When colour vision is defective each of the three attributes of hue, brightness, and saturation will be found to be defective in varying degrees, but the appropriate tests are laboratory procedures and are not usually suitable or necessary for clinical applications. Clinical tests are required for screening (has an individual normal or abnormal colour vision?), for determining the type of colour defect, and for assessing an individual's suitability for a vocation requiring some colour judgements.

For screening, pseudoisochromatic plates are the most useful and widely used, but they will not answer the other two questions. For precisely diagnosing a defect, the anomaloscope is the best test. Other tests, which involve hue discrimination of specially prepared coloured paper discs, are the Farnsworth-Munsell 100–Hue test and the Farnsworth Dichotomous Panel D-15 test (the latter is 'dichotomous' because it divides people into two groups, severe colour defectives, and mild colour defectives or normals). Lantern tests and colour aptitude tests are used for vocational testing.

Pseudoisochromatic plates, for example the Ishihara series, consist of numbers or symbols on a slightly different background. The test symbols and the background are made up of differently coloured spots and the hue, brightness, and saturation of the colours are chosen so that symbol and background are confused by colour defectives. In the Ishihara test two or three missed plates signify defective colour vision. The illumination for this, and for all other colour vision tests using pigments, is critical and should be diffused daylight or a special lamp of specified colour temperature.

Lantern tests are used as practical tests where recognition of colour signals is necessary, for example the armed services and railways. They are useless for diagnosing the type or degree of colour defect.

Defective Colour Vision

A commonly used classification of colour vision is based on the minimum number of primary spectral colours which an individual requires in a mixture to match any other spectral colour (including white). The normal individual requires a minimum of three primaries and is said to be a *trichromat*. Those few who require only two primary colours to match the spectrum are called *dichromats*. The very rare individuals who have no colour perception at all and can therefore match any colour with any other colour are called *monochromats*.

If an individual requires three primaries, but his colour mixtures differ from those of the normal he is called an *anomalous trichromat*. *Protanomalous, deuteranomalous* and *tritanomalous* trichromats are distinguished.

Four types of dichromatic defects are differentiated, namely *protanopia* and *deuteranopia* when there is confusion of the colours from green through yellow to red, and *tritanopia* and *tetartanopia* when there is confusion of the colours from blue through green to yellow. Protanopia, deuteranopia, tritanopia, and tetartanopia literally mean respectively, first, second, third, and fourth defect.

The commoner anomalous trichromasies and dichromasies are inherited as sex-linked recessive characteristics and therefore are manifested much more commonly in men than in women. Deuteranomaly is the commonest defect with an incidence in males of 5%. The incidence of protanomaly is about 1.5%, and that of protanopia and deuteranopia is about 1% each. The combined incidence of these defects in men is therefore between 8 and 9%. The other defects are very rare.

In practice protanopes confuse blue-greens (and greys) with red (and browns), deuteranopes confuse blue-greens with purple, tritanopes confuse yellow with violet, while tertartanopes confuse yellow with blue. Anomalous trichromats have difficulty in discriminating light tints and dark shades and can be dangerously uncertain of signal colours under adverse viewing conditions, for example in fog. For them the colour of anything stared at may rapidly fade and make them unable to name the hue accurately; this aspect of the disability may be lessened by looking briefly at the colour and looking away or closing the eyes.

Apart from certain occupations, such as some in travel and communications where only slight departures from normal colour vision are accepted, congenitally defective colour vision need not be a handicap for most occupations. It is important, however, that people know their type of defect, if any, so that they can avoid as far as possible having to rely on colour clues, for example in analytical chemistry or in histology.

Acquired Defects of Colour Vision

Colour vision may become defective as a result of lesions of the macula, optic nerve, or visual cortex, or because of changes in the optical media, for example cataracts. An acquired colour vision defect differs from a congenital one in that it is often asymmetrical in the two eyes, it may affect blue-yellow as well as red-green vision, it is associated with other defects of visual function, it is more variable, and it causes the patient to see the colours of objects differently and therefore to name them incorrectly.

ELECTROPHYSIOLOGY OF VISION

Methods Applicable to Human and Animal Subjects

Electro-oculography

There is a standing potential (6mV) of the eye such that the cornea is positive and the fundus is negative. It originates largely in the pigment epithelium and varies with the intensity of illumination. It can be used clinically to estimate the normality of the pigment epithelium.

As a result of this potential difference between the front and back of the eye, rotations of the eye induce a change in potential between electrodes placed on the skin at each side of the eye (Fig 3-19). A record of this is the electro-oculogram (EOG) and it can be used to detect and record horizontal eye movements, e.g. in nystagmus.

Electroretinography

Stimulation of the retina by a flash of light produces another action potential which is smaller (0.5mV) and briefer (0.5 sec.) and this can be detected between an electrode on the cornea and an indifferent electrode. This bulk response of the retina, the electroretinogram (ERG), in man is biphasic with a bright stimulus and monophasic with a dim stimulus (Fig 3-20). It may be used clinically to investigate the general state of the retina, e.g. when there is unexplained defective vision in infancy.

Visually Evoked Response

Visual stimuli influence the potentials recorded in an electroencephalogram (EEG) from the occipital region overlying the visual cortex. These visually evoked potentials (VEP) are disentangled from the other electrical activity of the brain by computer 'averaging' of the responses to repeated identical stimuli such as flashes of light or alternating checkerboard patterns. The latency of the response is a measure of the velocity of conduction along the visual pathways. Clinically a delay in conduction in an optic nerve may be the only detectable evidence of lesions such as patches of demyelination in multiple sclerosis or beginning compression by a tumour. The amplitude has been used experimentally as an objective means of estimating visual acuity and even of measuring refractive errors.

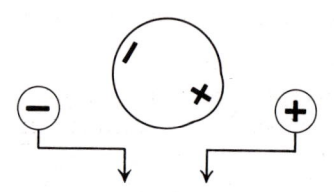

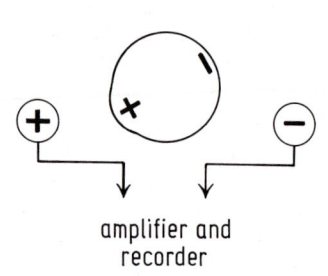

Fig 3-19 Electro-oculography. Electrodes below the inner and outer canthi record the potential difference between the front and back of the eye as it rotates from side to side.

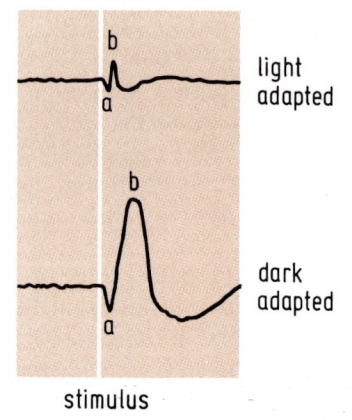

Fig 3-20 Components of a human ERG to a high intensity stimulus. The a-wave arises from the receptor cells and the b-wave from the Muller cells. The amplitudes of both waves are greater in a dark adapted eye.

Methods Applicable to Animal Subjects

Electrical Activity of Retinal Cells

While photoreceptors are unstimulated there is a constant external flow of current out of the inner segment and into the outer segment, the dark current. Absorption of light by the receptor outer segment reduces the dark current and there is a slow hyperpolarization of the photoreceptor graded according to the strength of the stimulus (analogue signals). In brief, photoreceptors are electrically active in the dark and light turns them off. The response of bipolar cells (and horizontal cells) is also graded and sustained; the cell is hyperpolarized or depolarized depending on whether the excitatory or inhibitory part of its receptive field is stimulated. In the ganglion cell the signal changes to propagated action potentials (digital signals). Nerve impulses in the optic nerve axons, like those in peripheral nerves, are thus in the form of spike potentials of constant amplitude but with the frequency of the spikes proportional to the intensity of the stimulus.

Receptive Fields. Effective Stimuli

The receptive field of a sensory neurone is the region in the periphery from which a stimulus will evoke a change in the firing of the neurone. The change may be an excitation or an inhibition of the neuronal activity. The receptive field of a *ganglion cell* or its axon is an area of the retina which consists of a central more or less circular zone surrounded by a concentric ring in which opposite changes in activity are induced (Fig 3-21). The size of the receptive field centres varies depending on the retinal location; for the fovea it is no wider than one foveal cone, while for the retinal periphery its diameter may exceed 1mm on the retina. For some ganglion cells stimulation of the centre of the field produces increased discharge (on-response) while stimulation of the periphery produces decreased discharge with a burst of firing on cessation of the light (off-response). This is called the *on-centre* type of field. Other ganglion cells have the *off-centre* type of field in which the responses are reversed. The net discharge rate of any ganglion cell is the result of an algebraic summation of the responses to stimulation of the two opponent regions of its receptive field. This explains the absence of response to uniform illumination of the whole receptive field. The significance of this arrangement for the enhancement of contrast is obvious. With dark adaptation the size of the on-centre receptive field increases at the expense of the inhibitory periphery. This fits in well with the reduced acuity and increased sensitivity found in dark adaptation.

The antagonistic centre-surround organisation of ganglion cell receptive fields also increases the dynamic range of the cells, that is, their ability to respond to small local changes in luminance throughout a wide range of background intensities of illumination. In other words, they *adapt* to whatever level of light prevails and continue to function whether it be dim or bright. Ganglion cells detect the small local changes by comparing the illumination on the centre with that on the surround of their receptive fields. The on-centre cells are excited when the centre of their field is brighter than the surround, the off-centre cells by the opposite configuration. Thus both local light increments and light decrements are signalled to the central nervous system by an excitatory process, and this means that the information is transmitted rapidly.

There are at least two *parallel systems* of ganglion cells called X and Y cells in the cat, the sustained response or slow-conducting and transient response or fast-conducting in primates. These two sorts of ganglion cells are anatomically and physiologically different and their axons go to separate parts of the LGB. The slow-conducting beta cells have small receptive fields, are mostly chromatically opponent and synapse in the four dorsal parvocellular layers of the LGB. They

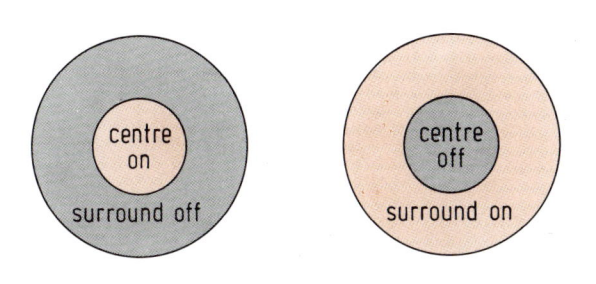

Fig 3-21 Concentric receptive fields of retinal ganglion cells.

transmit information about colour and fine high-contrast detail. The fast-conducting alpha cells have large receptive fields, little chromatic opponency and synapse in the two ventral magnocellular layers of the LGB. They may be involved in the detection of change, movement, and low contrast patterns. In effect there are several parallel channels or pathways which start in the retina and convey different sorts of information to different destinations in the central visual system.

Lateral Geniculate Body
Segregation of the parallel channels continues in the LGB where, as just described, there are different inputs into the parvo- and magnocellular layers. The different ganglion cell types, e.g. on- and off-centre, connect with counterparts in the LGB which have correspondingly similar receptive field behaviours. The inputs from the two eyes are also segregated in separate LGB laminae. However the LGB is more than a relay station. There are also large afferent connections from the visual cortex and the brain stem, and these modulate the onward transmission of information to the cortex.

Visual Cortex
Although the shape of the spread-out surface of the visual cortex is quite different from that of the retina (and its equivalent visual field) there is an ordered 'map' (cortical retinotopic map) of the retina (and field) on the cortex (p. 31). The basic spatial unit of the 2mm thick human visual cortex seems to be a block of tissue roughly 2mm square containing several hundred thousand cells. Each of these functional units or three dimensional modules, called cortical 'hypercolumns', corresponds to a unique location in the retinal peripheral receptor mosaic (and field), and this peripheral region is the receptive field of the cortical cells within the functional unit (Fig 3-22). The functional units are the same size throughout the cortex, but the sizes of the receptive fields increase with increasing eccentricity from the fovea (or centre of the visual field). This accounts for the relatively small area of cortex which represents the periphery of the retina (and visual field) compared with the large cortical area associated with the macula (p. 33).

When a recording electrode is inserted into the cortex at right angles to the surface it strikes a column of cells and in accordance with what has just been said, all the cells in a column have their receptive fields in more or less the same region of the visual field. Individual cortical cells respond optimally to certain features of a stimulus; they have a peak sensitivity to 'trigger' features such as the orientation, length, spatial frequency, direction and velocity of movement, and colour of the stimulus, and whether one or other eye is stimulated and, if both, the binocular disparity (p. 85).

There is a hierarchy of feature-detecting cells in a cortical column which corresponds to the layer of cortex in which the cell lies. There are six layers and the input from the LGB is to the stellate cells of the middle layer (layer IV). These cells have concentric circular receptive fields like those of the ganglion cells and the cells of the LGB.

The character of the receptive fields and trigger features of other cortical cells is unexpectedly different. For them the effective stimuli are specifically orientated straight lines or borders of light-dark contrast. Some, called *'simple' cells*, found superficially in layer IV, respond to a specifically orientated (horizontal, vertical, oblique) edge in a precise position within the receptive field (Fig 3-23). Like the concentric

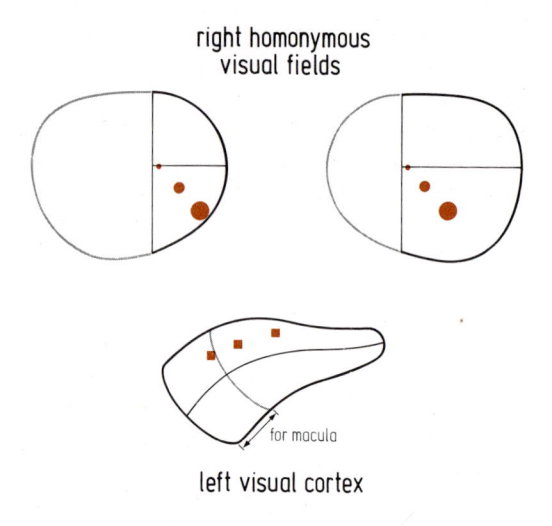

Fig 3-22 Receptive fields of three cortical modules or 'hypercolumns'.

PHYSIOLOGY

receptive fields of more peripheral visual cells, the receptive fields of simple cortical cells are divided into on- and off-areas. These may take different forms such as a central linear on-zone bordered on both sides by parallel off-zones, linear on- and off-zones lying side by side, or a linear off-zone centrally with an on-area on each side.

Another type of cell, called *'complex cells'*, are pyramidal neurones which occur in the layers superficial and deep to the middle layer, and they respond to the appropriate orientation of a linear stimulus anywhere within the receptive field or to one which moves in a particular direction (Fig. 3-24).

Some simple and complex cells have a *'hypercomplex'* property in that their receptive field is 'end-stopped', that is, the cell is inhibited by long lengths and is a corner detector (Fig 3-25). Initially it was thought that this hierarchy of cell types was serially connected but it is now appreciated that each type can have a direct input from the LGB via the parallel visual channels.

In addition to orientation and direction specificity some cortical cells respond optimally to a narrow band of spatial frequency. This is tested with sinusoidal gratings of selected frequencies at the appropriate orientation in the cell's receptive field. Many neurophysiological and psychophysical studies have tested the hypothesis that *frequency detecting cells* respond independently to the Fourier components of a stimulus pattern, that is, that there is a neural mechanism for an analysis of any complex stimulus into the set of sine waves which when added together reproduce the wave form of the spatial luminance profile of the stimulus. Although there is no direct evidence for this it is now customary and helpful to think of the spatial frequency content of visual stimuli. A sinusoidal grating is the simplest optical stimulus because it contains only one spatial frequency at one orientation. A single sharp spot of light is a complex stimulus in Fourier terms because it contains a wide band of frequencies at all orientations. There are high frequencies in the spectrum of Fourier components of a sharp edge whereas a gradual change in luminance is a low frequency stimulus. Focusing to get the sharpest image can be thought of as 'maximising the high frequencies'.

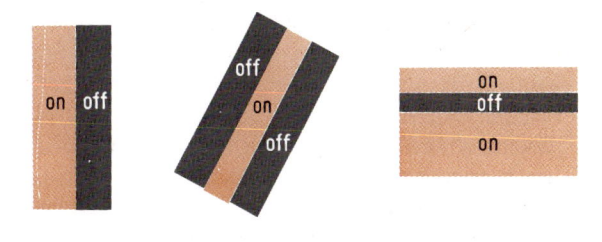

Fig 3-23 Linear receptive fields of a simple cortical cell.

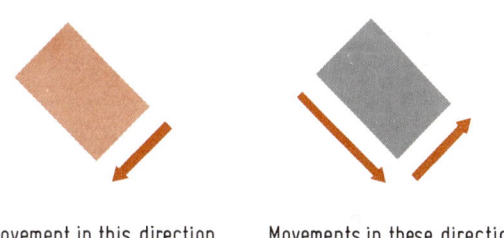

Movement in this direction anywhere within the field elicits a response.

Movements in these directions within the field, fail to elicit a response.

Fig 3-24 Linear receptive field of a complex cortical cell.

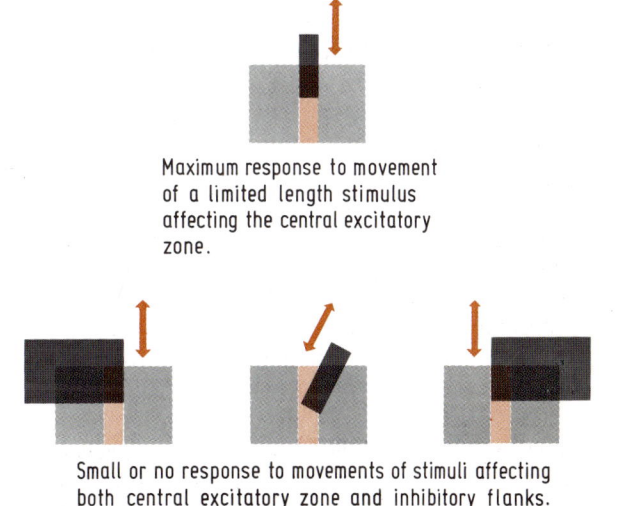

Maximum response to movement of a limited length stimulus affecting the central excitatory zone.

Small or no response to movements of stimuli affecting both central excitatory zone and inhibitory flanks.

Fig 3-25 Receptive field of a cortical cell with hypercomplex properties.

Colour Coding in the Visual System

There are potentially two kinds of information about physical light stimuli which an animal's visual system can extract and code, namely the intensity and the wavelength of the light from each point in its visual space. The mechanisms just described have dealt only with the relative intensities of light in a stimulus, that is with intensity coding in the visual system.

To extract information about the wavelengths in a stimulus an animal must have several different receptors (a minimum of two) with photopigments of different spectral sensitivities and a neural system so organized that it can detect different degrees of activation of the different types of receptors. A majority of animals have not evolved these two basic requirements for colour vision, but primates and some other animals satisfy the first requirement by having three types of cones and the second requirement by having two pairs of spectrally opponent cells, that is neurones which compare the extent to which one receptor type is more or less activated than another.

Human photoreceptors respond only to a restricted part of the visible spectrum and the wavelength of greatest sensitivity is different for different receptors, being 500nm for rods, 419nm for 'blue cones', 531nm for 'green cones' and 559nm for 'red cones'.

Spectrally opponent cells respond in one way, e.g. on, to some wavelengths and in the opposite way, e.g. off, to other wavelengths. In primates opponent colour cells are found among ganglion cells, lateral geniculate body cells, and cortical cells. There are two types of opponent cells, called single and double (Fig 3-26). In single spectrally opponent cells response to a particular wavelength is the same over the whole receptive field. Some single opponent cells have receptive fields arranged in a concentric centre-surround manner while others do not have a concentric arrangement. Slow-conducting ganglion cells can be subdivided into two pairs of spectrally opponent cells, namely red-on, green-off, and green-on, red-off which difference the outputs from the 'red' and 'green' cones, and blue-on, yellow-off and blue-off and yellow-on which difference the output of 'blue' cones and a combined output from 'green' and 'red' cones (yellow) (Fig 3-27).

In a double spectrally opponent cell the opponent colour arrangement in the peripheral surround of the receptive field is the reverse of that in the centre of the field. Such a cell will fire optimally, for example to a red spot on a green background whereas a single opponent cell with a red-on centre and a green-off periphery would be silent to this colour contrast. Double opponent colour cells of this type occur in clusters as 'blobs'

SINGLE OPPONENT CELL FIELDS

DOUBLE OPPONENT CELL FIELD

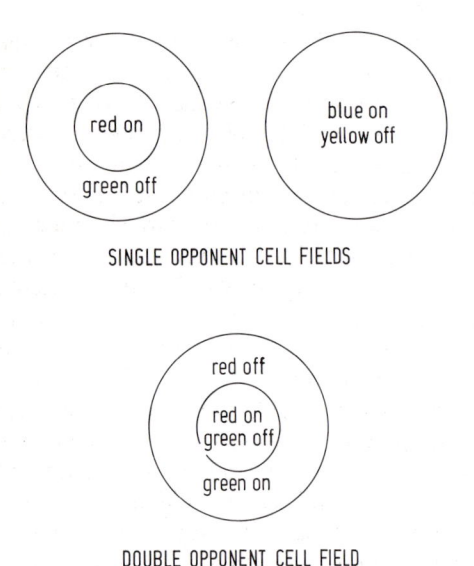

Fig 3-26 Examples of receptive fields of spectrally opponent cells.

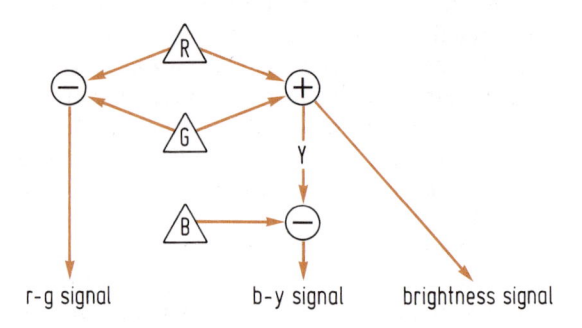

Fig 3-27 Possible model of opponent-colour process. The red-green opponent pathway conveys the difference in output of the R and G cones. The blue-yellow pathway conveys the difference between the B cone output and a combined output of the R and G cones (yellow). The achromatic brightness pathway conveys the sum of the output of the R and G cones.

or 'dots' in layers II and III of the visual cortex.

The same receptors act on both intensity-coding achromatic pathways and on colour-coding pathways. Spectrally opponent cells difference the outputs of different cone types whereas spectrally non-opponent cells sum the outputs. Spectrally opponent cells signal differences in intensity as well as differences in wavelength but spectrally non-opponent cells signal only differences in intensity.

Columnar Organization

The cells in a column of cortex pependicular to the surface all require the same orientation of the stimulus, except for those of layer IV which have no orientation preference. That is, cells with the same orientation specificity are all grouped together in a narrow (25-50 μm) vertical slab or column of cortex called an *orientation column*. The orientation specificity of cells in neighbouring columns changes in an orderly fashion so that within each functional unit ('hypercolumn') of the cortex, and therefore for each region of the visual field, there is a full set of orientation columns for orientations in steps of about 10° through 180° of orientation. This functional architecture of the cortex, detected initially by neurophysiological methods, has been confirmed anatomically by exposing monkey's eyes, immediately before they were killed, to only moving vertical contours and autoradiographically labelling active neurones with the C14 2-deoxyglucose technique, i.e. those which respond to a vertically orientated stimulus. In vertical sections of the visual cortex there were regularly spaced labelled bands perpendicular to the surface (except for layer IV which as would be expected was uniformly labelled) and in tangential sections there was a swirling meshwork pattern of labelled stripes.

A cortical cell may respond more to stimulation from the right eye or from the left eye, or respond equally to both eyes. The ocular dominance of a cortical neurone refers to the relative effectiveness of input from the right or left eyes. Cells in layer IV and simple cells are monocularly activated and are therefore right- or left-eye dominant. About half the complex cells are similarly dominated by the input from one eye while the other half are binocular. Monocular cells are grouped into more or less parallel vertical slabs which alternate between right- and left-eye dominance. These alternating bands in the cortex have been shown autoradiographically after tritiated proline was injected into the vitreous of one eye of a monkey. From here the labelled amino acid was transported axonally to the LGB and thence trans-synaptically to those cortical cells with input from the injected eye. These *ocular dominance columns* are estimated to be about 1.0mm wide in man so a pair, one for each eye, spans about 2mm. This pair of dominance columns together with a set of orientation columns subserving orientations through 180° make up a cortical 'hypercolumn', the functional unit of cortical architecture.

In the striate cortex there are four classes of binocular cells which code for stereoscopic *depth perception*. One class is excited when corresponding retinal points (p. 83) are stimulated, a second class is inhibited when this happens, the third class is excited by crossed disparities, i.e. when the stimulus is nearer than the fixation point common to both eyes, while the fourth class is excited by uncrossed disparities. Beyond this stage a computational process seems to use the information from these four cell types to give rise to depth perception.

Higher Cortical Areas

In addition to the striate cortex there are many visual areas not only in the occipital cortex (Brodmann's areas 17, 18 and 19) but also in the temporal and parietal lobes. In these extrastriate visual areas the field of vision is not usually represented topographically as it is in the striate cortex. There are many reciprocal connections between all visual areas and some have somatosensory or auditory inputs. Within this complex network there are two major pathways from the striate cortex, a dorsal one to the parietal cortex which is involved in processing information about space and movement, and may be the cortical counterpart of the fast-conducting system which starts in the retina, and a ventral pathway to the inferior temporal cortex which is concerned primarily with pattern, shape and colour, and which utilises information from the colour-opponent, slow-conducting parallel pathway which originates in the retina.

In the inferior temporal cortex there are feature-detecting cells each of which responds best to a unique combination of features. Some even appear to 'recognise' such features as a hand or a face. However, since it is now appreciated that many analytic processes, such as colour perception and stereopsis, do not depend on specific individual cells but on networks of many neurons, our perception of the visual world is likewise thought to be based on the action of networks and the computations they make.

Interference with Normal Development

The visual neurophysiological responses of newborn animals are similar to those of adult animals and therefore the complex anatomical connections in the visual pathway must be more or less fully developed at birth. But for a period after birth visual structure and function is 'plastic' and remains normal only if the young animal experiences conditions for normal seeing, essentially only if both retinas receive simultaneous patterned stimuli. For example, if one retina is deprived of pattern vision, e.g. by suturing the eyelids together, during the first few months of life the other retina becomes dominant so that few cortical cells respond to stimulation of the previously occluded eye, and in sections of autoradiographically labelled cortex there is a widening of the ocular dominance columns of the unoccluded eye at the expense of narrowed dominance columns of the occluded eye. These changes are largely irreversible. If patterned vision is prevented in both eyes ocular dominance is normal, but there is a reduction of the orientation specificity of cortical cells. If an artificial squint is produced at birth most cortical neurones are monocular and very few are binocularly driven. These findings in animals have implications for the development and maldevelopment of human binocular vision, not the least being the support they provide for preventive treatment of squint and amblyopia in infancy as opposed to ineffective treatment later (p. 182).

BINOCULAR VISION

Binocular vision is the fusion into a single perception of the two slightly different images from a pair of eyes. In addition to achieving single vision, this synthesis normally results in vision which is three dimensional and is called stereoscopic vision (literally, seeing solid). This ability to see singly and in 3D is learned during the first years of life and it cannot be acquired later.

Binocular vision requires
   reasonably clear images from both eyes,
   cerebral fusion mechanisms, and
   precise co-ordination of the movements of the two eyes for all directions and distances of gaze.

A basic requirement for single vision is that each object shall seem to be in the same place when seen with either eye. It is therefore useful to start by considering the reasons why things are seen where they are, first for one eye and then for two eyes.

Visual Direction

Each object seen within the field of vision is located at a position in visual space which is determined by its subjective direction and its distance from the self. The process whereby objects are given a subjective direction is called *visual projection;* we project a retinal stimulus in a certain direction. All directions are relative; one direction can be defined only by reference to another direction. Visual projection is made with reference to two directions, that of the visual axis of the eye (oculocentric direction) and that of the body as a whole (egocentric direction).

Oculocentric Direction

The sensation which results from stimulation of each point on the retina is projected in a particular direction in space. This is called the *visual direction* of the retinal point. The visual direction of the fovea normally coincides with the visual axis of the eye (the line from the fovea to the point of fixation), which is another way of saying that the sensation is projected towards the object looked at. This foveal visual direction, the *principal visual direction,* is the direction to which the visual directions of other retinal points are related — to the right, to the left, above, or below. The directions of objects relative to each

PHYSIOLOGY

VISUAL AXIS = principal visual direction

EGOCENTRIC DIRECTION of stimulated retinal point

Object straight ahead

a. eye looking straight ahead

egocentre

b. eye actively rotated

image / retina
+
eye / head

c. eye passively rotated

image / retina
eye / head nil

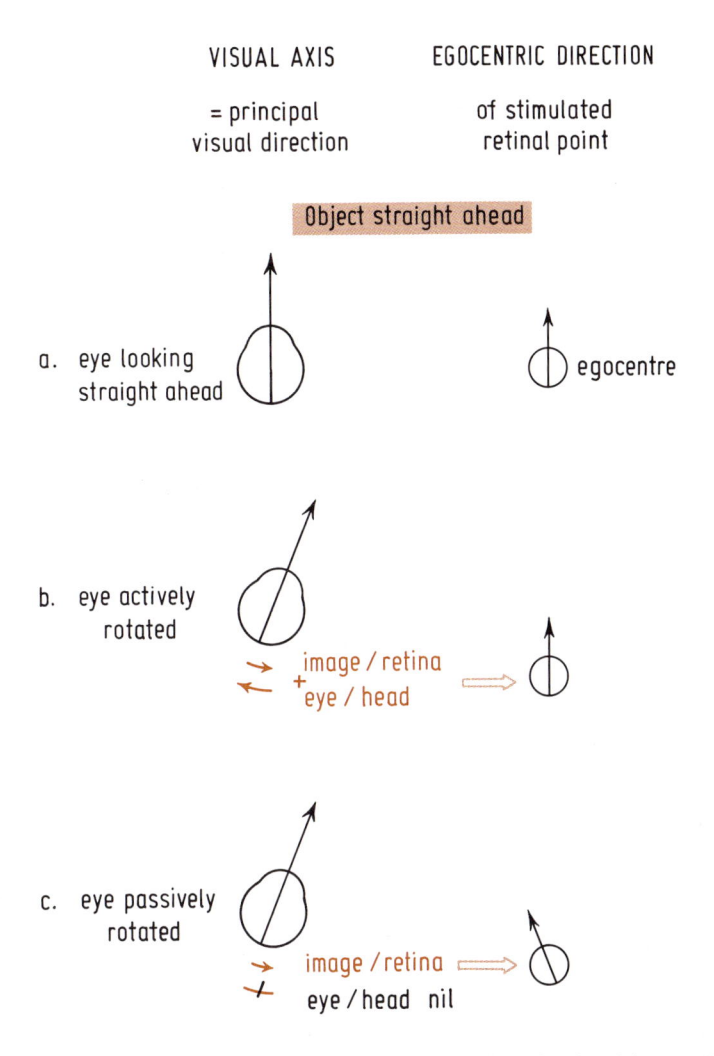

Fig 3-28 Relation of the egocentric direction of the retinal point stimulated by an object straight ahead, to the direction of the visual axis of an eye (a) in the primary position, (b) with active rotation of the eye, and (c) with passive rotation of the eye.

other are also derived from this relationship. This neural system, by which the visual direction imparted to a stimulus is determined by the part of the retina on which its image falls, has been called the *image/retina system*.

Egocentric Direction

A person's subjective visual space is the whole volume of his or her visual field and directions within it extend from a point within his or her body image, the visual egocentre (Fig 3-28a). This is located somewhere between the two eyes (perhaps eccentrically towards the side of the master eye) about the centre of the head.

Because the eye is free to move, the projections of all retinal points, including that of the fovea, with reference to the body image, must change when the eye moves. In general, no matter how the eye moves in the orbit, egocentric visual projection is effected as if the eye had remained at rest. This also applies to movements of the head on the body and to changes in the position of the body with respect to gravity, so that for all positions of the body, a stationary fixated

VISUAL AXIS   EGOCENTRIC DIRECTION

= principal   of stimulated
visual direction   retinal point

After image

a. eye actively rotated

image/retina nil
eye/head

b. eye passively rotated

image/retina nil
eye/head   nil

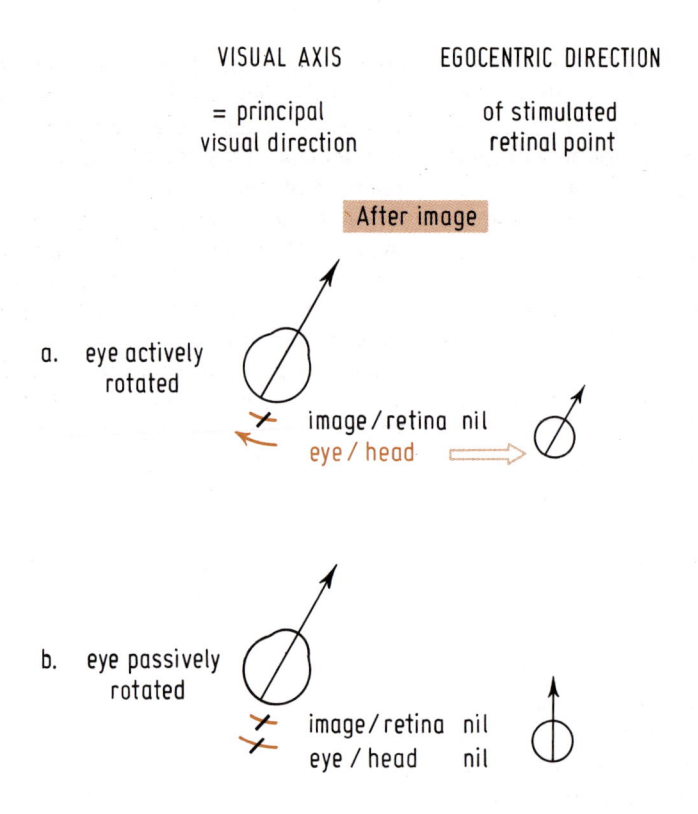

Fig 3-29 Relation of the egocentric direction of the fovea (stimulated by an after-image) to the direction of the visual axis of an eye (a) with active rotation and (b) with passive rotation.

object is unchangingly projected to the same gravitational co-ordinates in space. The neural system by which the visual direction of a retinal stimulus is determined by the position of the eyes in the head has been called the *eye/head system*.

This stability of the external world in spite of movement is achieved by the synthesis of proprioceptive and postural information with the visual information. It is as if changes in the image/retina and the eye/head systems cancel each other out (Fig 3-28b).

Human extraocular muscles have muscle spindles and feed-back from these could provide the signals indicating the position of the eyes. But, surprisingly, proprioception from the eye muscles plays no part in the corrections to projection which compensate for eye movements. This is simply demonstrated by the fact that passive movements of the eye cause stationary objects to appear to move. It is the innervational stimuli for active movements of the eye which provide the necessary correction, and it is the intention to move the eyes, rather than the actual movement, which seems to be involved. If an eye movement is 'intended' but does not occur, e.g. due to paralysis of an eye muscle, the postural correction takes place inappropriately and gives rise to a false projection.

Cover one eye and while looking straight ahead passively rotate the other eyeball outwards by gently pushing the outer part of the globe backwards with your finger at the outer canthus. Note that any object seen moves in the opposite direction to the movement of the eye. The image/retina system is functioning properly, but the eye/head system is not functioning (Fig 3-28c).

The image/retina system can be immobilized in the following way. In a room with no other light use a bare electric light bulb to produce an after-image in one eye by steadily fixing the centre of the lamp with one eye occluded for about 20 seconds. Immediately look towards a wall and note that as you look in different directions the after-image also moves. The eye/head system is functioning but is not cancelled by any changes in the image/retina system and therefore the sensation representing the exterior world changes position (Fig 3-29a).

Renew the after-image and this time passively rotate the stimulated eyeball outwards. Note that the after-image does not move so long as you 'intend' to look in an unchanging (straight ahead) direction. Neither the image/retina nor the eye/head system is functioning and therefore no movement is signalled (Fig 3-29b).

Binocular Vision

The visual fields of the two eyes overlap except for a peripheral crescent of each temporal field. The foveas of the two eyes have the same visual direction and all other visual directions in the common field of vision are subserved by a retinal point in each eye. Such retinal points in the two eyes which have a common visual direction are called *corresponding retinal points*. It follows that when corresponding retinal points are stimulated by images derived from the same point in space this is seen as one.

When the two eyes independently fix the same point nearer than 'infinity', the principal visual directions of the foveas are different. But in binocular vision the two principal visual directions become identical. This can be simply shown by a classic experiment of Hering. This experiment also demonstrates that subjective visual directions may differ from objective geometrical lines of directions and it also allows one to experience retinal rivalry.

Stand about two feet from a window giving a distant view. Keeping the head steady, close the right eye and look at a conspicuous distant object. On the window pane make a mark in line with the left eye and this object. Close the left eye, look at the mark on the window and note what distant object is in line with the mark and the right eye. Open both eyes and look at the mark on the window. This is seen singly and now both the distant objects previously noted will also seem to be in the same straight-ahead direction (Fig 3-30). The two objects will probably appear successively, appearing and replacing each other at intervals. This fluctuating behaviour is an example of retinal rivalry.

For any degree of convergence of the eyes only some points in space in addition to the fixation point will be imaged on corresponding retinal areas. The locus of these points in space is called the *horopter*. When some points in space are not imaged on corresponding areas, i.e. those points not on the horopter, one of two things happens, there is stereoscopic vision or there is double

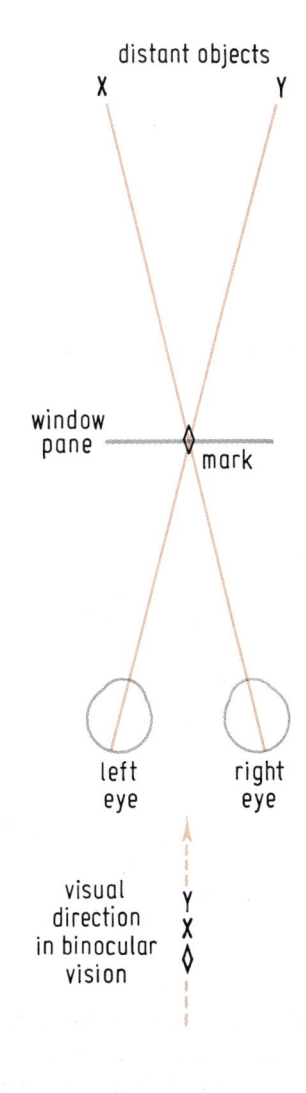

Fig 3-30 Hering's experiment.

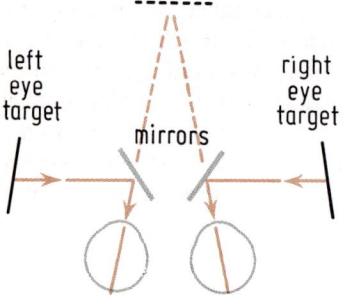

Fig 3-31 Principle of Wheatstone reflecting (mirror) stereoscope in which separate pictures can be simultaneously presented to each of the two eyes.

Fig 3-32 Principle of Brewster lens stereoscope in which convex lenses with focal lengths equal to their distance from the targets form images of the two targets at infinity. Each lens is decentred to produce a baseout prismatic deviation so that the images are appropriately positioned for eyes with more or less parallel visual axes. This permits the targets to be separated more widely than the interocular distance and hence larger pictures to be used.

vision. When corresponding retinal points receive quite dis-similar images there is suppression, retinal rivalry, or lustre.

One way of studying these phenomena is to use devices which present images separately to the two eyes, that is stereoscopes (Figs 3-31, 3-32) and haploscopes, e.g. a 'Synoptophore' (Figs 3-33, 3-34).

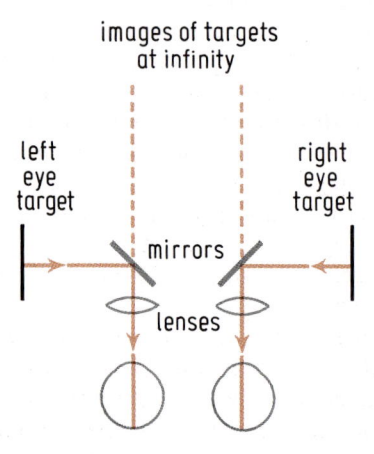

Fig 3-33 Principle of synoptophore. It is a Wheatstone mirror stereoscope with, in front of each mirror, a lens of focal length equal to the distance of the target. The images are therefore at infinity and no accommodation by the subject is required.

The target, mirror and lens for each eye is arranged on an arm which can be rotated about an axis that passes through the centre of rotation of the eye.

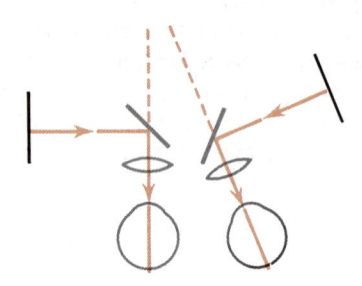

Fig 3-34 Rotation of one arm of the synoptophore in the case of a right convergent squint so that each eye is presented with its target at the same time. The arc through which the arm has to be rotated is a measure of the angle of squint.

Stereopsis

In normal seeing the images of an object received by the two eyes are not identical and this slight difference is called *disparity* (horizontal retinal-image disparity) (Fig 3-35). Disparity which mimics that occuring in normal seeing can be artificially created with pictures or transparencies in stereoscopes and haploscopes. Stereoscopic retinal photographs are especially useful for demonstrating differences in level in lesions of the optic disc or macula.

Because of disparity some points of the object are imaged on non-corresponding retinal points with their different visual directions. However, provided the disparity is not too great, *fusion* gives rise to a single compromise visual direction and the object is seen singly. In addition a sensation of depth is generated. In spite of disparity single vision occurs; because of disparity stereoscopic vision occurs.

Fusion and stereopsis are part of the same mechanism and both operate on the basis of a mosaic point-by-point or element-by-element correlation of the features of the left and right eye images. Stereopsis comes before perception of form. This follows from the demonstration (with random-dot stereograms) that recognisable features or contours in the targets are not necessary for the perception of stereopsis. The sense of depth has the same immediate perceptual quality as does colour.

Stereoscopic acuity is a measure of an observer's ability to detect the smallest difference in the distances of two objects from him or her. It is limited by the smallest amount of retinal disparity (measured as the angular subtense at the eye) which generates a stereoscopic perception. For trained observers this can be as small as four seconds of arc; the majority of people can detect a separation of 20mm at 6 metres distance.

Suppression, Retinal Rivalry, Stereoscopic Lustre

If the two eyes are artificially presented with patterns which are quite different a curious fluctuating effect may occur which is called *retinal rivalry*. The whole or parts of each picture are in turn not seen *(suppression)* so that various partial combinations appear and disappear. Fusion does not occur and both complete patterns are never seen simultaneously. If parts of the pictures have strong contours these may dominate so that there is constant suppression of those parts of the other picture which are adjacent to these contours. This is well seen when a black disc on a white background is superimposed on a larger black or coloured area; the disc is seen surrounded by a colourless corona or halo. This suppression of one of two dis-

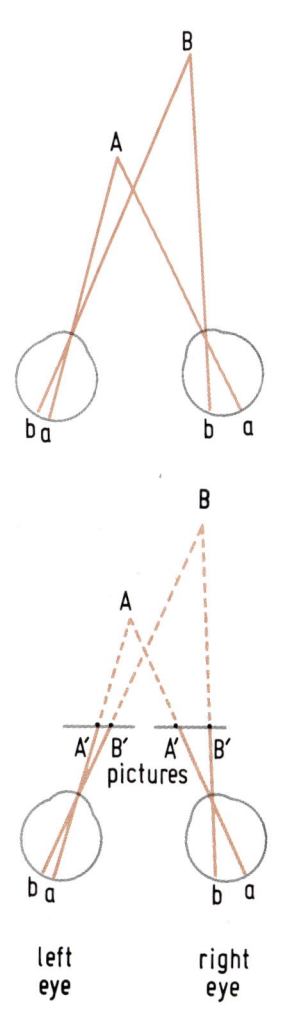

Fig 3-35 Stereopsis. **Upper** Objects A and B at different distances from the eyes produce disparate retinal images in the two eyes, the separation of a and b being greater in the right than the left eye.

Lower The disparity is reproduced when the appropriate pictures A' B' are presented to each eye; B' is seen as more distant than A'.

similar objects explains why the 'confusion' (p. 87) which occurs when there is a squint is rarely noticed.

Another artificial stereoscopic experience is that of *lustre* which occurs when the white parts of the picture for one eye are black in the picture for the other and vice versa. A real object has lustre because it reflects more light to one eye than the other. Again, fusion does not occur; simple fusion of black and white could produce only grey.

Diplopia

If the disparity of the retinal images of an object is too great, *double vision* occurs, i.e. seeing the same object in two places. This diplopia can be entirely normal.

Look at an object across the room and hold an index finger in line with your nose. The finger will appear double. Next look at the finger and the object in the distance will be double. This is *physiological diplopia* or *introspective diplopia* (Fig 3-36).

Pathological diplopia occurs when there is a squint, i.e. when the visual axis of one eye is not directed to the object being looked at by the other eye (Fig 3-37). The image of the object fixed falls on the fovea of the fixing eye and is correctly projected. In the other deviating eye the image

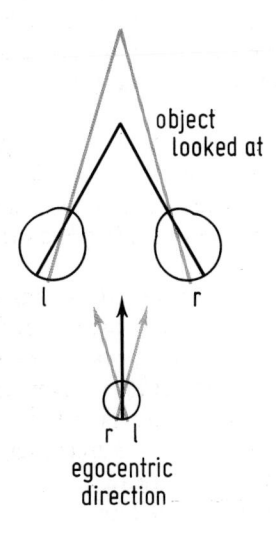

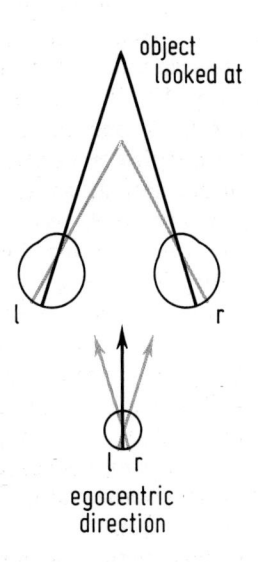

Fig 3-36 Physiological diplopia.

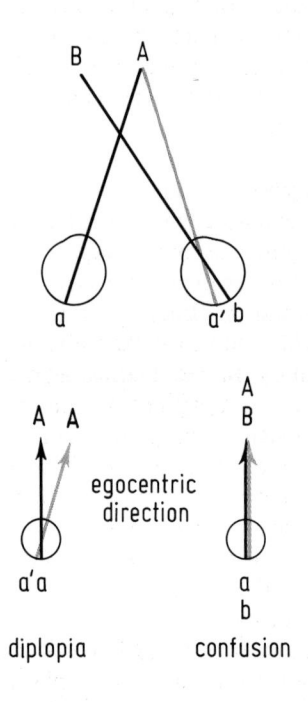

Fig 3-37 Diplopia and confusion from a right convergent squint.

of this object falls on a retinal area which has a different visual direction. Although the deviating eye is turned, the eye/head system is inoperative because the deviation is 'passively' produced. It is as if the central mechanism has not received a signal that the deviating eye is deviated. Therefore the image in the deviating eye is projected in accordance with the postural information from the fixing eye. When this is combined with the visual direction of the stimulated retinal area of the deviating eye, the object is projected in the direction this visual direction would have if the eye was not deviating. The result is that the same object is seen in two directions; the image of the deviating eye is displaced in the direction opposite to that of the deviation.

When there is a squint, diplopia results from the same image falling on non-corresponding points. But when this happens it must also happen that different images fall on corresponding areas, e.g. the two foveas. The resulting apparent superimposition of dis-similar objects is called *confusion* (Fig 3-37). However, as pointed out in discussing retinal rivalry, suppression of part or the whole of one of the images of dis-similar objects always occurs. In squints it is the foveal image of the deviating eye which is usually suppressed and therefore confusion is rarely troublesome.

The Synoptophore

The 'synoptophore' or a similar instrument is standard equipment for investigating the binocular function of patients in ophthalmic practice. The diagnostic tests routinely performed with it, on patients with squints for example, are commonly carried out by trained medical auxiliaries called orthoptists. It is a haploscopic instrument which can be adjusted to compensate for any deviation of the visual axes in a squint (Figs 3-33, 3-34). The angle of squint can be measured objectively by noting the adjustment needed to get the reflections of the instrument's lights from the subject's corneas placed centrally with respect to the pupils of his or her eyes.

Binocular sensory and central functions can be assessed with the synoptophore and it is customary to describe three 'grades of binocular vision' for which different styles of pictures are used.

These are traditionally called:

1 *'Simultaneous perception'*. For this, dis-similar but not mutually antagonistic pictures, e.g. an animal and a cage, are used and the subject 'puts the animal in the cage'. If the two pictures cannot be seen simultaneously there is (abnormal) suppression or there is defective sight in one eye.

The term simultaneous perception is misleading because, as discussed previously, two dis-similar objects are never seen simultaneously in the same position in space. With simultaneous perception slides one object, e.g. the animal, is smaller than the other, e.g. the cage, and while the smaller object is seen foveally the larger one is seen perifoveally.

3 *'Fusion'*. For this, each of the pair of identical pictures is incomplete in one detail, e.g. one cat without ears, the other without a tail. If sensory fusion is normal the complete picture is seen.

The 'range of fusion' is tested by making the subject's eyes converge or diverge and noting his or her ability to maintain fusion. Most people can 'hold fusion' over about 25° of convergence and about 3° of divergence. This is a test for sensory plus motor fusion – perceptual fusion plus corrective fusional reflexes.

When the arms of a synoptophore are moved to induce convergence of a subject's eyes the picture becomes both blurred and smaller. The blurring is due to the accommodation which inevitably accompanies convergence; it is inappropriate for the pictures because their images remain at optical infinity. The diminution in size, *convergence micropsia*, is due to a neuro-psychological mechanism which also accompanies convergence. In normal seeing, as an object approaches nearer to an observer its retinal image increases in size but the observer does not perceive a corresponding increase in size of the object. A compensatory reduction in apparent size more or less cancels out the effect of increasing image size to give *'size constancy'*. This mechanism must be initiated by convergence and when, as in converging with the synoptophore, the normal increase in image size is absent, the central mechanism is unopposed and gives rise to minification of what is seen.

3 *'Stereopsis'*. For this, pictures with stereoscopic disparity are used and the subject's ability to experience a sense of depth is noted.

Binocular Motor Co-ordination

Various reflexes control eye movements and hence the position of the eyes (p. 36). Postural reflexes arise from the labyrinths, the neck muscles, and the eye muscles (vestibular system). Visual information initiates other optomotor reflexes, namely fixation of an object detected in the periphery of the visual field (saccadic system), maintenance of fixation on the object of interest whether it is stationary or moving (smooth pursuit system), and corrective fusional movements to keep the visual axes of the two eyes on the object of interest in spite of varying vergences and versions (vergence and fusion system).

The simplest objective way to check that both eyes are directed to the same object is to have the subject look at a small light and note whether the reflections of light from the two corneas are more or less central. If one eye is not directed to the light the *corneal light reflex* of that eye will be displaced, e.g. temporally if the eye is convergent (p. 102).

A more accurate test is the *cover-uncover test*. In this while the subject looks at an object, one eye is quickly covered with the hand and the other uncovered eye is closely watched for any movement. If it moves it was not looking at the fixation object before its fellow was covered (p. 103).

Heterophoria

When the eyes are dissociated, i.e. when fusion is artificially prevented, the visual axes of both may continue to be directed precisely to the same point. This is called *orthophoria* and it is uncommon. More commonly, when freed of the need to maintain fusion, one eye deviates inwards or outwards and sometimes upwards or downwards. This is called *heterophoria* or a *latent squint*. Most of us are slightly heterophoric. In normal seeing this latent deviation is controlled by the binocular fusional reflexes. Sometimes, with larger degrees of heterophoria, these reflexes may be overtaxed with resulting discomfort or they may fail to control the deviation which then becomes a manifest squint and diplopia occurs.

The simplest way to dissociate the eyes is to cover one eye. The *alternate cover test* consists of covering alternate eyes while the subject fixes an object far or near from him or her. Larger degrees of heterophoria will show up as a movement to regain fixation as each eye is uncovered (p. 103).

The *Maddox rod test* is an ingeniously simple way of detecting and measuring the degree of heterophoria, usually for distant vision. The Maddox rod is a series of parallel red glass rods which when held before the eye converts a spot of light into a red line. The subject looks at a light with one eye and through the Maddox rod with

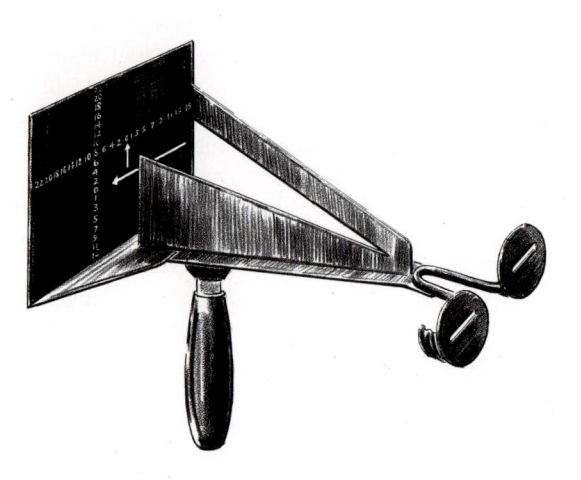

Fig 3-38 Maddox wing test.

the other. The same object then gives rise to dissimilar images and, because there is therefore no stimulus to fusion, the eye behind the rod assumes a 'fusion free' or dissociated position. If this is not orthophoric the red line will not coincide with the light. The amount of deviation, i.e. the degree of heterophoria, can be measured by determining the strength of prism required to make the line appear to touch the light.

Convergence and accommodation are linked so that for near vision the two occur together and normally it is impossible to converge without accommodating and conversely to accommodate without converging. This association between convergence and accommodation is one of the reasons why a person's heterophoria may be different for distant and near fixation.

The *Maddox wing test* is commonly used to measure a person's heterophoria when looking at near objects. In this hand-held instrument the subject looks through an aperture for each eye at a small black panel one-third of a metre distant (Fig 3-38). On the panel are a horizontal and a vertical scale of figures and a vertical and a horizontal arrow each pointing to the zero point of its respective scale. Baffles permit the right eye to see only the arrows and the left eye to see only the scales; because the two eyes can see nothing in common they are dissociated. While the right eye looks at an arrow the left eye will be directed at a figure on the corresponding scale according to the amount it has deviated from the position of orthophoria. To the subject the arrow will appear to be pointing at that figure and this number is a measure in prism dioptres of the subject's heterophoria for the distance of the test.

PART TWO

EXAMINATION AND INTERPRETATION

Chapter 4

EYE EXAMINATION BY THE GENERAL PHYSICIAN

OCULAR SYMPTOMS

Visual Symptoms
   Reduced vision
   Superimposed visual phenomena
   Diplopia

Abnormal sensation

Altered appearance

EXAMINATION OF THE VISUAL SYSTEM

Tests of function

Techniques of testing
   Visual acuity
   Visual field
   Binocular function
     Nystagmus
   Pupils
   Intraocular pressure
     Tonometry

Visual examination of ocular structure
   General observation
   Detailed inspection
     Lids
     Lacrimal sac
     Conjunctiva
     Cornea
     Sclera
     Anterior chamber
     Iris
     Pupil
   Differential diagnosis of the red eye

EYE EXAMINATION BY THE GENERAL PHYSICIAN

There are three reasons for examining patients' eyes. They are:
1. Complaint by the patient of symptoms which commonsense or experience suggests may be due to some ocular abnormality, e.g. pain in the eye, haloes around lights.
2. The fact that many ocular defects and diseases can be detected before they give rise to obtrusive symptoms and some of these can be successfully treated, e.g. amblyopia in infants, chronic glaucoma.
3. The fact that systemic diseases commonly have ocular manifestations and these may lead to the recognition of unsuspected disease, e.g. retinopathy in symptomless diabetes; or they may help in the diagnosis of the systemic disease, e.g. choroidal tubercles in an undiagnosed fever; or they may help in the management of the systemic disease, e.g. retinopathy in hypertension.

It will therefore be obvious that testing the functioning of the visual system and looking at the eyes is part of any full medical examination.

Clinical Method

The two-stage scientific approach of creating a hypothesis and testing it by experiment is applicable to medical diagnosis. Hypotheses are formulated to account for the symptoms and then are tested by further questioning or by examination. This is a continuous process in which the initial broad hypotheses are progressively amended and refined by the patient's replies to questions asked and by the findings on examination. These running hypotheses are guides to an interrogation and examination which is appropriate and economic. Application of this method requires some understanding of symptoms and how they are produced. For this reason ocular symptoms and their commoner causes are first reviewed.

OCULAR SYMPTOMS

Ocular symptoms can be classified into three groups. Patients can be aware of altered function (visual symptoms), of abnormal sensation (discomfort), or of altered appearance.

Visual Symptoms

Imperfections in the functioning of the visual apparatus consist of reduced vision, superimposed visual phenomena, and diplopia.

Reduced Vision

It is especially useful to think anatomically in ophthalmology and the *causes* of reduced vision can be classified into three *topographical* groups.
1. Defective formation of an image on the retina. This may be due to a refractive error or to impaired transparency of the transparent media of the eye, namely the cornea, the lens, and the vitreous.
2. A lesion of the retina or of the central visual pathway (optic nerve, optic chiasma, optic tract, lateral geniculate body, optic radiation, and visual cortex).
3. An abnormality of visual perception (agnosia).

Vision in man includes the perception of light, of movement, of space, of colour, and of form. Each of the three most highly evolved of these perceptions can be impaired more or less independently of the other two. The more primitive perceptions of movement and light, or of light alone, can survive when the others are lost.

Using this hierarchy of visual perceptions as a basis, the following *classification* of reduced vision into four types is clinically convenient.
1. *Reduced central vision* (impaired perception of form). This is manifested as a lowered visual acuity, a reduced ability to see details. *Distance* visual acuity alone can be defective, as in myopia; or *near* visual acuity alone can be defective, as in presbyopia; much more commonly both distance and near vision are impaired, as in macular degeneration. In general, reduced central vision with retained peripheral vision is caused by disorders peripheral to the optic chiasma.
2. *Reduced peripheral vision* (impaired perception of space). This is manifested as a defect in the visual field. There can be a partial or a total loss of vision in the affected area of the field and these defects are called respectively relative and absolute visual field defects. The defect may involve the outer margin of the visual field or it may affect an area entirely within the boundary of the visual

field. This latter type of defect in which there is a non-seeing area within a seeing area is called a *scotoma;* when a scotoma includes the fixation point at the centre of the visual field it is called a central scotoma and in this case central vision is also reduced. An arcuate scotoma (also called a nerve fibre bundle defect) is one in which the defect arches nasally from the blind spot above or below the fixation point. It is characteristic of some lesions of the optic disc (Fig 1-12).

Lesions peripheral to the optic chiasma produce defects in the homolateral visual field (Fig 1-36). Lesions of the chiasma itself or of the visual pathways central to the chiasma produce defects in the visual fields of both eyes. This bilateral defect resulting from a lesion in one region is called a *hemianopia.* A homonymous hemianopia is one in which the same side of each visual field is affected, e.g. a right homonymous hemianopia resulting from a lesion of the left suprachiasmal pathway. A bitemporal hemianopia is one in which the temporal side of each visual field is affected; this results from a lesion of the chiasma, as in pituitary tumours. A quadrant hemianopia or quadrantanopia involves the same quadrant of each field, e.g. an upper right quadrantanopia from a lesion of the lower left optic tract. Patients often erroneously describe a homonymous defect, especially if transient, as being due to interference with the vision of the eye on the affected side.

Patients are frequently unaware of visual field defects until questioned or until the field loss is demonstrated to them when testing their field. Loss of all peripheral vision with preservation of central vision is a much greater handicap than is the reverse pattern of lost central vision with retention of peripheral vision. Reduction of both central and peripheral vision is usual when retinal image formation is imperfect and it is also common with lesions of the retina or visual pathways.

3 *Impaired vision in dim light,* night blindness, results from malfunctioning of the peripheral retina or extensive loss of peripheral vision from other causes. When complained of, it is frequently due to psychological causes.

4 *Impaired colour perception,* colour 'blindness', is a common inherited defect (8% males, 0.5% females) of which the subject is naturally unaware. It may be noticed by the patient in some acquired conditions, e.g. macular lesions, digitalis toxicity.

The *onset* of reduced vision can be sudden or gradual. An abrupt or rapid onset suggests a vascular occlusion or a haemorrhage in the eye or the visual pathway. Patients can be surprisingly oblivious of considerable loss of vision, even to the total loss of sight in one eye, if the loss is very gradual, e.g. in chronic open angle glaucoma.

Superimposed Visual Phenomena

Floaters

Spots before the eyes of different sizes, shapes, and numbers are usually due to opacities in the vitreous. Small elusive specks (muscae volitantes, literally flying flies) are almost universal. Numerous or conspicuous floaters occur in inflammation of the uvea or retina and as a result of haemorrhage into the vitreous. This is therefore a symptom which demands respect, even though floaters are commonly the result of ageing of the vitreous and have no sinister significance.

Haloes

The appearance of rainbow coloured rings encircling bright lights is caused by alterations in the ocular media which give rise to diffraction. The most important cause is oedema of the corneal epithelium which occurs with a rapid increase in the intraocular pressure in acute angle closure glaucoma.

Photopsia

These are sensations of lights or luminous patterns which are experienced when the eyes are closed. They result form irritative stimulation of the retina or visual pathways. Unilateral photopsia are most commonly due to mechanical stimulation of the retina, as in retinal detachment. The commonest cause of photopsia experienced bilaterally in a homonymous visual field is vascular insufficiency in some part of the suprachiasmal pathway, as in the scintillating scotoma of migraine or in basilar artery insufficiency.

Metamorphopsia and Micropsia

Apparent deformation of objects looked at, e.g. kinking of lines known to be straight, is called metamorphopsia and an apparent minification of objects is called micropsia. These abnormalities of vision result from lesions such as oedema of the macular retina which disturb the normal spacing of the cones. If the cones are spread further apart a given retinal image covers fewer of them and therefore the object giving rise to the image is perceived as smaller than it actually is. Metamorphopsia is an important presenting symptom of senescent macular degeneration, especially of the type called disciform degeneration of the macula in which the macular retina is locally displaced by a small blister of fluid underneath the pigment epithelium (p. 194). Distortion can be confirmed or detected with an Amsler grid (p. 101).

Diplopia

Double vision is experienced whenever the visual axes of both eyes are not directed to the same object, provided that the vision of each eye is reasonably good and binocular vision has been normally developed. Young children rapidly suppress the second image.

Physiological diplopia (introspective diplopia) occurs in normal seeing but we are usually unaware of it because the confusing double images are suppressed. Occasionally patients are alarmed by the discovery of this normal diplopia.

Pathological diplopia is the result of weakness of one or more of the extraocular muscles. The diplopia is horizontal if one of the horizontal rectus muscles is affected and it is vertical and horizontal if a vertical rectus or an oblique muscle is affected. The separation of the images is characteristically greatest when looking in the direction in which the affected muscle has its principal action. The diplopia immediately ceases if either eye is closed.

There are many causes of paresis or paralysis of the extraocular muscles. Some affect the muscle itself as in myasthenia gravis (in which more than half the patients have diplopia and/or ptosis and which may affect only the ocular muscles), in thyroid exophthalmos, or in orbital injury. More commonly, the nerve supplying the muscle is affected. Examples are: a third cranial nerve lesion, in which there is also ptosis and mydriasis, due to pressure from an intracranial aneurysm or to a localized infarction of the brain stem near the cerebral peduncle so that pyramidal fibres are also involved and the ipsilateral third nerve palsy is therefore accompanied by a contralateral hemiplegia; a sixth nerve lesion due to a head injury, to raised intracranial pressure, to diabetes, or to a small vascular lesion; the brain stem focal lesions of disseminated sclerosis which cause slight and usually transient weakness of one or several ocular muscles, frequently as the initial symptom.

More rarely, diplopia (or even polyplopia) which is monocular in origin can occur as a result of an opacity in the lens.

Patients frequently describe indistinct or distorted vision as 'seeing double'. It is therefore wise not to accept such a complaint at face value but to confirm by questioning that objects are seen truly doubled.

Abnormal Sensation

Ocular discomfort may take the following forms
 deep pain in the eye
 foreign body pain in the eye
 superficial pain
 smarting, burning, scratching, 'aching behind the eyes', 'tired eyes'
 itching
 headaches
 photophobia
 dry eyes
 watery eyes

Deep pain in the eye if severe, and it may be very severe, occurs with inflammations of the iris and ciliary body, abrupt large increases in the intraocular pressure, scleritis, and herpes zoster ophthalmicus.

Tenderness, meaning pain or increase of pain on pressure, commonly accompanies pain. In scleritis the tenderness is localized to the affected area.

Foreign body pain or discomfort has numerous causes and may be quite misleading both as to cause and subjective localization of the source of the pain. As well as a foreign body on the conjunctiva or cornea some of the commoner causes are trichiasis (misdirected lashes which rub on the cornea) (Fig 4-1), entropion (inturning of lid margin) (Fig 4-2), conjunctivitis, corneal abrasion, corneal ulcer including dendritic ulcer, superficial punctate keratitis, actinic keratitis. A small perforating corneal wound with an intraocular foreign body may give rise to no more than a sensation of foreign body discomfort and is therefore a trap. If a patient felt something enter his or her eye while hitting metal on metal assume that there is an intraocular foreign body until this is disproved, e.g. radiologically.

Superficial pain in an eyelid is commonly due to infection, especially a stye.

The variously described minor *discomforts* (asthenopia) may result from inadequately corrected refractive errors or heterophoria. 'Eye-strain', although a commonly used expression, is undesirable because strain connotes damage and this does not occur from use of the eyes. In asthenopia the discomfort is almost always correlated with intensive use of the eyes and, in itself, the presence of a refractive error or a heterophoria does not mean that it is causing symptoms. This has to be determined largely on the history. This is especially so because nervous tension is a very common cause of ocular discomfort. Here the discomfort bears little relation to eye work. However, it may be related to the mental concentration required in a task which also involves using the eyes and therefore assessment of the relationship can require detailed interrogation.

Other causes of discomfort are blepharitis (inflammation of the lid margins), irritants such as smog, dust, sun, wind, and chlorinated swimming pools, and deficiency of tears as in Sjögren's syndrome.

Itching is characteristic of allergic conjunctivitis or dermatitis of the lids.

Headaches may occur as asthenopic symptoms and the history is all important in deciding if this is so. Contrary to popular opinion, ocular defects are not a common cause of headaches. Migraine is not caused by refractive errors.

Photophobia (ocular pain on exposure to light) most commonly results from light-induced movements of an irritated iris as in iritis or acute corneal lesions. Lesser degrees of discomfort in bright light may be normal for some individuals and it often seems to be of neurotic origin.

Photophobia in babies is a very important sign because it is normally the first evidence of congenital glaucoma.

Dry eyes, due to deficiency of tear secretion, is not often volunteered as a symptom by patients but on questioning they will state that they cannot weep.

Watery eyes may be due to over-production of tears (lacrimation) or to faulty drainage of tears (epiphora).

Lacrimation occurs with inflammations of the conjunctiva, cornea, iris or ciliary body.

Epiphora results from obstruction of the lacrimal passages anywhere from punctum to naso-lacrimal duct.

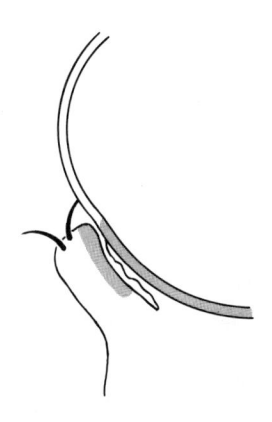

Fig 4-1   Trichiasis.

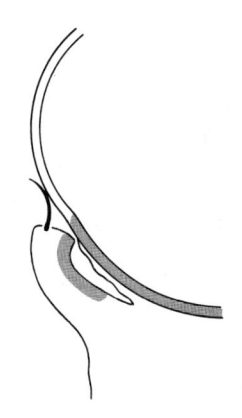

Fig 4-2   Entropion of lower lid.

Altered Appearance

Ptosis, drooping of the upper lid, is commonly congenital (Fig 4-3). It also results from third nerve lesions, orbital injuries, and abnormalities of the levator palpebrae muscle, e.g. myasthenia gravis. A slight degree of ptosis and miosis constitute Horner's syndrome signifying a lesion of the cervical sympathetic.

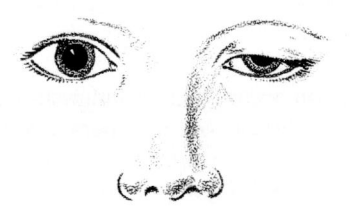

Fig 4-3 Ptosis of left upper lid.

Ectropion, drooping or eversion of the lower lid, brings patients because of the unsightliness, watering, and discomfort (Fig 4-4).

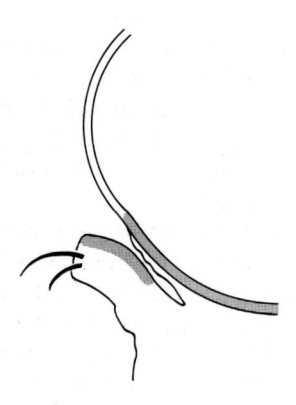

Fig 4-4 Ectropion of lower lid.

Retraction of the upper lid exposes a narrow rim of sclera above the cornea (Fig 4-5). Patients often say that their eye is bigger or they may describe their altered appearance as a stare. If it is not the result of proptosis it is most commonly due to thyroid disorders.

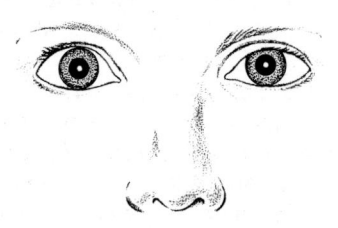

Fig 4-5 Retraction of right upper lid due to thyrotoxicosis.

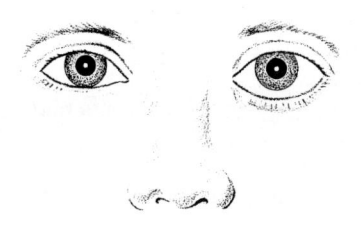

Fig 4-6 Proptosis of left eye due to an ethmoidal mucocoele.

Lagophthalmos, inability to shut the lids completely, may be noticed by the patient. It is due to weakness of the orbicularis oculi muscle, most frequently the result of a seventh nerve lesion.

Proptosis, by custom, is the term used for unilateral protrusion of the globe (Fig 4-6). It results from orbital injury, inflammation, or tumours.

Exophthalmos is used for bilateral protrusion of the eyes and it is most commonly due to thyroid disorders (Fig 4-7).

This usage of proptosis and exophthalmos is by no means universal and the words are synonymous. *Enophthalmos* is used for a sunken globe whether unilateral or bilateral.

Shutting one eye in bright light by infants is a common early sign of a divergent squint.

Squinting is used erroneously for screwing up the eyes as may happen with defective vision or with mild photophobia.

A *squint*, or *strabismus*, is an abnormal deviation of the eyes in that the visual axes of the two eyes are not simultaneously directed at the same object (Figs 4-8 and 4-9). Parents are commonly aware that something is awry with their child's eyes but without help may not notice whether the squint is convergent or divergent,

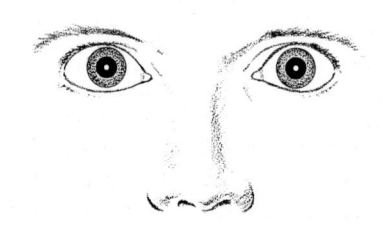

Fig 4-7 Bilateral exophthalmos in thyrotoxicosis.

EXAMINATION

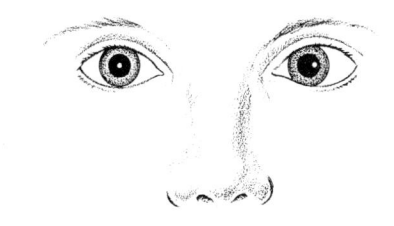

Fig 4-8 Convergent squint.

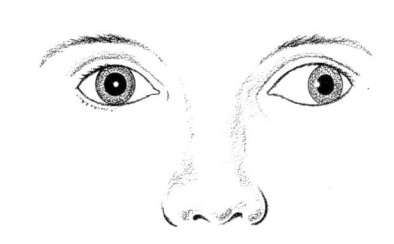

Fig 4-9 Divergent squint.

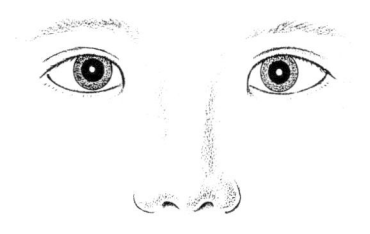

Fig 4-10 Pseudo-squint due to epicanthic folds.

monocular or alternating. The wide nasal bridge and epicanthic folds of some infants can produce a very good imitation of a convergent squint (Fig 4-10). No doctor, let alone parent, need be chagrined at having been fooled by such a pseudo-squint.

Discharge from the eye may be mucus or pus. It is evidence of conjunctivitis. With few exceptions it always occurs with conjunctivitis which should therefore rarely be diagnosed when there is no discharge.

Red rimmed eyes, often with crusting on the lashes, usually signifies blepharitis.

Swelling of the lids from oedema occurs readily because of the loose fatless subcutaneous tissue and thin elastic skin of the eyelids. It may be due to general causes, e.g. nephrosis, or to local causes, e.g. a stye, an insect bite.

A *localized swelling* of a lid is most commonly due to a Meibomian cyst which is usually painless but may become inflamed. A swelling just below the medial canthal ligament is likely to originate in the lacrimal sac.

Benign lid tumours include papillomata, which most commonly present as a wart at the lid margin, and xanthelasmata, which, as yellow intradermal plaques on the medial ends of the upper or lower lids can be disfiguring and occasionally are a manifestation of type II hyperlipidaemia.

A *malignant lid tumour* is most probably a basal-cell carcinoma (rodent ulcer) or a squamous-cell carcinoma (epithelioma). Rodent ulcers are common, curable if dealt with early, but may be unsuspected when they characteristically present as a small crusted nodular lesion on the lower lid or near the medial canthus.

Myokymia orbicularis may be seen as spasmodic fine contractions of part of an eye-lid. Subjectively the quivering and twitching sensation is obtrusive. It has no local significance and seems to be due to fatigue and perhaps anxiety; it occurs characteristically in students about exam time.

A *growth on the conjunctiva* is most likely to be a pinguecula or a pterygium. *Pingueculae* are small yellowish white lumps adjacent to the cornea in the region exposed in the palpebral opening (Fig 4-11). They are degenerative and almost universal in later life. A pinguecula may be more conspicuous when there is conjunctival hyperaemia in which it does not share or conversely when it alone is slightly hyperaemic. Treatment is unncecessary. A *pterygium* is a wing-shaped vascular thickening of the conjunctiva which gradually encroaches on to the cornea, usually from the nasal side, following degenerative changes in the surface of the cornea (Fig 4-12). Local drying of the tear film and long-term exposure to the ultraviolet component of sunlight are thought to be causative factors; it is common in those parts of the world with much sun and wind. The more aggressive pterygia which slowly advance towards the centre of the cornea will impair vision unless surgically thwarted.

CHAPTER 4

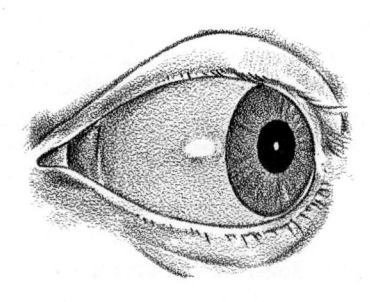

Fig 4-11 Pinguecula.

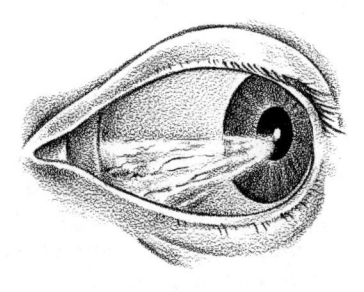

Fig 4-12 Large pterygium.

Arcus senilis is a complete or incomplete white ring encircling the cornea about 1mm within the limbus which is almost universal after the age of 60 years and may appear at a much younger age in some families and races. It is due to infiltration of the corneal stroma with lipids but it is not related to primary or secondary hyperlipidaemia and it never impairs sight.

Redness of the eye is due to hyperaemia of the conjunctival vessels or of the ciliary vessels or to a sub-conjunctival haemorrhage. The latter looks alarming but if spontaneous it usually has no local or general significance.

The differential diagnosis of the red eye is of great practical importance (p. 204).

EXAMINATION OF THE VISUAL SYSTEM

Medical examination is essentially a methodical search for physiological and anatomical deviations from the usual. In ophthalmology these twin explorations for altered function and altered structure can both be pursued by simple clinical means further than is possible in the examination of any other part of the body. Visual function can be adequately tested with simple apparatus and much of the eye can be seen under magnification with simple instruments. Ophthalmologists therefore have relatively little recourse to diagnostic laboratories because indirect tests of disturbed physiology are rarely needed and to pathology laboratories because pathological processes, almost to a histological level, can be seen in the eye as in no other part of the body. In two senses ophthalmology is a visual subject.

Tests of Function

Functional testing should usually precede anatomical testing.

Visual Function

Perception of *form* is assessed by testing distance visual acuity with a Snellen test-type chart and near visual acuity with a set of reading types. If the largest letters cannot be perceived, the ability to count fingers is tested.

If this is also defective, perception of *movement* is tested by determining if hand movements can be perceived. If this is also lacking, the most primitive of the visual perceptions, perception of *light,* is tested for.

Perception of *space* is assessed by testing the visual fields. Complete examination of the fields demands the use of a perimeter and perhaps a Bjerrum screen, but a surprising amount of useful information can be obtained very simply by confrontation testing of the fields with a small white-headed pin or with moving fingers.

Perception of *colour* is most simply tested with the Ishihara pseudo-isochromatic plates.

Binocular Function

The co-ordination of the two visual images can be assessed by a variety of specialized orthoptic tests. At the simple clinical level, observation of the *corneal light reflexes* will demonstrate the presence of a squint, the *cover-test* will reveal a latent squint or confirm a manifest squint, testing the *ocular movements* will permit study of nystagmus if present and will show up paralysis of one or more of the extraocular muscles, and *analysis of diplopia* if present will allow the detection of a paretic or paralysed extraocular muscle.

Pupillary Function

The relative sizes of the pupils and their reactions are tested by inspection.

Protective Function

The protective function of the *lids* is assessed by noting whether blinking occurs normally and whether the lids close completely on shutting the eyes. The protective function of *corneal sensation* is assessed by testing the corneal reflexes. The protective function of the *tears* is assessed by noting whether the eyes look moist and, if this is doubtful, by measuring tear production in response to irritation (Schirmer's test, p. 209). Malfunctioning of *tear drainage* is assessed by noting the position of the lower lid and by testing the patency of the lacrimal passages, e.g. by syringing saline through them.

Ocular Tension

Large derangements in the function of maintaining a normal intraocular pressure can be estimated by palpation of the globes but moderate and small increases in ocular tension cannot be detected without using an instrument called a tonometer.

Techniques of Testing Function

Distance Visual Acuity (VA) (p. 66)

Equipment:

Test;	Snellen letter chart, or
	Illiterate E, chart or single cards, or
	Letter-matching cards
Illumination;	60 watt bulb in a reflector directed on to the chart or card
	Normal room illumination
Occluder;	Card, envelope
Distance;	6 metres (20 feet) for a 6m test, or
	4 metres (13 feet) for a 4m test

Method:

With distance (not presbyopic) glasses, if worn. Test each eye separately. There is less to remember if the habit is adopted of always testing the right eye first and then the left eye. Ask the subject either to read the lowest line possible or to read from the top of the test chart.

When the patient stops, coax him or her to read more. The lowest line read more or less correctly is the 'denominator', and the distance at which the test is done, usually 6 or 4m, is the 'numerator' of the pseudo-fraction expressing acuity, e.g. 6/60, 6/5; 4/40, 4/4.

Record the results in the form:

VR =   VL =
   or, if glasses worn:
VR with glasses (or, with correction) =
VL with glasses (or, with correction) =
VA = (this is vision with both eyes).

If about half of the letters in the line are incorrectly read, record as 'partly' (p).
If a few of the letters are incorrect, record as (− number of incorrect letters).
If a few letters in the following line are correctly read, record as (+ number of letters in next line).
e.g. 6/18p, 6/5 (−2), 6/9 (+3).
If vision less than 6/60 or 4/40:
Reduce testing distance, e.g. from 4m to 2m.
CF at (X)m (counting fingers at number of metres distant).
HM (hand movements).
PL (perception of light).
No PL (i.e. blind − and only 'blind' if no PL).

Significance of results:

6/6 (4/4) is an arbitrary normal but vision as good as 6/3 (4/2) is possible for many young people.

An uncorrected vision of less than 6/6 (4/4) may be due to a refractive error. Therefore corrected vision needs to be known before deciding that a pathological lesion is lowering vision.

The pinhole test is an easy and useful screening test for retinal normality (p. 47).

Less than 6/9 (4/6) warrants referral.

6/18 (4/12) is the least with which reading is usually possible.

Near Vision

British Faculty of Ophthalmologists Reading Type is used (Fig 4-13). This consists of a series of

N5

An oculist and surgeon should
be descended from religious parents
be religious himself, and should have studied Latin,
anatomy, and the science of medicine

N8

Be a surgeon, having learned the barber trade from
youth on; not suitable are those that come to it
from the plough, manure waggon, or late in life
Have studied with an accomplished oculist and surgeon

N12

Have healthy and young eyes
Have fine, subtle, healthy hands and fingers, and
be nimble with both hands
Be able to draw and design in order to obtain
instruments

N18

Be married

N24

Not be greedy for money or be haughty

N36

Not be presumptuous

N48

Not be a drunkard

Fig 4-13 Reading type for testing near vision. The views are those expressed in 1583 by Georg Bartisch, one of the earliest European ophthalmologists. He went on to write, 'Very few such oculists exist.'

EXAMINATION

passages in 'Times Roman' print of sizes from 5 to 48 point. The notation used is N (for near) and type size, i.e. N5 to N48. Record each eye separately, with reading glasses if worn, e.g. VR with glasses = N5. (A point is 1/72 inch; the combined height of both ascending and descending letters in 5 point is just under 5/72 inch.)

Visual Field

Confrontation Testing

Seat yourself facing and on a level with the patient (Fig 4-14). Test the field of each eye in turn by having the patient cover the eye not being tested. Ask the patient to look at the bridge of your nose and watch that fixation is being maintained. As a test object use a small white-headed pin or, for gross defects, your moving fingers.

Bring the test object forward from behind the patient's head and note the point at which it is first seen by the patient. Repeat in other representative meridians. Judge the normal outline of the field in each meridian by the point where the test object is no longer obscured by the anatomical surrounds of the tested eye – the eyebrow above, the nose on the nasal side, the cheek below – or, on the temporal side, when it is level with the eye.

A useful alternative method is to ask the patient to say whether you are holding up one or two fingers in the periphery of each of the four quadrants of his or her field.

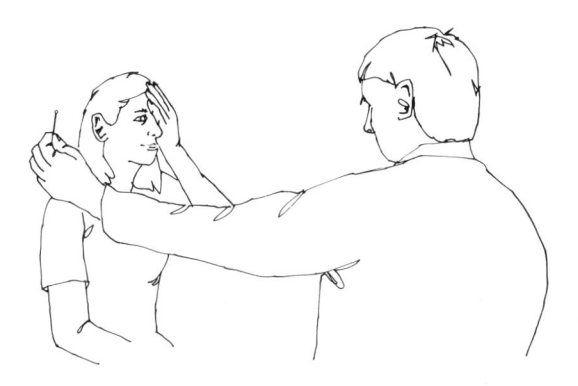

Fig 4-14 Confrontation testing of the right visual field.

Amsler Grid

This simple pattern of horizontal and vertical lines is a useful subjective test for disturbances of macular vision such as small scotomata or metamorphopsia (Fig 4-15). The patient, wearing his or her reading glasses if necessary, holds the chart in a good light and with one eye alone continuously fixes the central spot. He or she is asked to describe any gaps or kinks in the lines. Patients who have had a disciform degeneration of the macula of one eye may be given this type of chart to use at home in the hope of detecting involvement of their second eye should this occur at a stage early enough for possible treatment (p. 194).

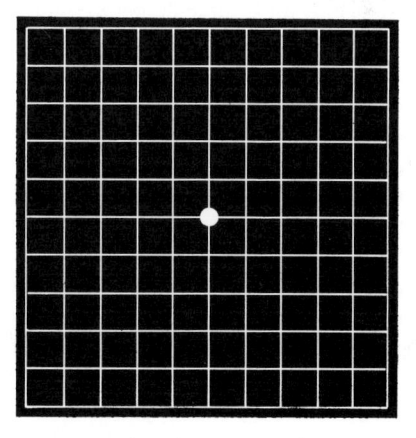

Fig 4-15 Central 10° of an Amsler grid. When the chart is held 30cm from the eye each small square subtends 1°. The usual complete chart subtends 20°.

Field Defects

There are four anatomical stages in the visual pathway with four corresponding types of visual field loss. These are (1) the retina and optic disc, (2) the optic nerve, (3) the optic chiasma and (4) the retro-chiasmal visual pathway (p. 31). Pre-chiasmal defects (1 and 2) are limited to the field of one eye but of course can be bilateral, while chiasmal (3) and retro-chiasmal (4) defects necessarily involve the fields of both eyes (Fig 4-16).

When a pre-chiasmal defect is due to a lesion of the *retina* or *optic disc* a corresponding lesion

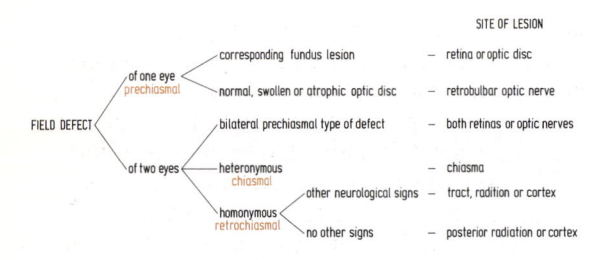

```
                                              SITE OF LESION
                   corresponding fundus lesion    — retina or optic disc
      of one eye
      prechiasmal  normal, swollen or atrophic optic disc — retrobulbar optic nerve
FIELD DEFECT       bilateral prechiasmal type of defect — both retinas or optic nerves
      of two eyes  heteronymous                   — chiasma
                   chiasmal
                              other neurological signs — tract, radiation or cortex
                   homonymous
                   retrochiasmal
                              no other signs     — posterior radiation or cortex
```

Fig 4-16 Topographical types of visual field defects.

can usually be seen with the ophthalmoscope, e.g. an area of choroidoretinal scarring; retinitis pigmentosa (which starts as a ring scotoma); glaucomatous cupping. The defect is not limited by the vertical midline between the nasal and temporal half fields and may therefore cross a line through the fixation point. It may correspond to the way the retinal nerve fibres run towards the optic disc, e.g. an arcuate defect in glaucoma, or to an area of retinal blood supply, e.g. loss of the inferior field nasal to the blind spot following occlusion of the superior temporal retinal artery.

Defects from lesions of the *retrobulbar optic nerve* tend to start as a central scotoma whether they are due to inflammation, e.g. optic neuritis; to compression, e.g. sphenoidal ridge meningioma, aneurysm of the anterior part of the circle of Willis; or to toxic or nutritional neuropathy, e.g. tobacco amblyopia, pernicious anaemia. Exceptions are the altitudinal or total loss in ischaemic optic neuropathy, and peripheral depression in tabetic syphilitic optic atrophy. They usually affect both nasal and temporal halves of the fields. Ophthalmoscopically, the optic disc may be normal, swollen or, eventually, atrophic.

Bitemporal (heteronymous) defects are the hallmark of *chiasmal* lesions. Often asymmetrical, they start in the upper or lower temporal quadrant and then affect the other temporal quadrant before crossing the midline to involve the nasal quadrants. Optic atrophy may take years to become apparent.

Retro-chiasmal lesions cause homonymous defects which may be hemianopic, quadrantanopic or scotomatous. Optic tract lesions are less common than lesions of the optic radiation or visual cortex, are incongruous and, after some months, are accompanied by bilateral optic atrophy.

When the optic tract or the anterior part of the optic radiation are involved there are usually other signs of brain damage, e.g. hemiplegic signs in lesions of the internal capsule which include the optic radiation, while there are no other signs with a lesion of the visual cortex, unless this is due to vertebro-basilar arterial disease which also causes mid-brain signs. Temporal lobe lesions cause an upper homonymous quadrantanopia. Vascular lesions of the optic radiation commonly cause an inferior homonymous quadrantanopia because the upper fibres are supplied only by branches of the middle cerebral artery whereas the lower fibres are supplied in addition by branches of the posterior cerebral artery.

Binocular Function

Corneal Light Reflexes (Reflections)

The pin-point reflection from each cornea of a fixated light should be symmetrically located in the two pupils (Fig 4-17). Asymmetry of the reflections usually signifies a deviation of one eye, that is one eye is failing to fix the light. This test is especially useful for babies who will normally look at a small light.

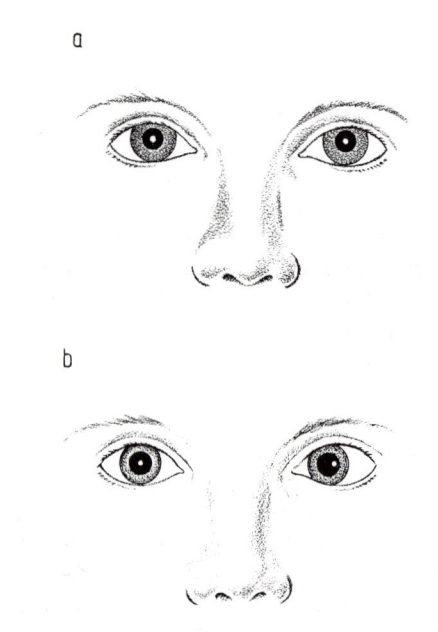

Fig 4-17 Corneal light reflexes
   a normal
   b with a left convergent squint.

Cover Test

The patient is asked to look intently at a small object, e.g. the light of a torch, held directly in front of him or her (Fig 4-18). While he or she regards this, one of the patient's eyes is obstructed by the examiner's hand which after a moment is then moved across to cover the other eye. Again, after a brief pause, the hand is moved across to cover the first eye, and the process of covering alternate eyes is continued while each eye is watched for any movement as it is **un**covered. This part of the cover test, *the alternate cover test*, will reveal any deviation of an eye because if such deviation occurs the eye will have to make a restitutory movement to regain fixation when it is freshly exposed (Fig 4-19). For example, if there is a convergent deviation, the eye while covered will be converged behind the covering hand. When the hand moves to cover the other eye, a movement outwards of the converged eye to correct this inturning is necessary to maintain fixation of the object of interest.

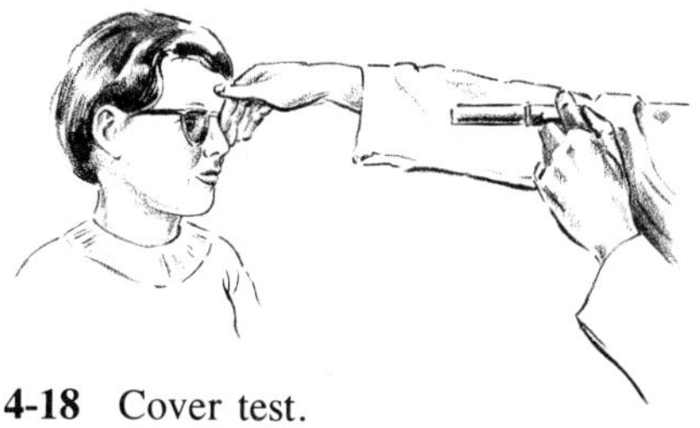

Fig 4-18 Cover test.

The alternate cover test does not distinguish between a manifest deviation (a squint) and a latent deviation (a heterophoria). The second part of the cover test, the *cover-uncover test,* is necessary to make this important distinction (Fig 4-19). In the cover-uncover test one eye is momentarily covered and then uncovered. After studying the response to several coverings and uncoverings of the first eye, the procedure is applied to the second eye. While covering, the unobstructed eye is observed. If any movement of this uncovered eye occurs, it obviously had not been fixing the test object and therefore there had been a *manifest* deviation of this eye. While uncovering, the obstructed eye is observed. If there was no manifest deviation of the uncovered eye, any movement of this covered eye reveals that there is a *latent* deviation. Often this recovery of fixation is rapid but it may be delayed. Sometimes after several interruptions of binocular fixation recovery is long delayed because, as a result of the test, a latent deviation has become manifest.

The cover-uncover test also distinguishes a unilateral from an alternating squint. In a *unilateral* squint covering of the deviating eye produces no movement of the preferred fixing eye, while covering of the fixing eye produces a straightening movement of the deviating eye on applying the cover and a movement of reversion to the original deviation on removing the cover. This latter movement will, of course, be accompanied by a recovery movement of the dominant eye. In an *alternating* squint fixation is happily maintained by whichever eye is not being repeatedly covered.

Ocular Movements

While the patient intently fixes an object, e.g. a torch light, moved in turn into each of 'the six cardinal directions' of gaze (Fig 1-30), lagging of either eye is looked for. Small defects in eye movement are readily shown up by performing the alternate cover test with the fixation object held in these directions of gaze.

If nystagmus is present, its behaviour is noted as the patient follows an object moved to either side and up and down.

Nystagmus

Nystagmus is an involuntary rhythmic oscillatory movement of the eyes from side to side (horizontal nystagmus) or up and down (vertical nystagmus). The to-and-fro movements may be either equal in speed and amplitude (pendular nystagmus) or consist of slow drifts in one direction alternating with rapid refixation saccades in the opposite direction (jerky nystagmus). In jerky nystagmus the direction of the nystagmus is conventionally named according to the direction of the fast phase. Pendular nystagmus often becomes jerky on lateral versions of the eyes.

Pendular nystagmus (ocular nystagmus) with few exceptions is due to loss of central vision of both eyes before the age of two years from such causes as congenital cataracts or maldevelopment of the macula in albinism, or it is a congenital nystagmus with no other defect. Pendular nystagmus cannot be acquired after the age of six years.

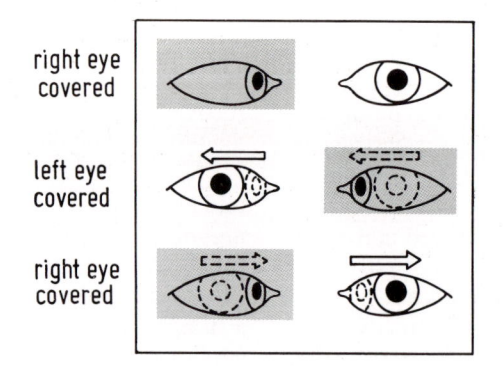

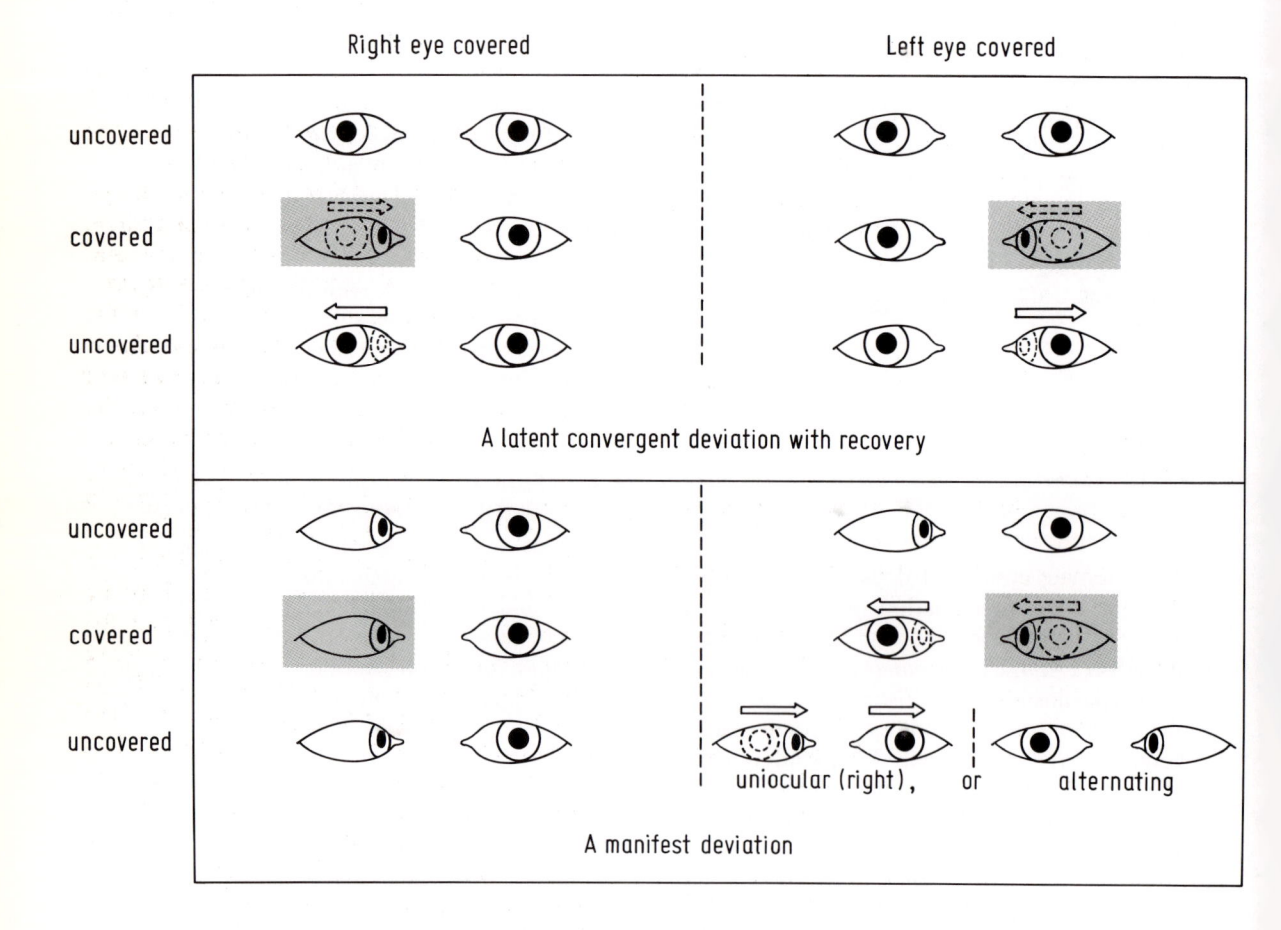

Fig 4-19 Interpretation of the cover test
  Upper Alternate cover test
  Lower Cover uncover test
Horizontal arrows represent the eye movements which occur when the cover is applied or removed.

The eye movements in *jerky nystagmus* may be purely horizontal or vertical (fixation nystagmus) or they may have a rotatory component combined with the horizontal or vertical movements (vestibular nystagmus).

Fixation nystagmus is seen physiologically as optokinetic nystagmus (p. 39) and as the nystagmoid jerks of end-position nystagmus which occur in most people on extreme version to either side and which are more marked in debility, fatigue, or as a result of drugs such as alcohol, barbiturates, and phenytoin. *End-position nystagmus* occurs pathologically, that is nystagmus occurs on gaze up, down, to the right, or to the left before the normal limits of the eye movement are reached, when there is a neuro-muscular insufficiency of ocular movement such as a gaze paralysis or weakness of an extraocular muscle. *Latent nystagmus* is an uncommon type of fixation nystagmus, usually associated with a convergent squint, which occurs in both eyes when one eye is covered. As a result monocular visual acuity when tested in the ordinary way is much worse than the acuity with both eyes together. In some patients with congenital nystagmus the movements are jerky rather than pendular.

Vestibular nystagmus occurs physiologically when endolymph is caused to flow in the semicircular canals as by rotation of the body or by caloric irrigation of the external auditory meatus (COWS: cold opposite, warm same). For example, cold water in the left ear induces a nystagmus (with the rapid phase) to the right, while warm water in the left ear causes a left nystagmus. Pathological vestibular nystagmus results from either peripheral lesions of the labyrinth or from central lesions involving the vestibular nuclei or their connections.

Peripheral vestibular nystagmus, due for example to labyrinthitis or Ménière's disease, is accompanied by other labyrinthine symptoms such as vertigo and tinnitus and recovers within weeks.

Central vestibular nystagmus may occur without acoustic symptoms and persist. The fast phase of the nystagmus is towards the side of the lesion. More common causes are multiple sclerosis, vascular lesions such as postero-inferior cerebellar artery occlusion, cerebellar and cerebello-pontine lesions, and drugs.

Unless due to drugs such as sedatives and anticonvulsants, *vertical nystagmus* signifies pathology of the mid-brain, brain stem, or upper cervical cord. *Ataxic nystagmus,* in which on lateral version there is nystagmus of the abducting eye and incomplete movement of the adducting eye, is seen in internuclear ophthalmoplegia and is caused by a lesion of the medial longitudinal bundle (p. 38).

Analysis of Diplopia

The separation of the two images is greatest when the eye turns in the direction of maximum action of the paretic muscle.

1. Find the direction of gaze in which the separation is greatest. In the case of vertical diplopia consider only the vertical separation and ignore any horizontal separation.
2. The more peripheral image belongs to the eye with the paretic muscle. This is determined by a cover-uncover test on one eye and eliciting which of the two images disappears.
3. In vertical diplopia, to determine which of the pair of elevating or of depressing muscles is at fault, find whether the eye with the affected muscle is abducted or adducted when the vertical separation (ignore horizontal separation) is greatest. If it is greatest in abduction, a rectus muscle is paresed. If it is greatest in adduction, an oblique muscle is faulty.

For example, a patient experiences diplopia in which one image is higher and to one side of the other image. On testing it is found that the vertical separation between the images is greatest when he is looking downwards and to his left and that on covering his right eye the lower of the two images disappears. In laevodepression it is the lower of the two images which is the more peripheral one. The weak muscle therefore belongs to the right eye and it must be one of the two depressor muscles of the right eye (superior oblique and inferior rectus). In laevodepression the right eye is adducted (so that its visual axis is close to the axis of its oblique muscles) and therefore it is a weakness of the right superior oblique muscle which is causing his double vision (Fig 1-33).

Pupils

The integrity of the two pupillary reflexes, constriction with light and with near vision, in both their afferent and efferent pathways is tested by noting whether the pupils are equal and round and whether they react normally to light and to accommodation.

Small inequalities (anisocoria) of the pupils are frequently found in the normal population. This is called *benign anisocoria*. The inequality may be greater in dim light than in bright light. So long as both pupils react normally to light, to dark, and to near stimuli an anisocoria is almost certainly of this type.

If a pupil is not circular the cause is usually in the iris itself.

When testing the pupillary reactions remember that there are two afferent and two efferent (parasympathetic and sympathetic) pathways and that the aim is to test them separately. To this end only one stimulus, light or accommodation, should be changed at a time. The *light reflex* is tested, preferably in dim light, with the patient *fixing on a distant object* and a bright light is shone into each eye in turn. Constriction of each pupil, both directly and consensually is noted and compared.

Any prechiasmal lesion of the afferent visual/pupillary pathway will result in reduction of the direct pupillary response to light, but the consensual response of the involved eye is retained (the consensual response of the uninvolved eye is also impaired). There is no anisocoria with afferent pupillary defects. Prechiasmal afferent pupillary defects will be associated with abnormalities of vision although these latter may be too subtle to be detected by the usual clinical tests.

A useful variation of technique is the *swinging flashlight test* which aids comparison of the right and left afferent pathways. A small light held just below and midway between the subject's eye is shone for about five seconds alternately into each eye and the size of both pupils noted while the patient looks at a distant object. When the eye on the affected side is illuminated both pupils are larger than when the unaffected eye is illuminated. Put another way, the pupil of the affected eye is seen to dilate when the light is shone into it (Marcus Gunn sign). This test detects subtle asymmetrical afferent defects and is most helpful when vision is reasonably good, e.g. after retrobulbar neuritis.

The *near reflex* is tested by having the patient, in unchanging illumination, look from a distant object to a small target held just below and midway between his or her eyes and then continue to concentrate on the target as it is moved closer until he or she can no longer follow it. Constriction of the pupil with the near reflex will be greater than constriction with the light reflex when there is a defect of the afferent light pathway. This is called *light-near dissociation*. It is also found, even though the afferent pathway is intact, i.e. vision is normal, with an Adie's myotonic pupil (p. 34), Argyll Robertson pupils (p. 34), and occasionally with diabetes and tegmental pretectal lesions. Usually when there is a defect of the common efferent pathway constriction to light and near are equally affected.

Efferent pupillary defects are due to a lesion of either the parasympathetic or the sympathetic pathway and in each case there is anisocoria. With a *parasympathetic* defect the pupil is larger and the inequality is greater in bright than in dim light. Constriction to light and to near is reduced or absent. With a *sympathetic* defect the pupil is slightly smaller and the inequality is greater in dim light. The light and the near responses are intact but there is delayed and incomplete dilatation in dim light. There is commonly an associated slight ptosis (Horner's syndrome, p. 35).

A parasympathetic defect is commonly due to a third nerve lesion, e.g. intracranial aneurysm; *Hutchinson's pupil,* which is a fixed dilated pupil due to increased intracranial pressure in which either an ipsilateral lesion, e.g. a subdural haematoma, compresses the third nerve against the dorsum sellae, or bilaterally, when a tentorial pressure cone causes brain stem compression.

When confronted by *anisocoria* the cause of which is not obvious, first check whether it is due to a local ocular cause, such as constriction from iritis or the use of miotic eye drops, or dilatation from angle closure glaucoma, trauma or the use of mydriatic eye drops. Next determine whether the light reaction is obviously impaired in one eye. If it is, there is probably a parasympathetic lesion and the larger pupil is the abnormal one. If it is not, there is probably a sympathetic lesion and the smaller pupil is the abnormal one. Look for confirmation by noting whether the anisocoria is greater in bright light (probably a parasympathetic defect) or in dim light (probably a sympathetic defect or benign anisocoria).

Intraocular Pressure

Digital Estimation

The patient must look down and keep looking down but not actively close his or her eyes. The tips of the examiner's two index fingers feel the sclera through the upper lid above the upper border of the tarsal plate. Gentle pressure of the alternate finger tips is applied towards the centre of the globe. Feel for and estimate the sense of fluctuation imparted to the stationary finger or estimate the rebound of the sclera as the indenting finger is relaxed.

Small deviations from normal will not be reliably felt, but it is worth developing the feel of the normal so that pronounced alterations will be detected.

Tonometry

Tonometry is the instrumental estimation of the intraocular pressure (IOP) which is often referred to clinically as the ocular tension. Ideally it should be part of any routine full medical examination of persons over 60 years. Because direct measurement of the IOP is not clinically possible, an indirect method is used in which a force is applied to the cornea and the resulting deformation is measured. Two types of deformation are used, indentation or denting of the cornea and applanation of flattening of the cornea. *Indentation tonometry* is done with a Schiötz tonometer in which, with the subject lying down, a weighted plunger of 1.5mm diameter is rested on the cornea and the depth of indentation is measured. *Applanation tonometry* is usually done with a Goldmann applanation tonometer attached to a slit-lamp microscope in which, with the subject seated at the slit-lamp, a plane surface is pressed against the cornea and the force required to flatten a standard area of cornea is measured (Fig 4-20). Although indentation tonometry is less accurate than applanation it does not require such elaborate equipment or special skill and it remains a valuable clinical tool for non-specialists.

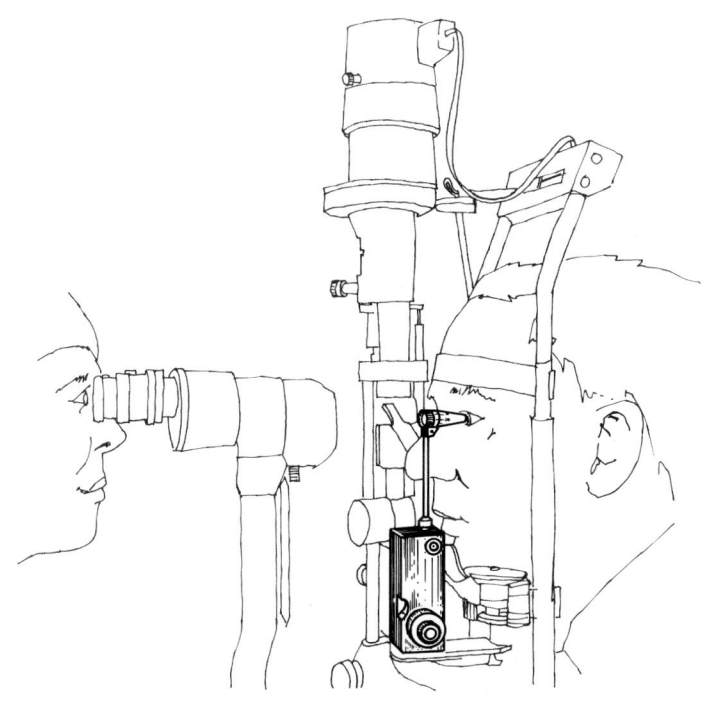

Fig 4-20 Applanation tonometry.

The *Schiötz tonometer* consists of a cylinder with a concave foot-plate through which passes a plunger, the upper end of which works against one arm of a lever, the other arm being a pointer (Fig 4-21). The radius of curvature of the foot-plate is flatter than that of the cornea (15mm compared with 8mm) so that only a portion of the foot-plate immediately surrounding the plunger hole is in contact with the cornea; the foot-plate acts as a reference point from which movements of the plunger are measured. The tip of the plunger has a concavity of similar radius to that of the foot-plate. The test block provided with the instrument is part of a metal sphere of radius 16mm so that with the instrument on the test block and a scale reading of zero, the plunger is 0.05mm beyond the foot-plate. This is because in use the plunger sinks into the corneal epithelium for 0.05mm before indenting the cornea as a whole.

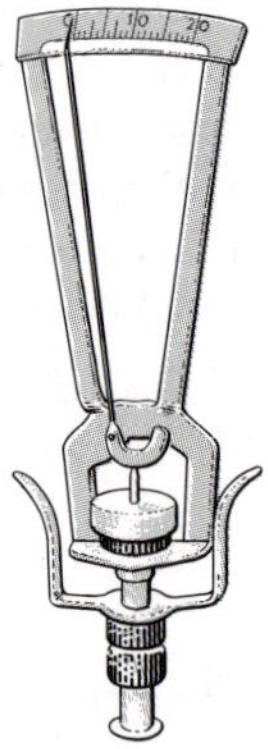

Fig 4-21 Schiötz tonometer.

The scale over which the pointer moves is graduated so that each division represents a displacement of 0.05mm of the plunger relative to the foot-plate. In some instruments there is a mirror surface behind the pointer immediately below the scale so that parallactic errors in reading the position of the pointer on the scale can be eliminated.

The weight of the plunger is 5.5g and this can be increased by additional weights to give total plunger weights of 7.5g, 10g and 15g. These different weights have several uses, but the most important in using the tonometer is to select that weight which results in a deflection of about five scale divisions because it is in this range that the instrument is most accurate. The heavier weights are required only for eyes in which the pressure is pathologically increased.

The scale reading on the tonometer may be translated into mm Hg by reading from a conversion table supplied with the instrument.

Use of a Schiötz Tonometer
Before 'taking the tension' check that there is free movement of the plunger and clean it with isopropyl alcohol on a swab if there is not. Check the zero position of the pointer with the test-block.

Explain simply to the subject the purpose of the test. Have him lie comfortably on his back on a couch. Instil one drop of proxymetacaine (proparacaine) eye-drops 0.5% in each eye. Prepare the patient adequately by insuring that he is not apprehensive, that his collar is not tight, that his neck is not awkwardly flexed, that he is not holding his breath, and that he does not squeeze his lids.

The subject is asked to keep both eyes open and to keep his eyes in the primary position by fixing a spot directly in front of his face on the ceiling.

Carefully apply the tonometer to the right eye so that it is vertical, the foot-plate is resting evenly on the cornea, the plunger is central on the cornea and so that you are not pressing on the orbit or the eyeball. Check that the pointer is pulsating freely with the subject's heart beat before taking the reading. If the tonometer has a mirror use it to avoid parallactic error in reading the scale. Repeat the procedure for the left eye. Use the conversion table to obtain the IOP of each eye in mm Hg.

After use the foot-plate and end of the plunger of the tonometer is cleansed with a 70% isopropyl alcohol swab.

With the Schiötz tonometer the instrumental error is half a scale-division and the reading error is also half a scale-division. Together with errors due to individual variation in the distensibility of the sclera these result in an accuracy of no better than ± 3mm Hg. The calibration table gives the figures for IOP to two decimal places but this obviously suggests a spurious level of accuracy.

The mean IOP of a large number of apparently healthy subjects is 15 ± 3mm Hg.

EXAMINATION

Visual Examination of Ocular Structure

General Observation

Just as the inexperienced microscopist tends to miss things by using too high a magnification too soon, so the learner clinician tends to overlook the value of a preliminary low power examination. In ophthalmology there is a tendency to immediately concentrate on the details of the eye itself without preliminary observation of the whole patient and especially the surrounds of the eye.

Obvious changes which can in this way be overlooked are an abnormal head posture; exophthalmos or enophthalmos; ptosis or retraction of the upper lid; ectropion or entropion of the lower lid; incomplete closure of the lids; the colour of the irides.

Detailed Inspection

Many important changes can be seen in a good light with just the naked eye. Non-specialists often miss quite gross abnormalities because they do not realize this and, in fact, do not even try to look at their patients' eyes.

To do this well requires some experience and the understanding gained from seeing abnormalities with magnification and special methods of illumination, e.g. with the slit-lamp microscope. For this reason students are encouraged to examine patients at every opportunity with the slit-lamp. Prepared in this way, it is much easier to look for and interpret the abnormalities which may be encountered when specialized methods of examination are not available.

The only equipment needed is a clinical torch. *Oblique or lateral illumination* is more useful than frontal illumination and this is especially so when examining the cornea. Always direct your light from several directions; you will often discover that one particular direction of illumination shows up a detail which is not seen with the light coming from other directions.

As always, it is sensible to systematize one's inspection on an anatomical basis and to work from the surface inwards.

The following is a brief list, for each structure in turn, of the major abnormalities to be on the alert for.

Lids
Ectropion, ectropion of the lower lacrimal punctum, entropion, trichiasis; discharge, blepharitis; swellings.

Lacrimal sac
Swelling, tenderness; regurgitation from the punctum on applying pressure over the sac.

Conjunctiva
The bulbar conjunctiva may be seen by separating the lids with your fingers taking care to apply pressure only over the bones of the orbital margins. To examine the tarsal conjunctiva of the lower lid, pull down the lid while the patient looks upwards. To see the conjunctiva of the upper lid it is necessary to *evert the lid*. The simplest way to do this is, with the patient looking far downwards but not shutting his or her eyes, to apply a cotton-tipped applicator (swab-stick) to the skin of the lid centrally just above the upper margin of the tarsal plate. This acts as a fulcrum about which to rotate the lid by gently pulling on some central eye lashes first slightly downwards, then slightly away from the eye and finally upwards. The applicator is then slid out from behind the everted lid which can be held in this position by gentle finger pressure of some central lashes against the skin below the eyebrow. To restore the lid to its normal position simply ask the patient to look upwards and the lid will flip over.

Hyperaemia superficial, as in conjunctivitis, or deep (circumcorneal or ciliary injection or hyperaemia), as in iritis.

Discharge.
Foreign body.

Sclera
Localized hyperaemia with tenderness localized to the area of hyperaemia means episcleritis.
Lacerations (should be specifically looked for in injuries).

Cornea
Take particular note of the brilliance and regularity of the surface as a mirror by directing the light in different directions in turn so that its reflection from all parts of the corneal surface enters your eye.
General loss of lustre, e.g. epithelial oedema, as shown by irregularity of the image of a spot of light.

Localized imperfections of the mirror surface, e.g. abrasions and ulcers.
Foreign body.
Grey spots or areas, i.e. ulcers, infiltrates.
Perforating wounds and lacerations.
Opacities.
Vascularization.
KP (keratic precipitates, which are small clumps of inflammatory cells sticking to the mesothelial surface and signify iridocyclitis).
Staining with sterile 2% fluorescein solution is a useful adjunct in examining the cornea because areas of epithelial loss retain the green dye.

Anterior Chamber

Depth — Shallow with a perforating wound; shallow in potential or actual angle closure glaucoma.
Deep in aphakia (absence of lens, as after removal of a cataract) or subluxation of the lens.
Iris bombé (doughnut-like bulging of mid iris due to total block of the pupil from adhesions).

Hyphaema (blood in anterior chamber).
Hypopyon (pus in anterior chamber).
An aqueous flare (Fig 5-4) if dense can be seen with a narrow focused pencil of torch light.

Iris

Hyperaemia and oedema (muddy iris) such as may occur in iritis are difficult to detect.
Iridodonesis, a jelly-like tremulousness of the iris on movement of the eye, signifies absence of support of the iris by the lens as in subluxation of the lens and in aphakia.
Irido-dialysis (tearing of part of the peripheral attachment of the iris to the ciliary body).
Loss of colour compared with the other eye (heterochromia iridis) may be congenital or atrophic, e.g. from cyclitis.

Pupil

Small and reduced mobility in *iritis*.
Dilated and immobile in acute *glaucoma*.
Irregularity: Posterior synechiae (adhesions of pupil margin to lens capsule).
Injury — rupture of sphincter; D-shaped pupil with irido-dialysis.

DIFFERENTIAL DIAGNOSIS OF THE RED EYE

	Conjunctivitis	Corneal lesion, e.g. abrasion, foreign body, ulcer	Acute iritis	Acute angle closure glaucoma	Episcleritis
Symptoms	Discomfort	Pain, photophobia	Pain, photophobia	Severe pain	Aching pain; tenderness localized to affected area
Discharge	Mucopurulent	Watery discharge	Watery	Slight watering	Slight watering
Vision	**Never impaired**	May be impaired	**Impaired**	Severely **impaired;** haloes	Normal
Hyperaemia	Generalized	Ciliary (may be localized to region nearest to lesion)	Ciliary	Ciliary (surprisingly little in early stages)	Predominantly area affected
Cornea	Normal	Alteration of surface reflection; ± opacity	Normal	Steamy, loss of lustre	Normal
Pupil	Normal	May be irritative miosis	**Small** and may be irregular	**Dilated** and non-reacting	Normal
Ocular tension	Normal	Normal	May be secondary glaucoma	Raised	Normal

Chapter 5

INSTRUMENTAL EXAMINATION OF THE EYE

SLIT-LAMP MICROSCOPY

Principle
Use of the slit-lamp
Ocular anatomy as seen with a slit-lamp microscope
  Conjunctiva and sclera
  Cornea
  Anterior chamber
  Iris
  Lens
  Vitreous

OPHTHALMOSCOPY

Principle
Use of the ophthalmoscope
  The red reflex
  Dilatation of the pupils

INSTRUMENTAL EXAMINATION OF THE EYE

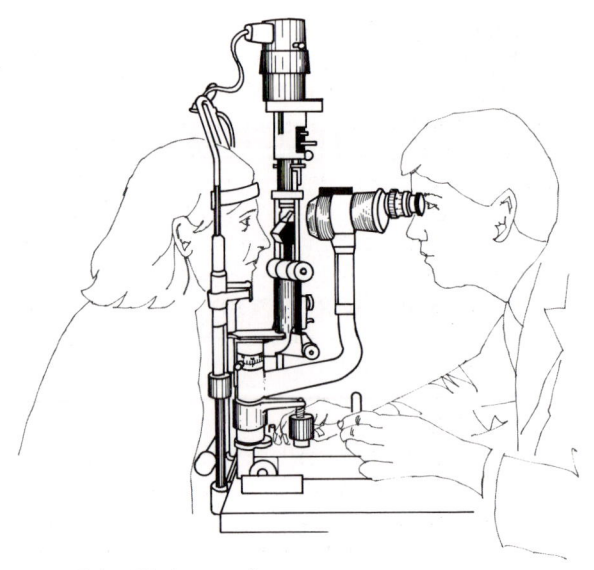

Slit-Lamp Microscopy and Ophthalmoscopy

The ophthalmologist's two basic instruments for looking at eyes are the slit-lamp microscope and the ophthalmoscope. The former is primarily used to examine the anterior part of the eye as far in as the vitreous immediately behind the lens. With the aid of a flat-surfaced contact lens to neutralize the refraction of the cornea, it is also used to examine the interior of the globe, the fundus. The ophthalmoscope is used to see the fundus and to detect any loss of transparency of the tissues anterior to the fundus.

The ophthalmoscope is also an essential instrument for all physicians and therefore mastery of its use is an obvious necessity. Although slit-lamp microscopes are usually available only in ophthalmologists' rooms and in hospital departments of ophthalmology and casualty departments, the experience and understanding gained from seeing abnormalities with this instrument make it much easier to examine and interpret changes in the eye in clinical practice when a slit-lamp microscope is not available.

The ability to use a slit-lamp microscope and an ophthalmoscope is also needed for an important part of practical ocular anatomy because with these two instruments a student is able to see a surprising amount of the living anatomy of the eye.

Fig 5-1 Slit-lamp microscopy.

SLIT-LAMP MICROSCOPY

Principle

The slit-lamp microscope is a low power binocular microscope coupled with an illuminating system mounted on a table which also has a head-rest to steady the patient's head (Fig 5-1). It is colloquially called a slit-lamp.

Light which is brought to a focus in a vertical line (a 'slit') is directed into the eye so that the beam of light cuts a slice through the transparent and semi-transparent structures (Fig 5-2). In this way a section, an *optical section,* is cut through the tissue. The directions of the light and of the axis of the microscope are at a variable angle (0° to 70°) to each other. The illumination is

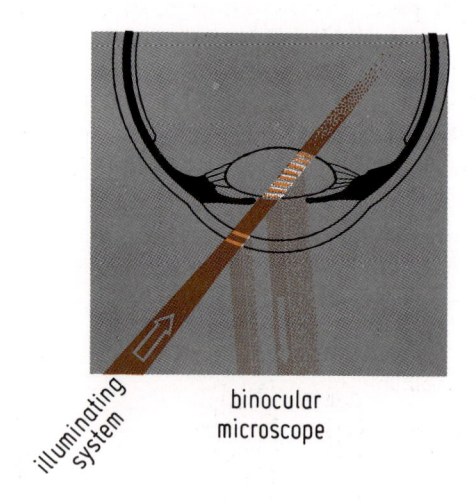

Fig 5-2 Principle of slit-lamp microscopy.

usually directed obliquely into the eye from one or other side while the microscope is usually directed more or less straight at the eye. With this arrangement it is easy to see the shape and thickness of transparent structures and to localize the position (the depth) of any alterations in these structures.

SLIT-LAMP

Even though tissues such as the cornea are very highly transparent a small fraction (1%) of light passing through is scattered or diffracted and it is this scattered light which makes it possible to see transparent tissues with the slit-lamp microscope. The essential feature of such optical arrangements is that they permit visualization of faint scattered light without its being overwhelmed by the much brighter light reflected from parts of the eye other than that being examined. Light is scattered in different degrees by different tissues and therefore microscopic differences in structure smaller than the resolving power of the low power microscope which is used can be detected. For example, in an optical section of the cornea the tear film is faintly seen, the epithelial layer is not seen, Bowmann's membrane is brightly seen, the stroma is well seen, and Descemet's membrane and mesothelium together are brightly seen (Fig 5-3). Normally the aqueous scatters insufficient light for it to be seen but if there is any increase in its protein, as occurs in inflammation of the iris or ciliary body, a beam of light passing across the anterior chamber is visible, as are individual leucocytes or other cells which may be abnormally present floating in the aqueous (Fig 5-4). Of course reflected light from opaque tissues, e.g. iris, sclera, can also be seen and examined with the slit-lamp microscope.

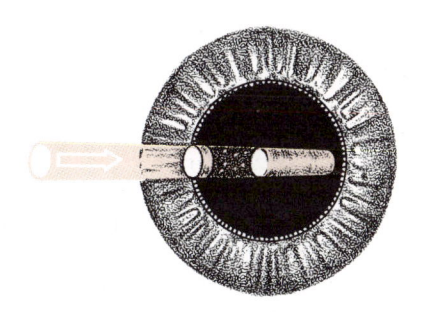

Fig 5-4 A small pencil of light is seen as it crosses the anterior chamber from the left side. This is abnormal and is called an aqueous flare. A few cells of an inflammatory exudate are spot-lighted by the beam as they float in the aqueous.

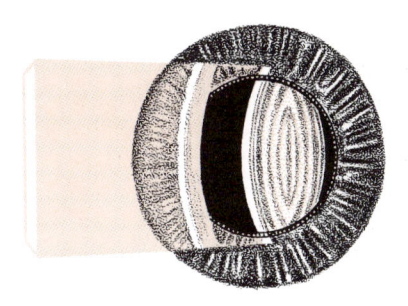

Fig 5-5 Cornea and lens seen in optical section with a slit-lamp.

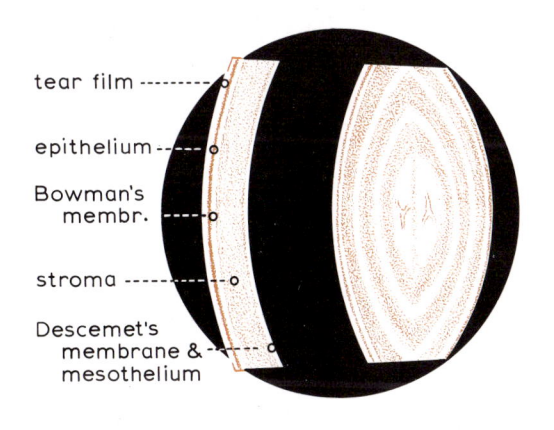

Fig 5-3 Optical sections of the cornea and the lens obtained with a narrow beam of light coming from the left side. In practice all depths of the cornea and lens will not be simultaneously in focus as is shown in this composite diagram.

The width of the slit can be varied. When it is narrow an optical section of the anterior part of the eye is seen; from the exterior inwards this consists of the cornea, a dark interval corresponding to the anterior chamber, and either the iris or the lens and the anterior part of the vitreous (Fig 5-5). When the slit is wide, blocks of the transparent tissues are illuminated; in the case of the cornea this block is a parallelopiped and the external epithelial surface and the internal mesothelial surface can be distinguished with the stroma in between them (Fig 5-6).

All levels are not simultaneously in focus and therefore, as in using any microscope, focusing movements must be made to build up a composite mental picture of the tissues in depth. In the slit-lamp the light and the microscope are usually linked so that they are both focused on a common spot.

Use of the Slit-Lamp

The subject is seated and the heights of the stool, table, and head-rest are adjusted so that he or she is comfortable. The light is switched on and the position of the subject's eyes is controlled by having him or her look at the fixation light which is appropriately positioned.

Use a moderately narrow slit and direct the light obliquely from the side on to the subject's eye. Swing the microscope aside and observe the image of the light in the subject's eye with your naked eye. Use the antero-posterior (focusing), lateral, and vertical controls to position and focus the light. For a start it may be easier to see when the light is focused if it is directed on to the iris.

When you understand the naked-eye appearances and the focusing controls, move the microscope back into position so that it is directed straight at the subject's eye. Again, it may be easier to start by looking at the iris. Adjust the separation of the oculars to your own interpupillary distance.

First use the low power and, when you understand what you see with this, change to high power. Continually adjust the focus and vary the obliquity of the light and the height as required.

Switch the light off as soon as the examination is finished.

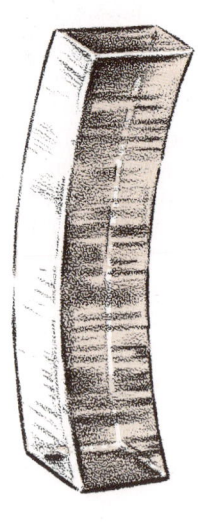

Fig 5-6 Block of illuminated cornea seen with a broad beam of light coming from the left side.

Ocular Anatomy as seen with a Slit-Lamp Microscope

Structures to Examine

Bulbar Conjunctiva and Underlying Sclera
   Conjunctival and episcleral vessels.
      Streaming of blood will be visible in the smaller vessels due to a granular appearance of the blood.
      In some capillaries, clumps of red cells can be seen moving jerkily.
      Aqueous veins may be found.
      The tear film meniscus along the margin of the lower lid.
      The junction of conjunctiva and cornea, with capillary loops on the surface.

Cornea
Broad beam:
   Tear film, with dust and cellular debris on the anterior surface which move slightly due to gravity or partial blinking.
   Anterior, lateral, and posterior surfaces of the corneal parallelopiped (Fig 5-6).
   Corneal nerves in the anterior ⅔ of the stroma can usually be seen at the periphery where for about 1mm they have a myelin sheath.

Narrow beam, optical section:
   The anterior surface is bounded by a pair of bright lines, the anterior line being the tear film while the posterior line is Bowman's membrane (Fig 5-3). The intervening dark interval represents the corneal epithelium. The stroma has an opalescent texture. Posterior to the stroma is another bright line representing Descemet's membrane and mesothelium. If the tear film is lightly stained with fluorescein it is more readily seen.

Anterior Chamber
   Note the depth, centrally and peripherally.
   Note that the angle is invisible unless a gonioscopy contact lens is used to overcome the total internal reflection at the corneal-air-interface of light from this peripheral region (Fig 1-22).

Iris
   The open sponge-like texture and the colour of the stroma.
   Vessels are visible in light-coloured irides.
   The collarette may have embryonic remnants (pupillary membrane) attached to it.

OPHTHALMOSCOPY

The pigmented pupillary margin (ectodermal layer) is quite distinct.

The sphincter pupillae muscle can be seen in light-coloured irides by indirect illumination.

The pupil is continually moving even with unchanging illumination. Note its reaction to light.

Lens (not fully seen with undilated pupil)

In a narrow beam the zones of optical discontinuity give it a layered, onion-like appearance. The nuclei, cortex, and Y sutures are readily seen (Fig 5-3).

Anterior vitreous (not easily seen with undilated pupil)

With the slit-lamp this gel is seen as wavy, opalescent, gossamer folds which oscillate with movements of the eye.

OPHTHALMOSCOPY

Principle

The optics of the eye are such that light rays entering it through the pupil are, after reflection, returned back along the same path. This is why the illuminated pupil is normally black and nothing is seen of the interior of the globe. To see the interior, the fundus, it is necessary to be able to look along a beam of light which is directed into the pupil. An ophthalmoscope is simply an instrument which enables one to look in almost exactly the same direction as a shaft of light which it projects (Fig 5-7).

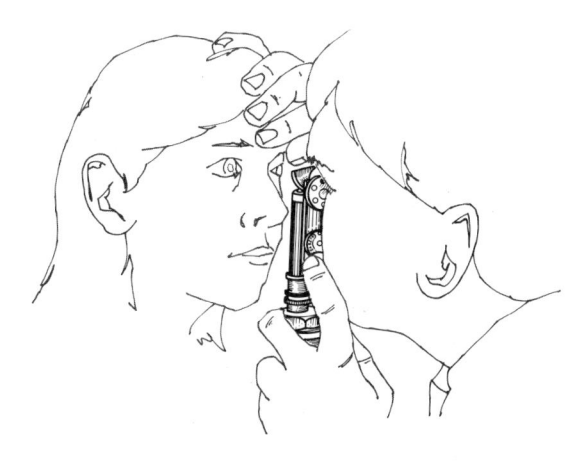

This principle is incorporated in a number of optical systems to give different types of ophthalmoscopes (and also retinal cameras). One type is a binocular indirect ophthalmoscope which is worn on the observer's head and with which he or she obtains a stereoscopic, slightly magnified view of a relatively large area (30° diameter) of the fundus. A standard retinal photograph also encompasses a field of about 30° of the fundus. Wide angle photographs cover an area of up to 60° horizontally and 45° vertically but the magnification is of course less.

The most widely used instrument is the *monocular direct ophthalmoscope* (Figs 5-8, 5-9). Essentially this consists of a mirror (or a reflecting prism) on to which light from a low voltage lamp is focused by condensing lenses and is then

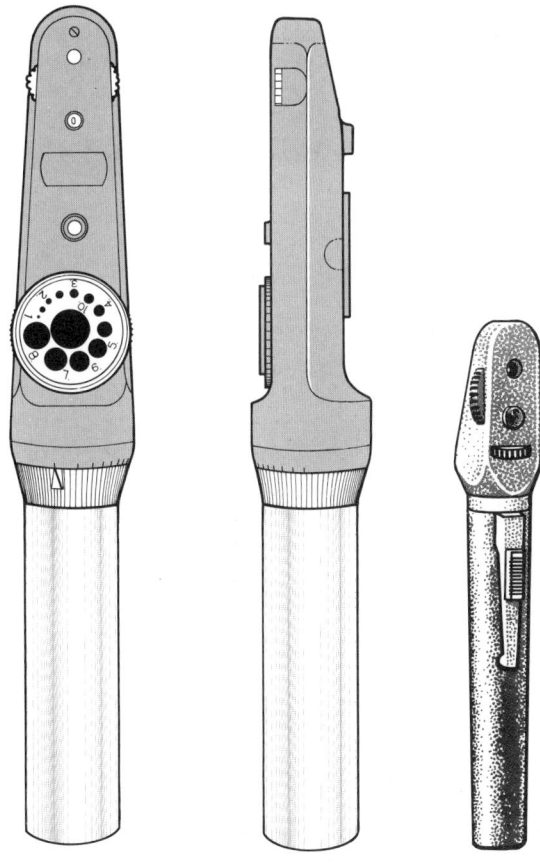

Fig 5-8 One type of (monocular direct) ophthalmoscope.

Fig 5-7 Ophthalmoscopy.

Fig 5-9 Pocket ophthalmoscope.

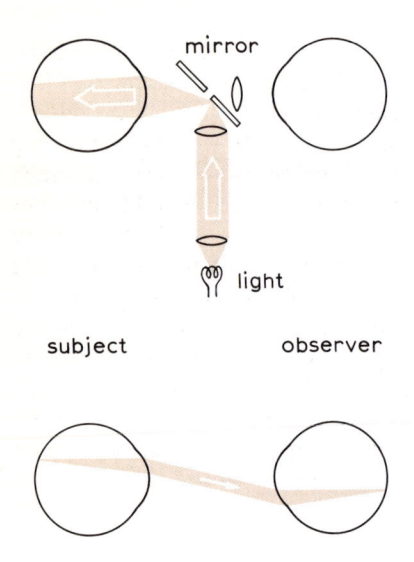

Fig 5-10 Principle of ophthalmoscopy. Ray diagrams show the illumination entering the subject's eye and the reflected light passing from the subject's fundus to the observer's eye.

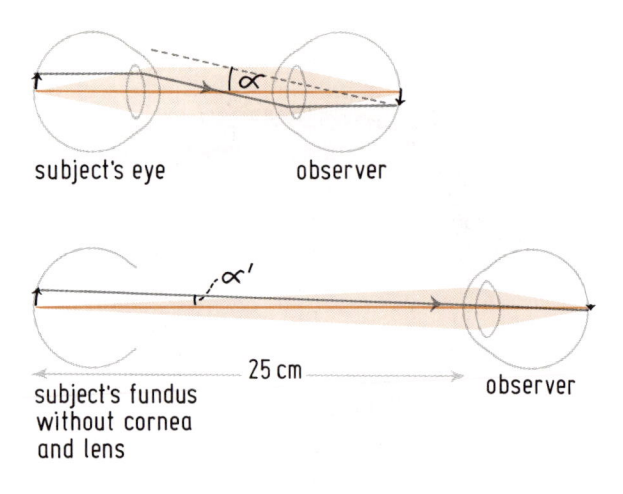

Fig 5-11 Magnification in ophthalmoscopy.
Upper The cornea and lens of the subject's eye act as a simple convex magnifying lens for the fundus by permitting the observer to approach close to the fundus and still see it clearly because the image is at infinity.

The (angular) magnification obtained with a magnifying lens is the ratio of the visual angle (α) subtended by the image seen through the lens to the visual angle (α') the object would subtend at the naked eye if viewed at a (arbitrarily chosen) distance of 25cm **(lower)**.

Details of the fundus appear 15 times larger through an ophthalmoscope than they would look from a distance of 25cm with the cornea and lens removed.

reflected as a slightly diverging beam out of the instrument (Fig 5-10). A small central hole in the silvering of the mirror is the sight hole through which the observer looks from immediately behind the mirror along the beam of light. The ophthalmoscope has a battery of small correcting lenses, both convex and concave, and the appropriate lens can be moved into position behind the sight hole to compensate for refractive errors of the subject and/or the observer by rotating with finger or thumb the milled edge of the lens wheel. These lenses are for focusing, not for magnification.

The 15x *magnification* with which the fundus is seen with a direct ophthalmoscope is due to the subject's cornea and lens acting like a strong (60 D) simple magnifying glass placed in front of the retina and optic disc (Fig 5-11). This magnification makes it possible to resolve details in the fundus as small as 20 μm.

If the subject is emmetropic the light reflected from each point on his or her fundus emerges from his or her eye as a parallel bundle of rays (Fig 5-10). This follows from the reversibility of light pathways in optical systems and from emmetropia being the optical state of an eye in which parallel rays from infinity entering the eye come to a point focus on the retina. If the observer is also emmetropic the parallel light rays coming from the subject's eye will be focused on his or her retina without any accommodation. In other words, the *image* seen when using an ophthalmoscope is optically *at infinity* and not as close as four or five centimetres from the observer's eye. In beginners the sense of nearness often overrides the absence of a true stimulus for accommodation with the result that inappropriate accommodation occurs and the fundus is not clearly seen. This is readily corrected by using a negative (concave) lens in the ophthalmoscope until the observer learns to relax his or her accommodation.

As with looking through any restricted aperture the nearer the observer's eye is to the aperture, in this case the subject's pupil, the larger will be

OPHTHALMOSCOPY

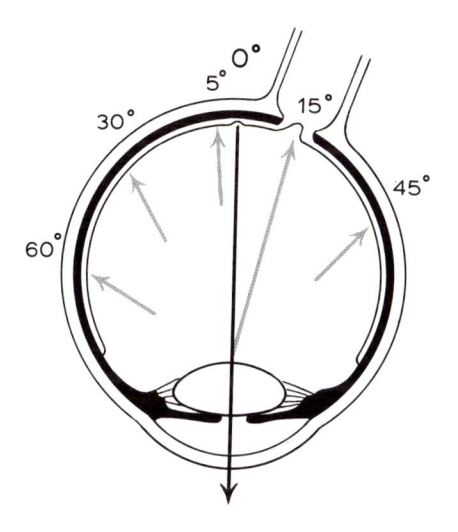

Fig 5-12 Horizontal section of a right eye viewed from above showing perimetric degrees from the fovea on the fundus.

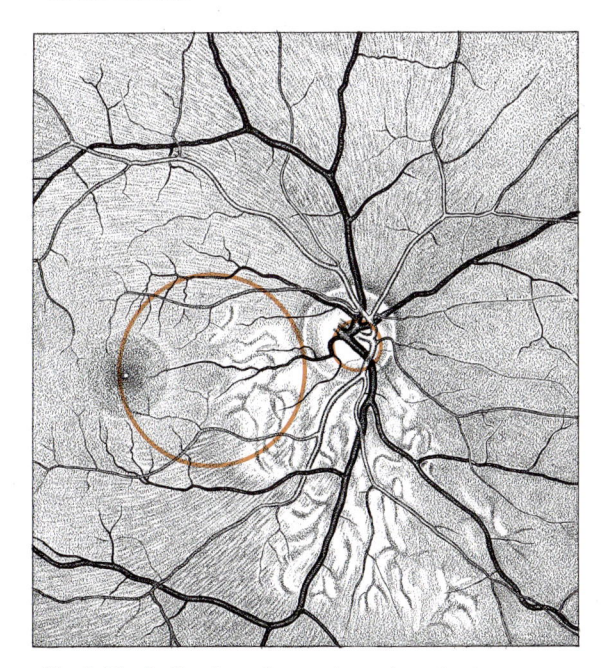

Fig 5-13 Indication of areas in perimetric degrees on the fundus. The smaller circle outlines an area with a diameter of 4°, the larger circle one of 13°.

the *field of view*. The field of view obtained with a direct ophthalmoscope also varies with the refraction of the subject's eye (large in hypermetropia, small in myopia), and with the size of the subject's pupil. With a small pupil of 2mm diameter the field is limited to about 4° (Fig 5-12).

This is not large enough to include all of the optic disc (Fig 5-13). With a dilated pupil of 7mm diameter a field of view of about 13° is obtained. This larger area which can be seen without having to move the ophthalmoscope makes it much easier to find one's way about a fundus, but it is of course still necessary to look in many directions to cover the whole fundus and build up a continuous complete mental picture of all that can be seen. In whatever direction the ophthalmoscopist looks into an eye his or her light and line of sight must always pass through the subject's pupil and in changing direction the pupil should be thought of as a centre of rotation for the movement (Fig 5-14).

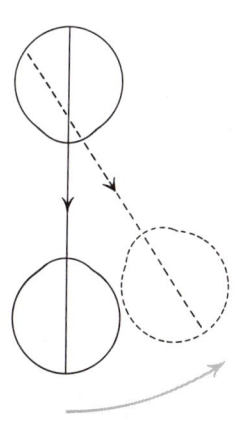

Fig 5-14 Movement from one part of the fundus to another with an ophthalmoscope has to be centred on the pupil.

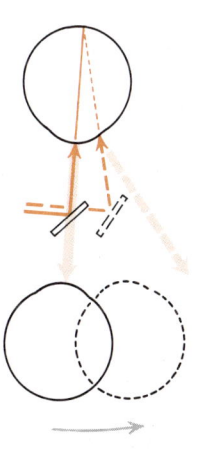

Fig 5-15 Looking eccentrically through the subject's pupil avoids dazzle from the corneal light reflex.

Some of the light from the ophthalmoscope will be reflected from the convex mirror surface of the subject's cornea back to the instrument where it may pass through the sight hole to dazzle the observer. The glare of these corneal *light reflexes* is one of the greatest difficulties in learning to use an ophthalmoscope. The reflection can often be displaced to where it is less of a nuisance and can be more readily ignored by very slightly tilting the ophthalmoscope mirror in one or other direction. If the line of sight of the ophthalmoscope is directed slightly eccentrically through the subject's pupil so that the optical axes of the instrument and the cornea do not coincide, the reflex will be displaced away from the sight hole (Fig 5-15). This applies especially when looking at the macular area and there is therefore the likelihood of looking along the optic axis of the subject's eye. This manoeuvre is fully effective only if the subject's pupil is dilated.

In using the monocular ophthalmoscope the observer is deprived of stereoscopic vision. In order to detect differences in level of parts of the fundus, that is elevations forwards or depressions backwards from the general plane of the fundus, it is necessary to rely on *parallactic movement* (Fig 5-16). This is looked for by moving with the ophthalmoscope from side to side and/or up and down within the limits imposed by the size of the subject's pupil. If parts of the fundus are not on the same level, the nearer part will seem to move in the direction opposite to that made by the observer while the more distant part will move in the same direction. This important test is easier when the subject's pupil is dilated and so allows larger movements to be made.

For the three reasons already given, namely to secure a large field of view, to enable the corneal light reflex to be better avoided, and to facilitate eliciting parallectic movement, and for the two further reasons that a large pupil is necessary for inspection of the anterior periphery of the fundus and that a small pupil reduces the amount of light available for illumination of the fundus, it will be apparent that dilatation of the subject's pupils with *mydriatic eye drops* greatly facilitates and is a necessary part of ophthalmoscopy.

Most ophthalmoscopes are equipped with a range of apertures and filters to alter the size or colour of the projected beam of light. The *aperture stop* which reduces the diameter of the light to a small spot on the subject's fundus is useful when the pupil is small or there are opacities in the optical media, because less light will be scattered from the narrower beam. It is used also when some feature is indirectly illuminated by shining the light adjacent to rather than on to what is being looked at, e.g. colloid bodies (p. 144). A *green (red-free) filter* is particularly useful for detecting subtle changes in retinal blood vessels such as arterial calibre variations, capillary changes such as focal dilatations and microaneurysms, or small haemorrhages. Blood anywhere in the retina is darkened more than the fundus background with a consequent increase in contrast. Similarly, more vascular detail is seen in black and white retinal photographs taken with a red-free filter than is possible with colour photographs of the fundus (Figs 7-7, 7-9).

Use of the Ophthalmoscope

1. Ask the subject to look straight ahead and to keep both eyes open.
2. If you have a refractive error and are not wearing your glasses, select the appropriate correcting lens in the ophthalmoscope and use this as equivalent to zero lens power. Otherwise start with 0 lens in the ophthalmoscope.
3. Use your right hand and right eye for the subject's right eye, and your left hand and eye for the subject's left eye.
4. Hold the sight hole of the ophthalmoscope

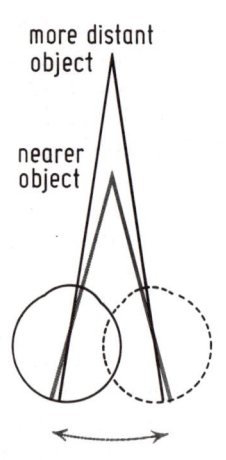

Fig 5-16 Principle of eliciting parallactic movement.

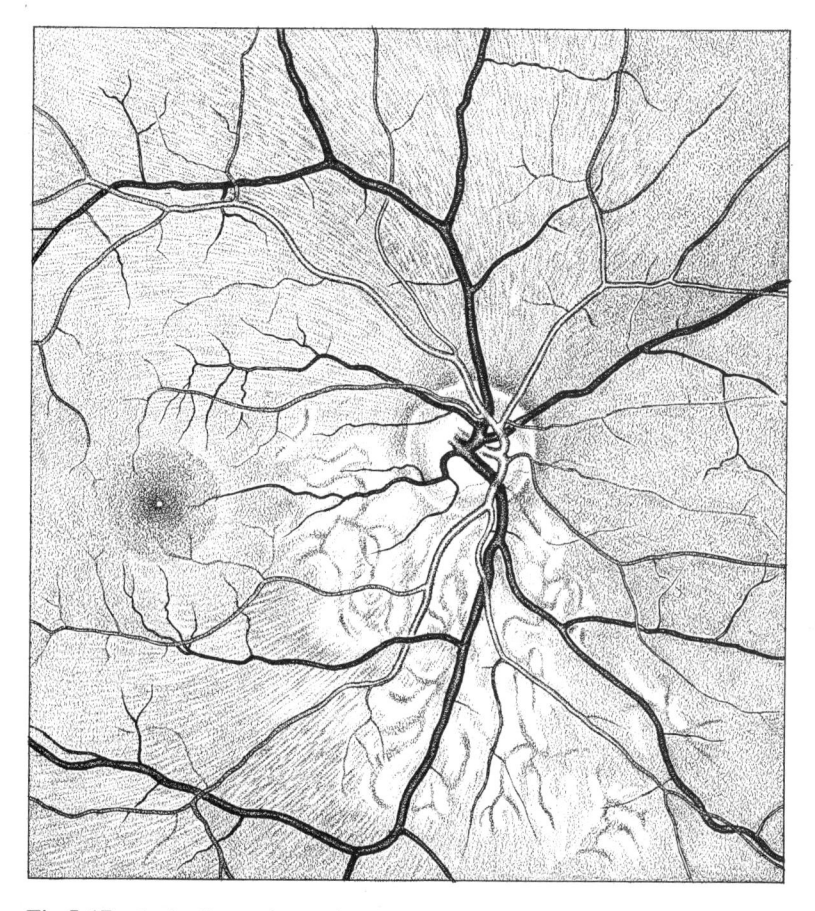

Fig 5-17 Optic disc and macula of a normal fundus of a right eye. Below the optic disc there is a blonde area in which the larger choroidal vessels are vaguely seen because of a relative paucity of pigment in the retinal pigment epithelium.

as close as possible to your eye. Steady the instrument by resting it firmly against your nose and/or your superior orbital margin. Find this position by looking through the sight hole across the room at some distinctive object. The ophthalmoscope should remain fixed in this position so that it moves with you as if attached to your head.

5   Rest the thumb of your other hand on the subject's superior orbital margin and gently raise his or her upper lid clear of his or her pupil.
6   Start with the ophthalmoscope 20 to 30cm away from the subject's eye and direct the light into the patient's pupil which should glow uniformly red. (The *red reflex,* red reflection or RR.)
7   Move closer to the subject's eye looking for opacities or shadows silhouetted in the RR. If any are seen they may be made more defined by using plus lenses (+5 to +12) in the ophthalmoscope. Request the subject to look in turn up, down, right, and left and watch for movement of any opacities in the RR.
8   With the subject again looking straight ahead, move towards his or her eye until your forehead is touching your thumb or the subject's forehead, that is approach as close to the subject's eye as is possible without touching his or her eyelashes or cornea.
9   Find and study the optic disc (OD) which is slightly (15°) to the nasal side of the optic axis of the eye (Fig 5-17). If necessary follow a blood vessel, all of which converge on the OD.

10 Try altering the lens in the ophthalmoscope until the clearest view is obtained; it is probable that you will see better with a negative lens (−) because most beginners over-accommodate. Throughout the examination vary the focus as necessary by turning the lens wheel with the forefinger or thumb.
11 Follow the main vessels out from the OD into each of the four quadrants in turn and study the vessels and the adjacent retina.
12 Find and study the macula. In looking at the macula it is always necessary to dodge reflections of light from the cornea and this can be difficult if the subject's pupil has not been dilated. The macula is a relatively avascular area, about the size of the OD, two disc diameters (dd) temporal to the OD. The fovea is a minute pit at the centre of the macula which in young people acts as a concave mirror and so is seen as a small glistening spot of reflected light, the foveal reflex (reflection).
13 Examine the periphery in all quadrants by having the subject look in the direction of the quadrant which is being inspected and move yourself and ophthalmoscope, with the subject's pupil as a centre of rotation, to look in the same direction.

The Red Reflex

Imperfections in the red reflex signify opacities in the media (cornea, aqueous, lens, and vitreous) (Fig 5-18). When the cornea is normal, a dull or absent RR is most commonly due to a cataract or to blood in the vitreous.

Localize opacities by having the patient look in different directions; opacities in front of the pupil appear to move in the same direction as the eye moves while those posterior to the pupil appear to move in the opposite direction. Opacities in the vitreous continue to move after the eye has stopped moving.

Alterations in the RR may well explain your inability to obtain a clear view of the retina and so it is wise to observe the RR before trying to see the fundus. Dilatation of the pupil often enables a view to be obtained in spite of opacities in the media.

Dilatation of the Pupils

Dilatation of the subject's pupils is necessary for any full ophthalmoscopic examination. Especially in the early stages of learning to use an ophthalmoscope, always dilate the pupils. The only *contra-indications* to this are:
1 When the patient is known to have glaucoma.
2 When the pupillary reactions are being used in the clinical management of the patient, e.g. some neurological conditions.
3 When the patient is too ill to be unnecessarily disturbed or should the patient refuse.
4 When one type of intraocular lens (iris fixated) has been inserted after removal of a cataract.

In a very few patients an attack of *acute angle closure glaucoma* will be precipitated by dilating the pupils (p. 176). This is a rapidly blinding condition but with prompt recognition and treatment it can be completely controlled. In fact, if and when this happens to a patient already in hospital and therefore optimally placed for speedy treatment, it is a service to that patient. Although unplanned, a provocative test will have revealed the vulnerability of his or her eyes to this type of glaucoma and this can then be treated to prevent any further attacks. Without this treatment these would sooner or later occur spontaneously and probably under less favourable circumstances.

The mydriatic drops most commonly used to dilate the pupils for ophthalmoscopy are tropicamide (Mydriacil) 0.5% eye drops or cyclopentolate (Mydrilate) 0.5% eye drops. One drop produces adequate dilatation in about 15 to 20 minutes. An alternative is phenylephrine (Neosynephrine) 2.5% or 10% eye drops.

It used to be orthodox practice when the examination was finished to instil a miotic such as pilocarpine 2% eye drops to antagonise the mydriatic and hasten the return to normal size of the pupils. In fact, this is rarely helpful or necessary.

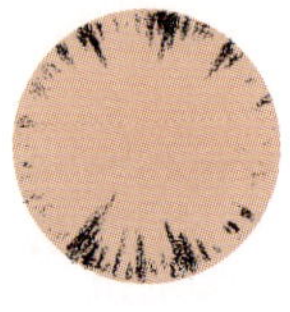

Fig 5-18 Lens opacities of an early cuneiform cataract silhouetted in the red reflex.

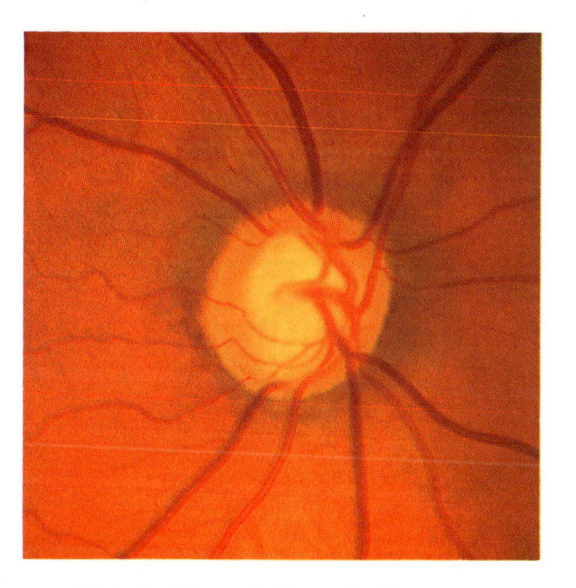

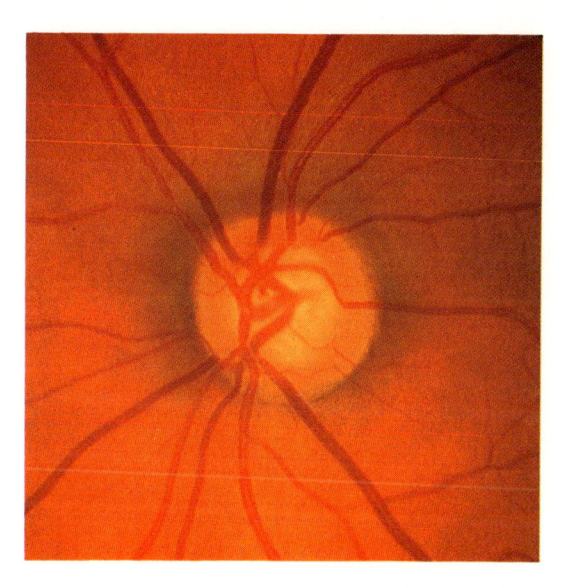

Plate 1 The optic discs of a 54 year old man with an early stage of chronic open angle glaucoma. The cup of the right disc *(left)* is larger than that of the normal left disc *(right)*. It is vertically ovoid because the lower and upper margins of the cup are nearer to the edge of the disc as a result of local loss of disc tissue. A superior arcuate scotoma in the right visual field confirmed damage to axons which entered the disc inferiorly.

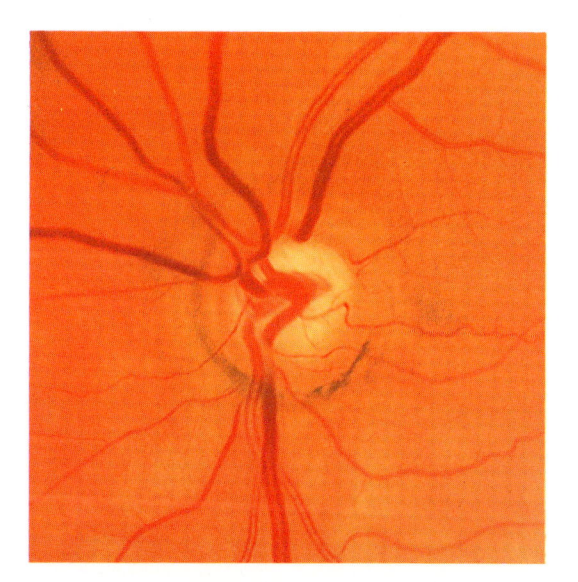

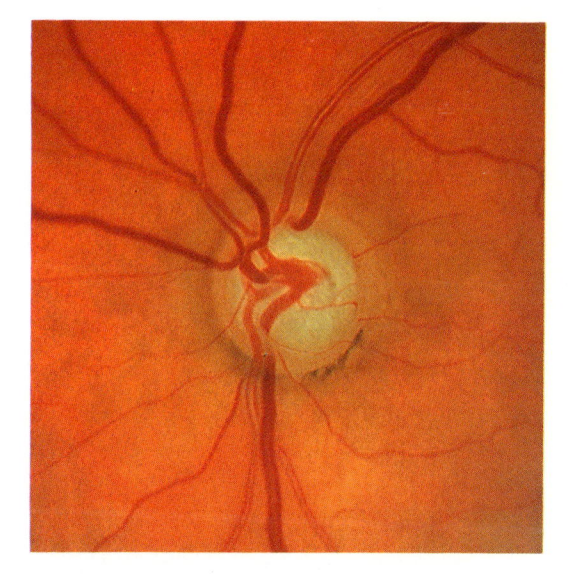

Plate 2 Change in an optic disc cup in steroid glaucoma. The *left* photograph of a left optic disc shows a large physiological cup. In the *right* photograph of the same disc taken four years later the cup has enlarged towards the temporal margin of the disc. The small vessel which crosses the disc margin at 2 o'clock is no longer covered by a rim of disc tissue. In the interval between the photographs steroid eye-drops had been used frequently and had caused an irreversible abnormal increase in the intraocular pressure.

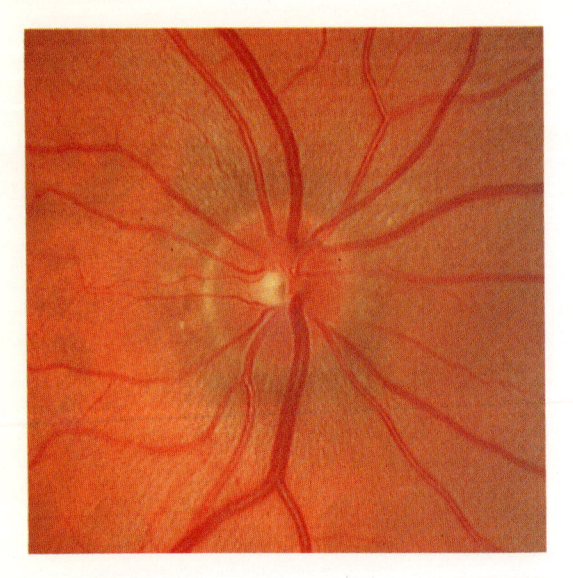

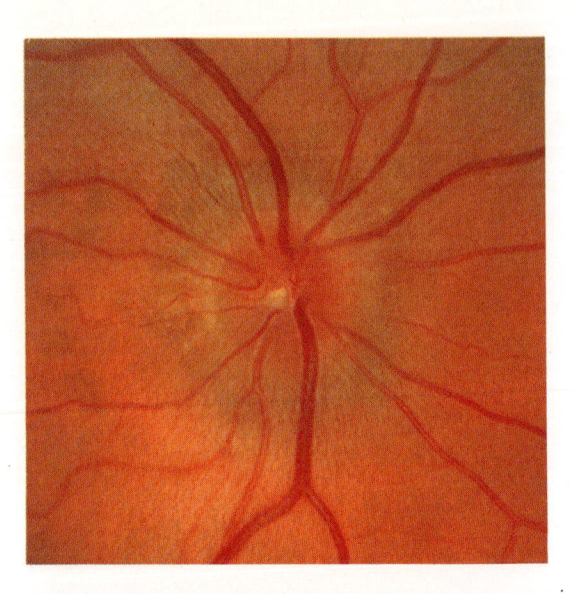

Plate 3 The *left* photograph was taken when the (right) optic disc was normal. It has a small physiological cup and a relatively obscure nasal margin. The *right* photograph of the same disc was taken some months later after papilloedema from raised intracranial pressure had just become detectable. There is now a loss of transparency of the superficial tissues of the disc and surrounding retina so that the margin of the disc and some parts of some vessels are less clearly seen. The elevation of the swollen disc is not apparent in this single photograph but it was obvious in a stereoscopic pair of photographs and also ophthalmoscopically when parallactic movement was looked for.

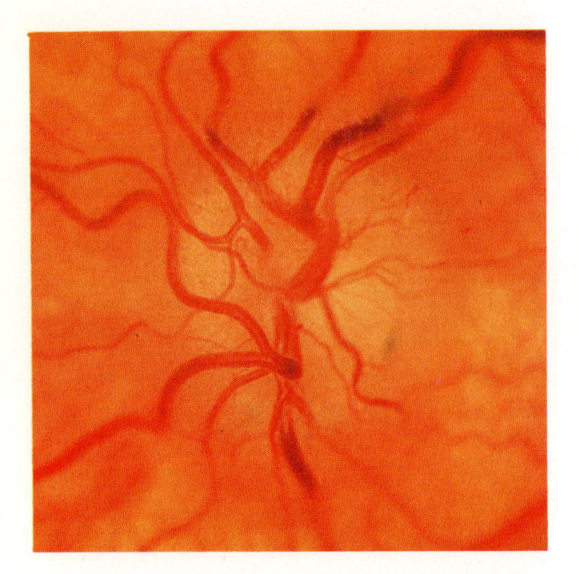

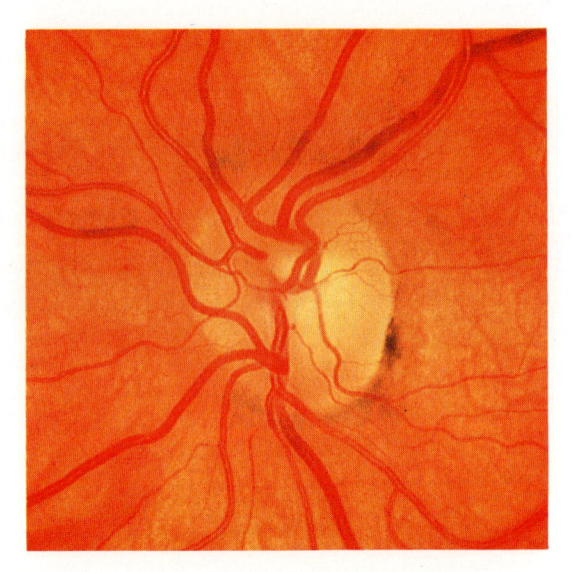

Plate 4 The (left) optic disc of a 21 year old woman in the *left* photograph is obviously swollen and the retinal veins are dilated. Since the vision of this eye had fallen rapidly to the perception of hand movements and there was an afferent pupillary defect, papillitis was diagnosed. When the *right* photograph of the same disc was taken one month later the vision had recovered to 4/5 and the disc appeared to be normal. The relative temporal pallor of the disc is similar to that of the right disc and so cannot be considered to be abnormal.

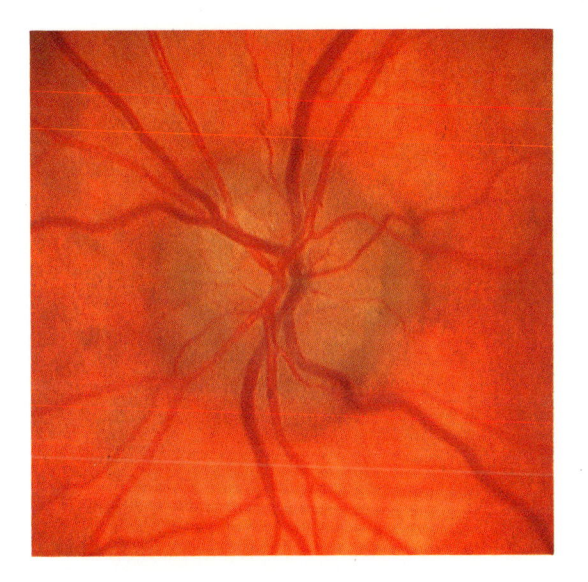

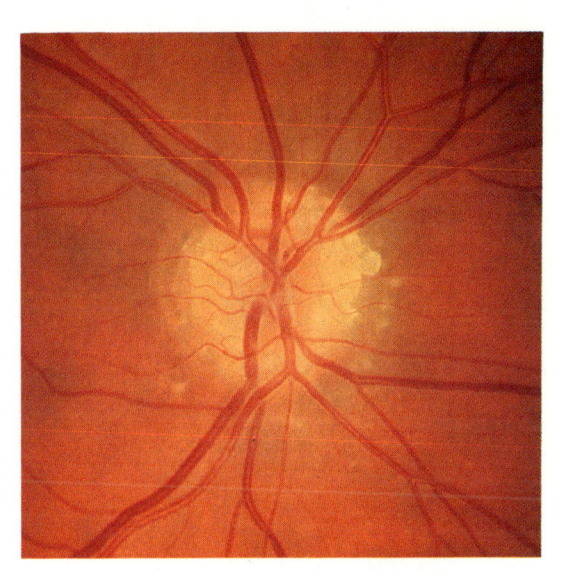

Plate 5 The 17 year old woman whose left optic disc is shown in the *left* photograph underwent extensive neurological investigations when she complained of headaches, because she was thought to have papilloedema. The elevation and unclear margin of her disc is in fact pseudopapilloedema due to buried drusen, one of which can be faintly seen deep to the vessels between 10 and 11 o'clock, and another at 3 o'clock. More obvious drusen, some of them on the surface of the disc, are seen in the *right* photograph of the right disc of an older man.

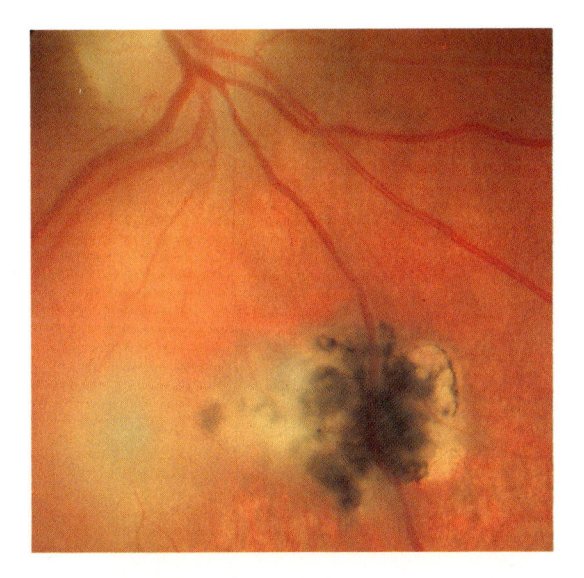

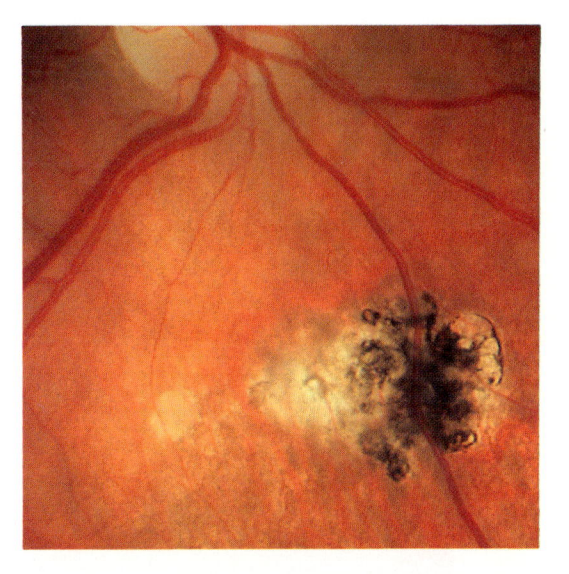

Plate 6 Toxoplasmic choroidoretinitis in a 31 year old woman during a recurrence *(left)* and after the inflammation had subsided *(right)*. The diffuse pale area to the left of the larger area of pallor and pigmentation is a focus of active inflammation. This has impaired the transparency of the neural retina so that it reflects light and looks pale.

The small pale spot seen after the inflammation had resolved is due to local exposure of the sclera as a result of loss of the pigment of the retina and choroid at the centre of the lesion. There had been similar loss of pigment together with clumping of pigment and possibly proliferation of retinal pigment epithelium in the earlier, larger lesion.

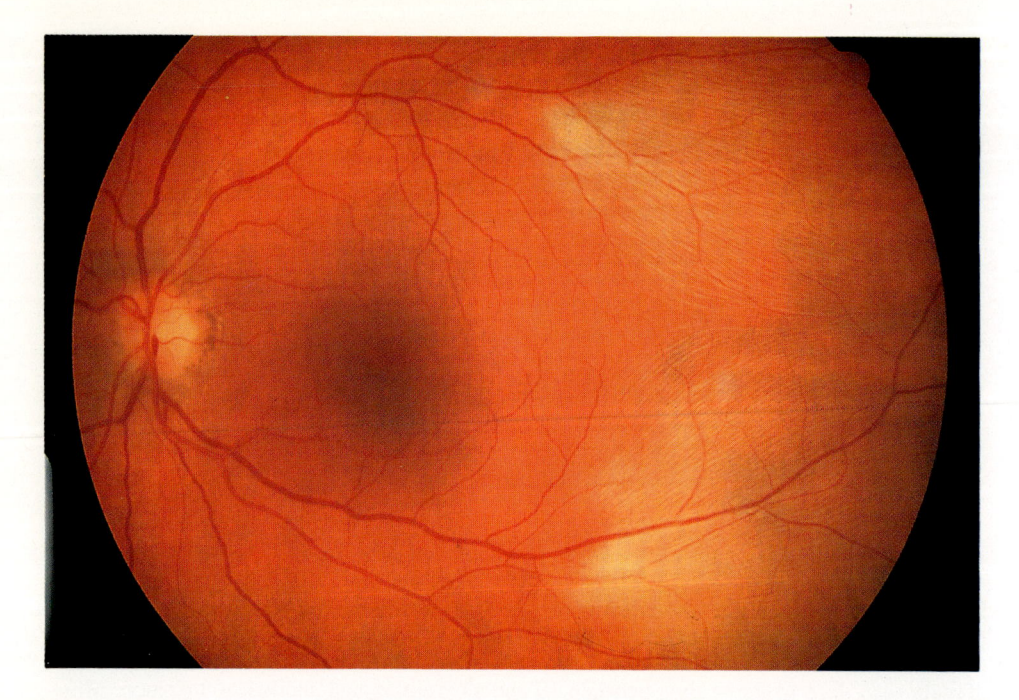

Plate 7 Opaque nerve fibres. This rare example of myelination of the axons of some ganglion cells so far from the optic disc shows the beginning of the arcuate course of axons from the temporal periphery of the retina and the temporal raphe between those from the upper and lower halves of the retina.

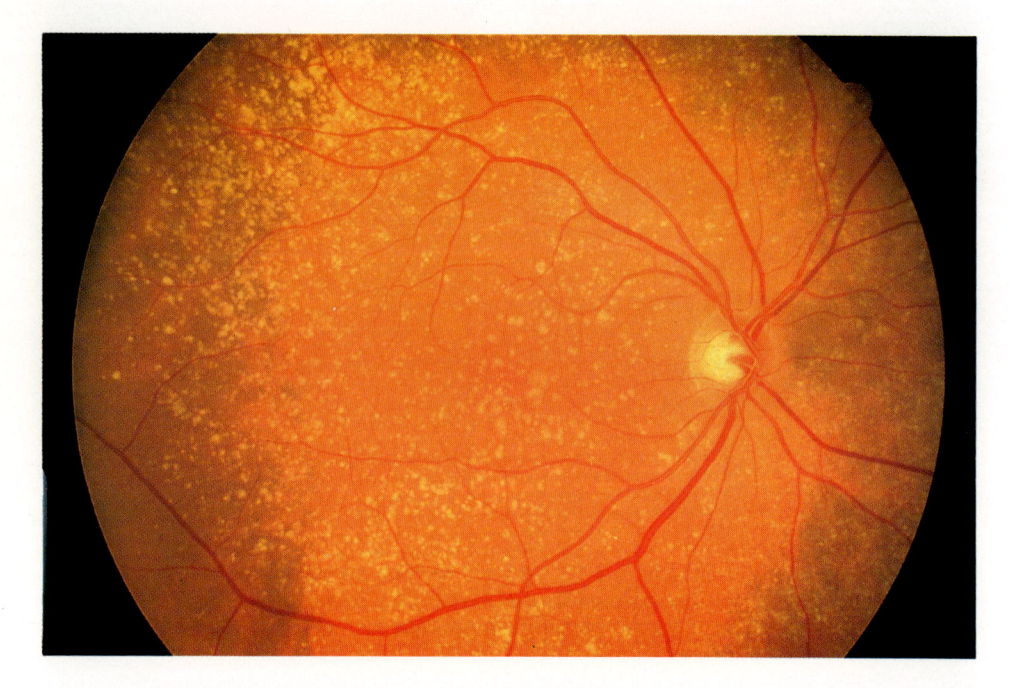

Plate 8 Colloid bodies or retinal drusen which individually look like hard exudates. But exudates would be in rings, fans or confluent patches and accompanied by other vascular abnormalities. The vision of this eye of a 70 year old man was normal.

125

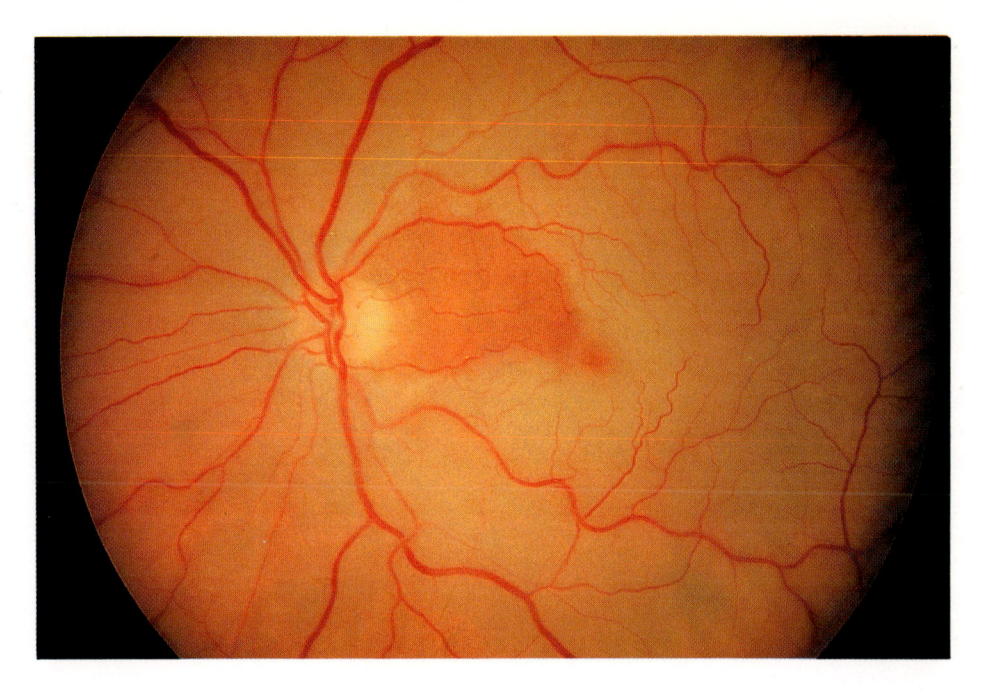

Plate 9 Occlusion of the central retinal artery in a 63 year old man. An area of retina between the optic disc and the macula is not opaque and therefore not pale because it is supplied by a separate cilioretinal artery. The macula itself also retains its transparency because it is not supplied from the central retinal artery.

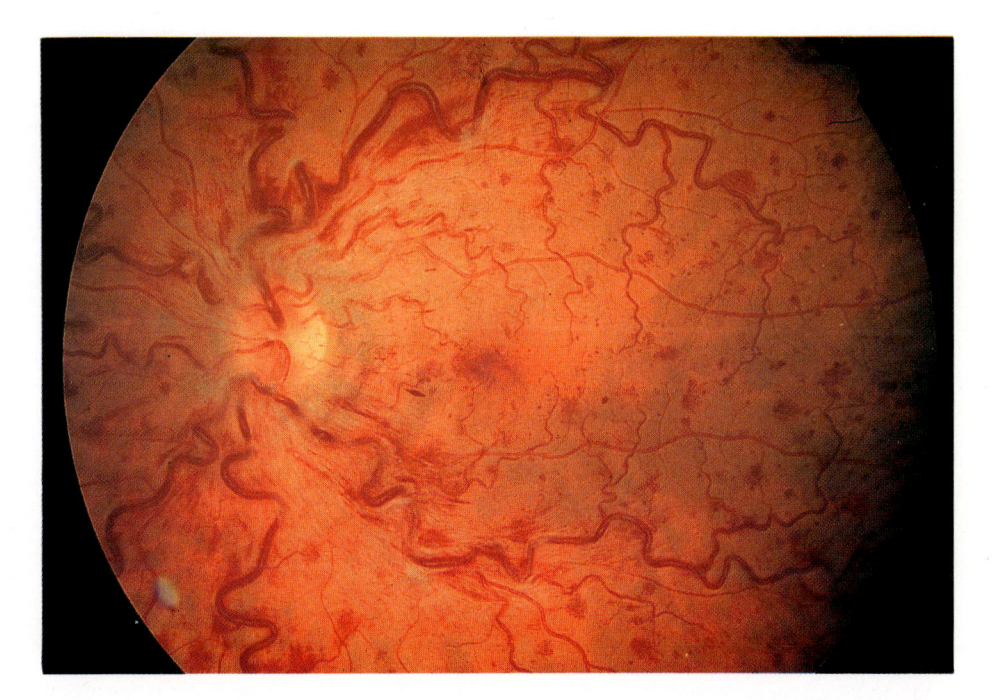

Plate 10 Occlusion of the central retinal vein in a 31 year old woman who was using an oral contraceptive. The vision of the eye was never worse than 4/8 and recovered fully after this medication was stopped.

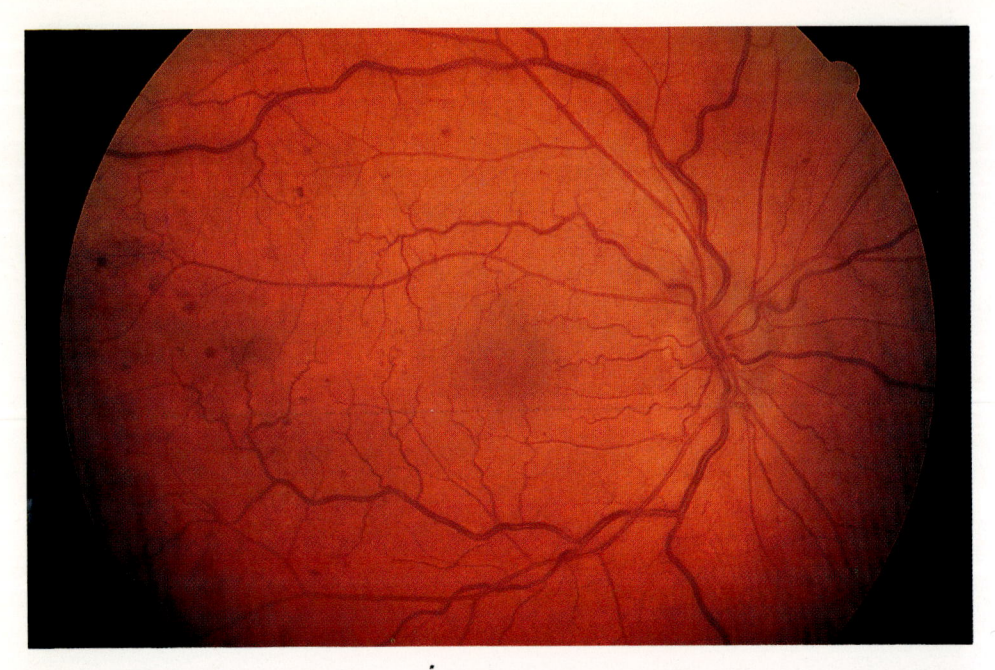

Plate 11 Carotid artery insufficiency retinopathy (venous stasis retinopathy). The scattered microaneurysms and small blot haemorrhages in the right fundus of a 53 year old man are inconspicuous. Even when the retinal veins are not dilated, as in this example, these easily overlooked changes suggest lowered central retinal artery pressure due to stenosis of the right internal carotid artery, as was the case in this patient.

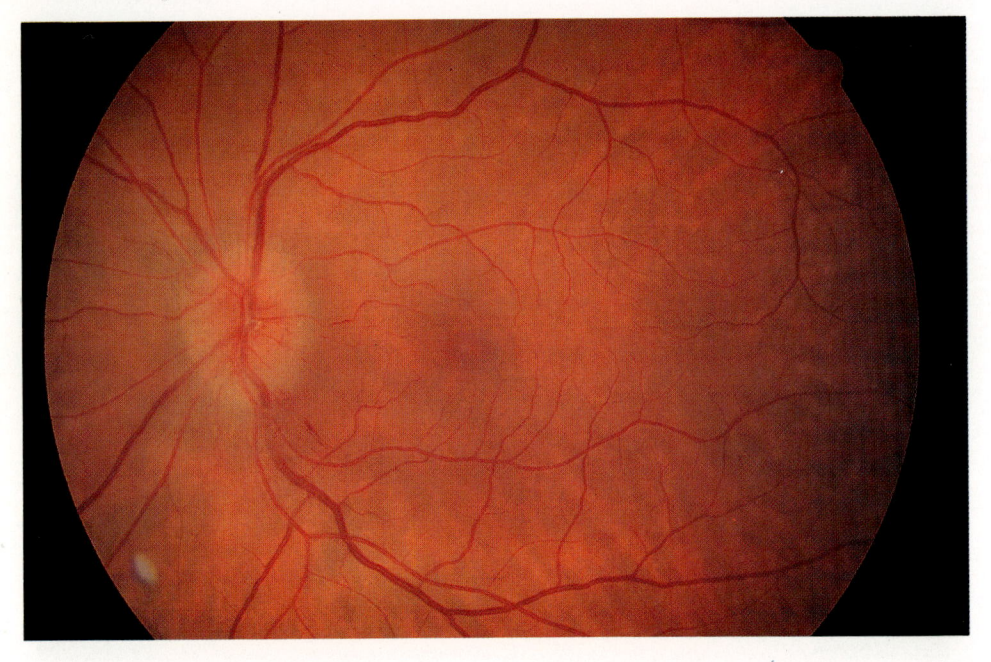

Plate 12 Ischaemic optic neuropathy in a 73 year old woman who lost all vision in this eye overnight. The infarcted optic disc is pale and swollen and there is one small linear haemorrhage in the retina. The retinal circulation is unimpaired. The inconspicuous changes in appearance do not match the total loss of function.

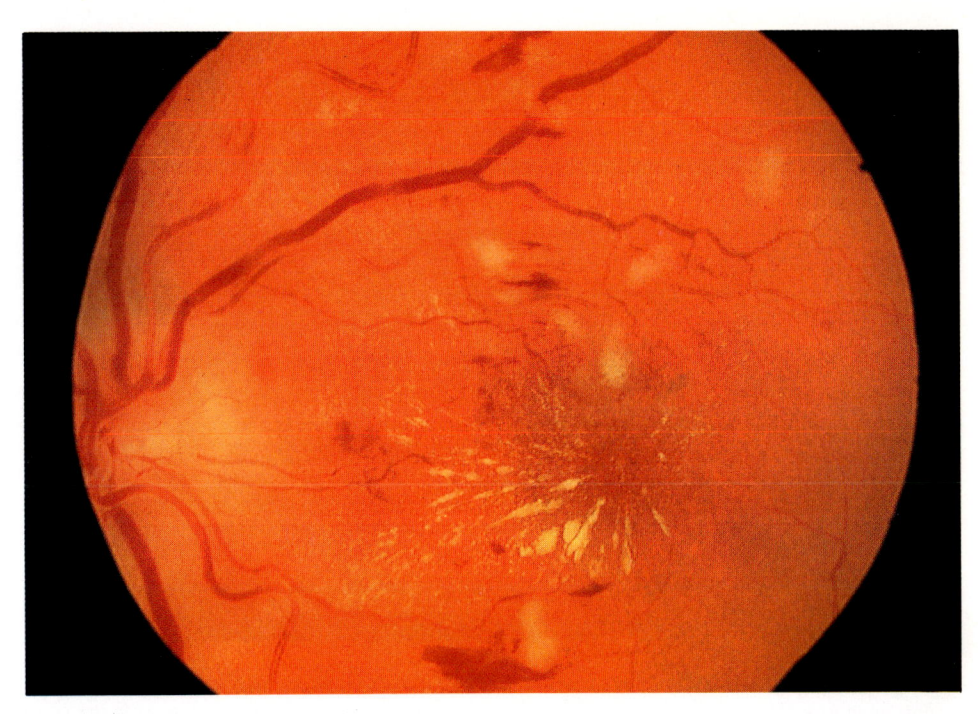

Plate 13 The left fundus of a 23 year old woman who presented because of reduced vision (4/12) and was found to have a casual blood pressure of 200/140. This combination of superficial retinal haemorrhages, cotton wool spots, a macular star of hard exudate and disc oedema can only be due to a severe hypertensive retinopathy.

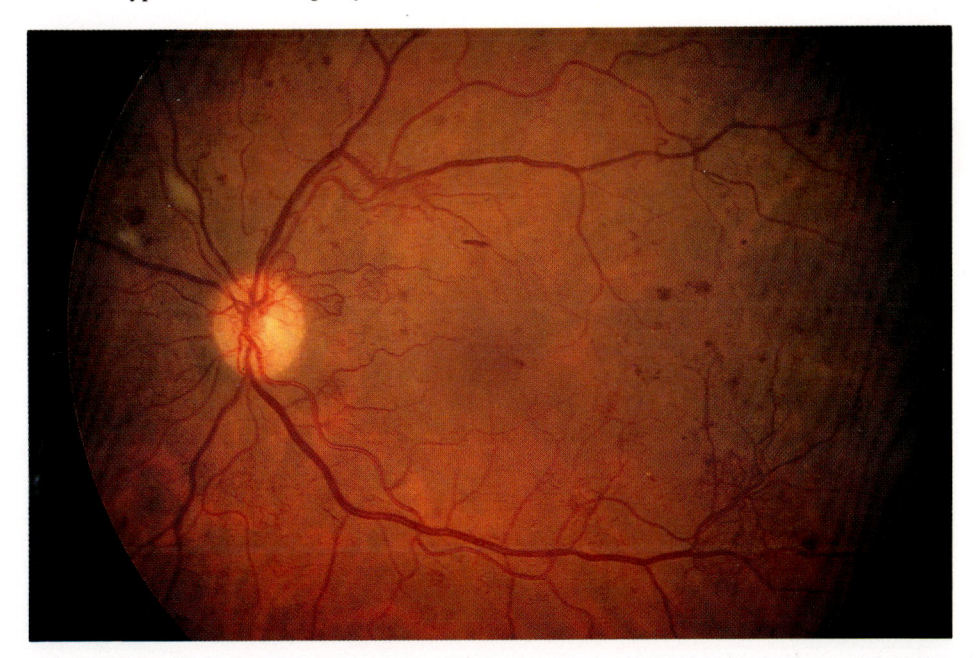

Plate 14 Proliferative diabetic retinopathy in a 47 year old man who had been diagnosed as diabetic four years previously. In this fundus there are dot and blot haemorrhages and microaneurysms, two cotton wool spots, irregularly dilated capillaries (IRMA) and patches of new-formed vessels, but no hard exudate.

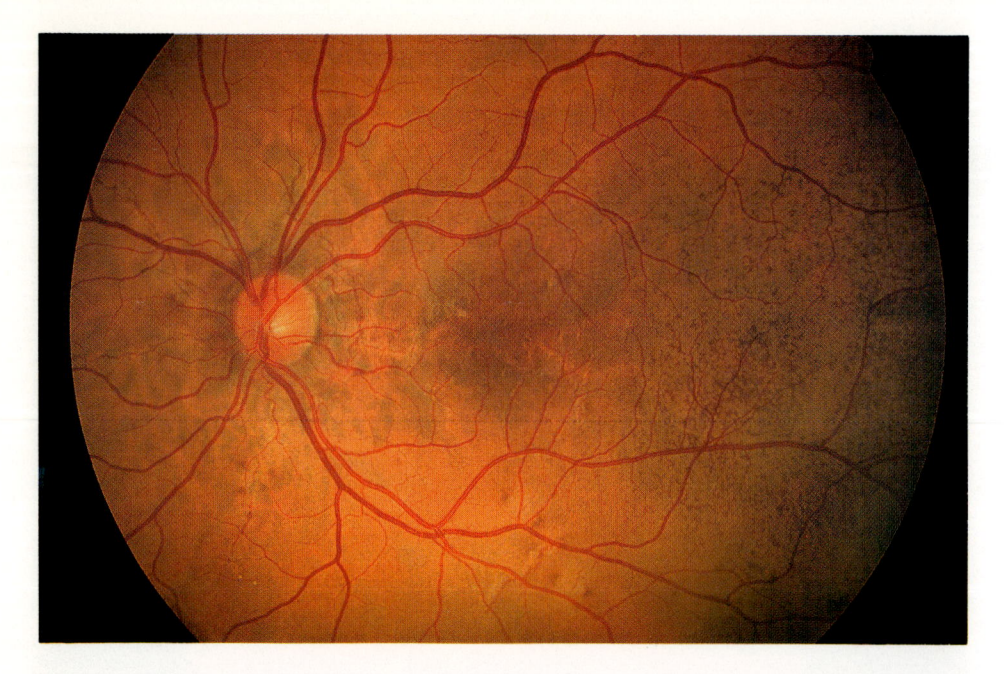

Plate 15 Angioid streaks around the optic disc and one inferiorly in line with the macula, and a stippled peau d'orange appearance temporal to the macula in a 21 year old man with the Grönblad-Strandberg syndrome. There had been a choroidal rupture with haemorrhage underneath the macula of his other eye after a trivial blow to his head.

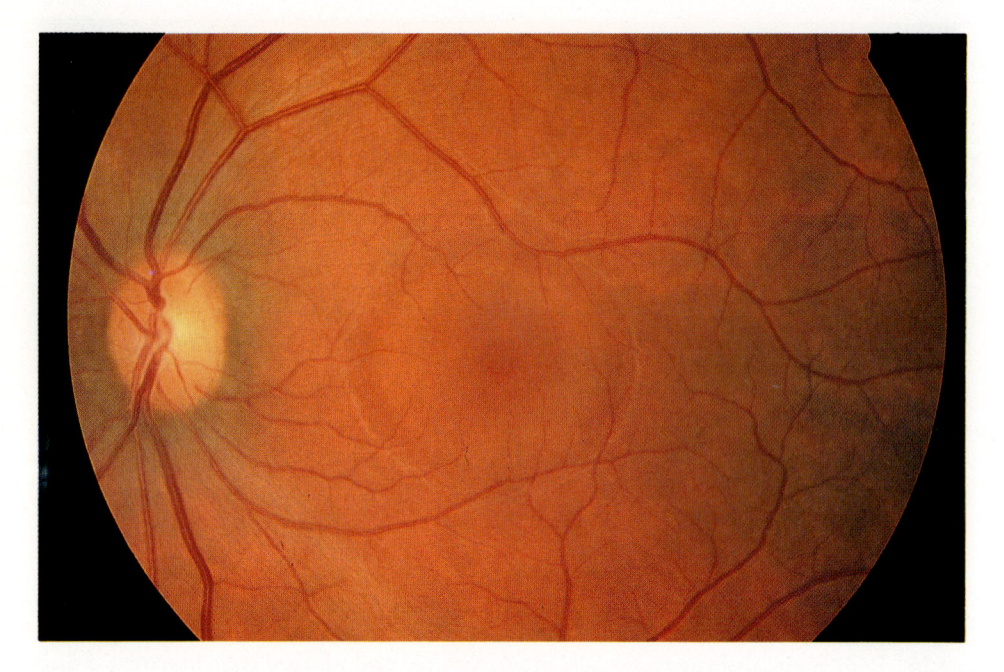

Plate 16 Central serous retinopathy in a 31 year old man. A ring of light reflected from the internal surface of the retina surrounds the dome of elevated retina. The vision of the eye which had been reduced to 4/6 returned to normal in two months without treatment.

Chapter 6

INTERPRETATION OF OPHTHALMOSCOPIC CHANGES

**INTERPRETATION OF
OPHTHALMOSCOPIC CHANGES**

Optic disc changes
   Cupping
   Elevation
   Visability of disc margins
   Hyperaemia
   Pallor

Vessel changes
   Arterial
   Capillary
   Venous
   Neovascularization

Fundus background
   Normal
   Pale areas
   Red areas
   Black areas

INTERPRETATION OF OPHTHALMOSCOPIC CHANGES

A good programme for examining the fundus of the eye is to start with the optic disc and then to inspect the retinal vessels by following them into each of the four quadrants in turn. Next, the fundus background in each of the quadrants is observed and finally the macula is studied. During this systematic survey the subject keeps his or her eyes still in the straight ahead position. The optic disc serves as a reference from which to take bearings and each exploratory movement along vessels, into the quadrants generally and to the macula, should start from the disc. To examine the periphery of the fundus it is necessary to have the subject turn his or her eyes in the direction of the area being examined so that it is possible to look quite obliquely through the pupil.

This order of examination — optic disc, vessels, fundus background — will be followed in describing the things to look for.

The most useful way to interpret what is seen with an ophthalmoscope is to translate the ophthalmoscopic appearances into anatomical structure both normal and pathological. To do this it is necessary to understand the structural basis and optical mechanisms involved. The following guide as to what to look for contains more explanation of these factors than is usual because in the long run this makes ophthalmoscopy more intelligible and easier.

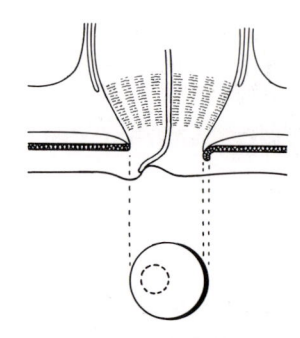

Fig 6-1 Correlation of ophthalmoscopic features and underlying structure of a normal optic disc with a moderate sized cup and a temporal pigment crescent.

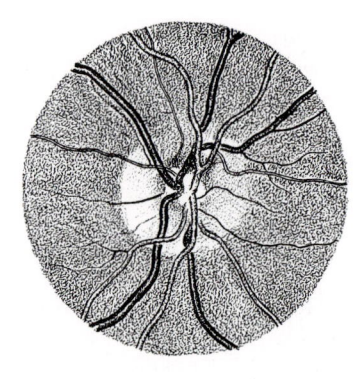

Fig 6-2 Normal right optic disc with a small cup. The temporal part of the disc is paler than the other parts.

Optic Disc Changes

The three things to look for in an optic disc are
- differences in level, i.e. the degree of excavation (cupping) or of elevation (swelling),
- the visibility of the disc margin, and
- colour, i.e. hyperaemia or pallor, haemorrhages.

Differences in level of parts of the fundus are detected by parallactic movement when the observer moves the ophthalmoscope from side to side or up and down within the limits imposed by the size of the subject's pupil. This is a more sensitive technique than looking for differences in the ophthalmoscope lenses required for clear focus of adjacent parts.

Pigment in the retina at the disc margin (pigment crescent) (Fig 6-1), exposure of a crescent of sclera at the disc margin (scleral crescent) (Fig 6-4), and visibility of the grey holes in the lamina cribosa (Fig 6-6) are common variations of normal anatomy.

Unless there is a large difference in the refractive errors of the two eyes, a person's two optic discs are usually similar in appearance.

Cupping

Most optic discs have a central depression, the diameter and depth of which vary greatly from individual to individual (Figs 6-1, 6-4). This *physiological* cupping can take the form of a small dimple (Fig 6-2), a slender funnel, a shallow hollow, a deep cup at the bottom of which the

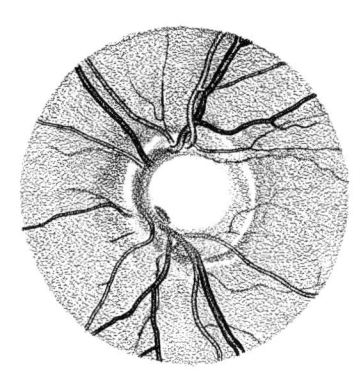

Fig 6-3 Normal left optic disc with a large physiological cup.

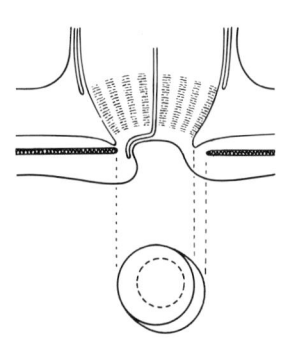

Fig 6-4 Correlation of ophthalmoscopic and structural features of a normal optic disc with a large physiological cup and a temporal scleral crescent.

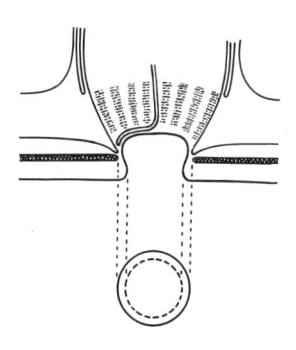

Fig 6-5 Correlation of ophthalmoscopic and structural features of an optic disc with advanced pathological glaucomatous cupping.

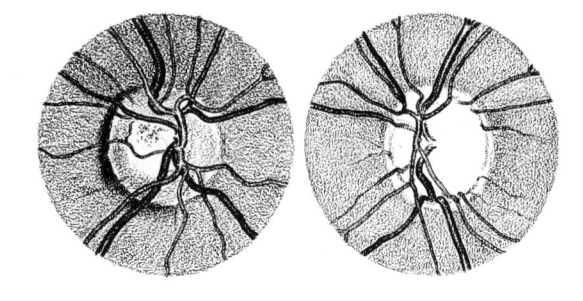

Fig 6-6 Optic discs of a patient with open angle glaucoma. The right optic disc is normal with a moderate sized cup in the floor of which the stippled appearance is due to the lamina cribrosa. The left optic disc shows gross glaucomatous cupping and optic atrophy of the narrow rim of remaining disc tissue.

lamina cribrosa is visible, or a large excavation with overhanging edges which occupies up to 70% of the area of the optic disc (Fig 6-3).

Pathological cupping occurs in chronic open angle glaucoma (p. 178) and its recognition is the commonest way in which this insidious disease is detected (Fig 6-5). Glaucomatous cupping results from loss of glial and nerve tissue which leads to an enlargement of the physiological cup and its appearance in the early stages will therefore be determined by the type of cup which the individual initially had. Enlargement is greater in diameter than in depth and when it occurs in a disc with a small, shallow physiological cup glaucomatous cupping need not be deep. One eye is commonly affected before the other, and therefore a definite difference in the cups of the two eyes should be assumed to be pathological (Plate 1, p. 121).

The enlargement of the cup is commonly first localized to the lower or upper margin; a cup with a vertically ovoid outline is usually pathological. Eventually the margin of the cup approaches the margin of the disc so that only a narrow rim of disc tissue remains (Fig 6-6). The wall of the cup becomes steep and vessels crossing the cup margin bend abruptly as they reach the level of the surrounding disc. The greatest diameter of the cup may be posterior to the actual margin of the cup so that the edge is overhanging. In this case the vessels will be lost sight of until they appear over the edge of the cup. As they cross the cup edge the vessels are naked, whereas in deep physiological cupping when the margin is undercut the vessels appear through the rim of disc tissue or are covered by at least a thin layer of glial tissue (Plate 2, p. 121). Developed glaucomatous cupping is always associated with the pallor of glaucomatous optic atrophy.

The distinction between a large physiological cup and early glaucomatous cupping can be very difficult and may be impossible on ophthalmoscopic appearances alone. However, the early detection of glaucomatous cupping is so important that there should not be any hesitation in referring for specialist assessment any patients in whom the suspicion arises.

Elevation

The tissue of some normal optic discs is elevated above the level of the retina and this *physiological* protrusion is called *pseudopapilloedema* (Fig 6-7). This variant of normal anatomy is more common in small hypermetropic eyes (Fig 6-8).

Pathologically, oedema, whether active as in inflammation of the optic nerve or passive as in raised intracranial pressure, produces swelling of the optic disc tissue and this is visible ophthalmoscopically as an elevation of the optic disc (Fig 6-9). A deliberate attempt to elicit parallactic movement will reveal a slight elevation of the disc more surely than attempts to find differences in focus between the disc and its surrounds.

With lesser degrees of oedema the optic cup is still present and may look like a crater on a volcanic summit. With much oedema the cup becomes obliterated and the stage at which this happens is influenced by the original size of the cup.

The swelling of an optic disc due to local inflammation of the optic nerve is called *papillitis,* while oedema of the disc from any other cause, e.g. raised intracranial pressure, hypertensive retinopathy, acute ischaemia of the optic nerve, is called *disc oedema,* disc swelling or *papilloedema* (Chapter 8). (The terms papillitis and papilloedema are derived from the old anatomical name for the optic disc of optic papilla.)

Just as with physiological and pathological cupping, the distinction between physiological and early pathological elevation of the optic disc can be very difficult and may be impossible on ophthalmoscopic appearances alone.

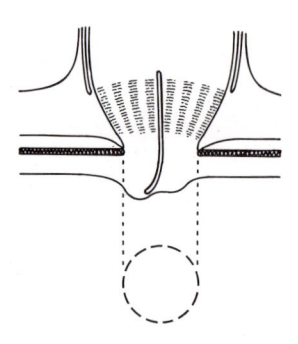

Fig 6-7 Correlation of ophthalmoscopic and structural features of a normal optic disc with the appearance of pseudopapilloedema.

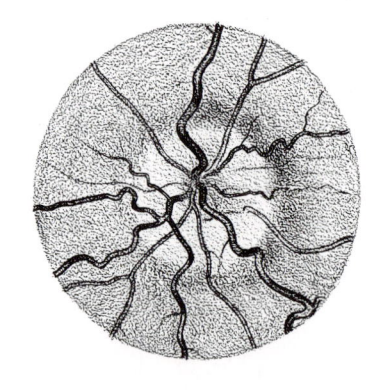

Fig 6-8 Pseudopapilloedema, a variation of normal anatomy.

Visibility of Disc Margin

The boundary of many optic discs can be clearly seen around its whole circumference, but in other normal discs the edge is more or less obscured by glial tissue especially on the nasal side.

When oedema of the optic disc affects its edge and the adjacent retina, the swollen tissues lose their translucency and make the disc margin indistinct or invisible (Fig 6-10; Plate 3, p. 122). Blurring of the disc margin also occurs with the gliosis which may follow papilloedema or papillitis.

OPHTHALMOSCOPIC CHANGES

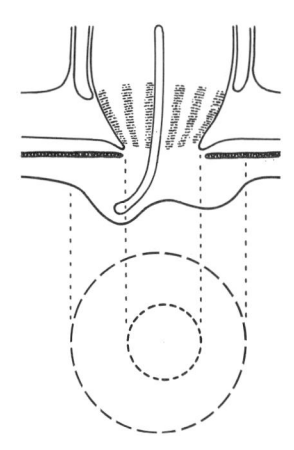

Fig 6-9 Correlation of ophthalmoscopic and structural features of papilloedema. The inner circle corresponds to the normal disc outline, the outer to the extent of adjacent retinal oedema.

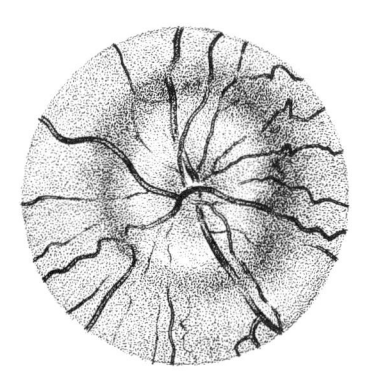

Fig 6-10 Early papilloedema. The vessels crossing the disc are obscured in places due to the loss of translucency of the prelaminar tissue in which they lie.

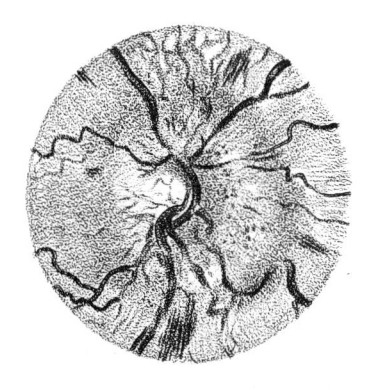

Fig 6-11 Established papilloedema with haemorrhages.

Hyperaemia

There is considerable variation in the *normal* yellowish red *colour* of the optic disc, often described as pink. The colour is due to a network of capillaries among the translucent nerve fibres overlying the white lamina cribrosa. In contrast to the retina there is no layer of pigment to impart a dusky shade to the red colour. There are few nerve fibres and consequently few capillaries covering the lamina cribrosa in the optic cup which therefore looks whiter than the rest of the optic disc. (Do not make the mistake of judging the colour of a disc by the colour of the cup in the disc.) The temporal part of an optic disc usually looks paler than the nasal side.

The capillaries of the disc come mainly from small arteries (posterior ciliary) which pass through the adjacent sclera to the choroid and, contrary to expectation, they receive little blood from the central retinal artery. The venous drainage of the disc on the other hand is mainly into the central retinal vein. This explains why increase in venous pressure in the central retinal vein, e.g. from raised intracranial pressure, leads to hyperaemia of the optic disc. Conversely, swelling of the disc can compress the central retinal vein and lead to engorgement of the retinal veins.

Dilatation of the optic disc capillaries increases the red colour of the disc and individual, radially running, fine vessels may become visible. This hyperaemia can be either active as a result of inflammation, or passive as a consequence of obstructed venous drainage. Hyperaemia of any severity or of some duration results in leakage of red blood cells as well as leakage of oedema fluid, and these are seen as *haemorrhages* on or near the disc (Fig 6-11). While hyperaemia and oedema usually go together, occasionally compression of the disc capillaries by oedematous tissue pressure produces a swollen disc which is pale. Pallid oedema also results from an ischaemic infarct of the disc as in the ischaemic optic neuropathy caused by giant cell arteritis or by atherosclerosis.

Dilatation of the retinal *veins* commonly occurs with hyperaemia of the optic disc, either as a result of a venous obstruction central to the disc which is causing the disc hyperaemia or secondarily to the associated disc oedema.

Because of the range of normal variations of disc colour and because of the difficulty of being sure that retinal vessels are altered in calibre, it can be very difficult to decide that slight degrees of hyperaemia and venous engorgement are definitely pathological.

Pulsation of a retinal *vein* or veins on the optic disc, in contradistinction to retinal arterial pulsation, is normal (p. 15). If it is present there is not papilloedema (the converse is not true).

Pallor

Reduction of the capillary network of the disc allows the white lamina cribrosa to show through the translucent nerve fibres and glia, and the disc therefore looks unusually pale or even white. This appearance is called *optic atrophy* (Fig 6-12). The reduction in blood supply may result from atrophy of the nerve fibres (e.g. following optic neuritis), or the ischaemia may cause the atrophy (e.g. following ischaemic optic neuropathy), or both the ischaemia and the atrophy may result from a common cause (e.g. unrelieved papilloedema). Oedema cannot occur in a disc which is atrophic.

The atrophy can be limited to only a part of the disc. Because of the common relative pallor of the temporal rim of disc tissue, temporal pallor must be striking or unilateral before it is considered to be pathological (Plate 4, p. 122).

The margin of an atropic optic disc will retain its sharpness unless the cause of the atrophy, e.g. unrelieved papilloedema, has also caused proliferation of glial tissue.

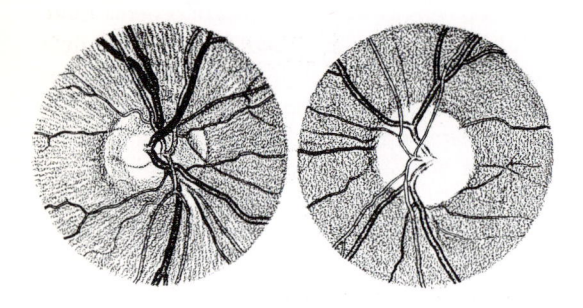

Fig 6-12 Optic discs of a patient with traumatic optic atrophy of his left eye. In the right fundus the streaky pattern of nerve fibres converging on the normal optic disc can be detected. The left optic disc is white and flat and the nerve fibre pattern is not seen in the surrounding retina.

Unless one of the two discs is normal for comparison, it may be impossible to diagnose slight degrees of optic atrophy on ophthalmoscopic appearance alone. However, with adequate tests some defect in the visual field will be found in all cases of optic atrophy.

Vessel Changes

Physicians and ophthalmologists describe a number of changes in the retinal vessels which are traditionally thought to have diagnostic value. Unfortunately, because of the difficulty of assessing them and because of the uncertainty as to their significance, some of these vessel changes are quite unreliable. Formal studies have confirmed that there are large within- and between-observer errors in assessing most of these changes. In the following, an attempt has been made to select those changes which are useful. This also has the effect of simplifying a confused and confusing topic.

Arterial

CHANGES WHICH CAN BE ASSESSED AND ARE SIGNIFICANT

1 Irregularity of Calibre; Localized, Segmental, or Focal Arterial Narrowing

This is usually due to focal or segmental narrowings of the arteries but localized widenings also occur. Ophthalmoscopically they appear as abrupt or tapered narrowing of the blood columns for some length especially of the major arteries, sudden invisibility of terminal arteries before their expected natural termination, and abrupt narrowing of smaller branches which do not regain their original width (Fig 6-13). Another type of irregularity is a fine rippling of one or both sides of an arterial blood column; the significance of this appearance is unknown. Changes in vessels within ½ dd from the optic disc should usually be ignored because they may be due to glia covering the vessel.

Pathologically this change is due to either the involuntarily sclerosis of age or the arteriolar sclerosis and possibly arterial hypertonus of hypertension.

The probable significance of irregularlity of calibre is that age can cause slight irregularity of calibre in one or two branches but more than this is a reliable sign of hypertension.

OPHTHALMOSCOPIC CHANGES

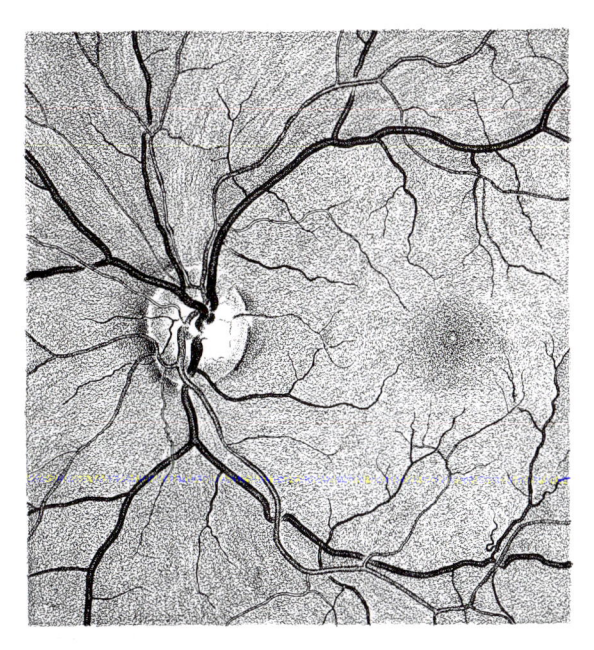

Fig 6-13 Segmental narrowings of the major retinal arteries and narrowing of some terminal branches in the left retina of a 49 year old man with treated hypertension. At two infero-temporal AV crossings there is deviation of the vein and at two superior AV crossings there is concealment of the vein.

2 Arterio-venous Crossing Changes

It is necessary to define what appearances at AV crossings are to be regarded as pathological. For example, slight apparent nipping of the vein where it is crossed by the artery is probably not pathological. At a normal AV crossing the venous blood column is visible right up to the arterial blood column on either side and it can usually also be seen dimly behind the artery (Fig 6-14a). Histologically there is often slight (20%) narrowing of the vein deep to the artery at normal crossings.

Pathological AV crossing changes are

  i Concealment of the vein
The venous blood column appears to stop a short distance from the arterial blood column (Figs 6-14b, 6-13). This appearance is due to obscuration of the blood in the vein by thickening of the common adventitial and glial sheath of the AV crossing.

  ii Deviation of the vein
A kink occurs in the course of the vein from just before to just after it crosses behind the artery

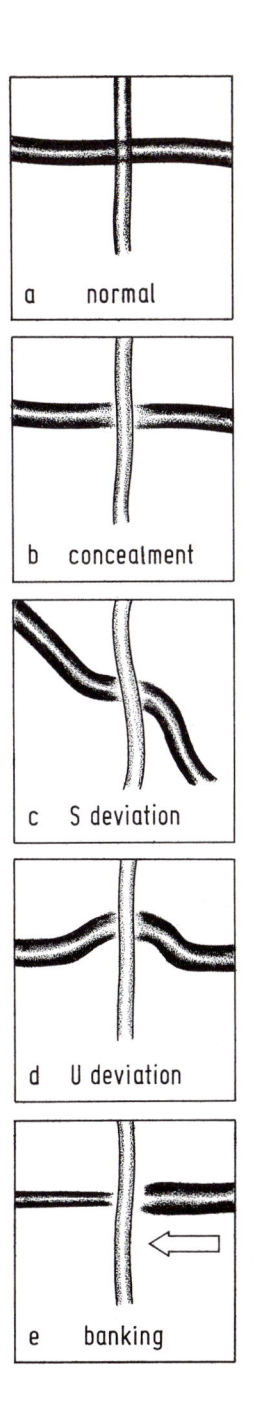

a normal

b concealment

c S deviation

d U deviation

e banking

Fig 6-14 AV crossing changes.

(Figs 6-14c and d, 6-13). This deviation will be in the form of a U if the general direction of the vein is at right angles to that of the artery, or in the form of an S if the crossing is oblique. The altered course of the vein looks as if it could have been produced by a longitudinal movement of the artery dragging the underlying part of the vein along with it.

iii Banking of the vein

This uncommon change consists of a widening of the vein distal to the crossing (Fig 6-14e). It probably signifies an impediment to venous flow at the crossing.

The significance of AV crossing changes has caused much disagreement. It is suggested that minor changes, or definite changes at only one or two crossings, occur in normotensive, ageing (60 plus) people, whereas generalized definite changes are a reliable sign of hypertension.

3 Opacities of Vessels

Opacities may be within the vessel lumen (emboli) or in the vessel wall (sheathing).

Emboli

Several sorts of emboli are occasionally seen in retinal arteries. *Cholesterol* emboli are bright, lustrous spots or specks which appear to be on the vessel walls (Fig 6-15). They may be inconstantly visible and commonly they do not obstruct the blood flow. They are flat crystals of cholesterol from atheromatous ulcers in a carotid artery. A *platelet* embolus looks like a small white blob in an artery and usually obstructs the blood flow (Fig 6-16). A *calcific* embolus, which is very rare, also obstructs blood flow and comes from a mitral valve vegetation. Fat emboli are usually too small to be seen.

Sheathing

Arteries on or near to the optic disc may have a filmy covering of glial tissue as a normal variation.

Parallel white lines bordering the blood column of an artery or vein are due to opacification of the vessel wall. If the opacification is complete the blood column is hidden and the vessel looks like a white line; this is called pipe-stem sheathing (Fig 6-17). Opacification may be due to advanced arteriolar sclerosis as in hypertension, to fatty deposits around veins as in venous occlusion and diabetic retinopathy, to infiltration with inflammatory cells in vasculitis or to perivascular infiltration with leucocytes in leukaemia.

Atherosclerosis does not occur in vessels of the size of the retinal arteries.

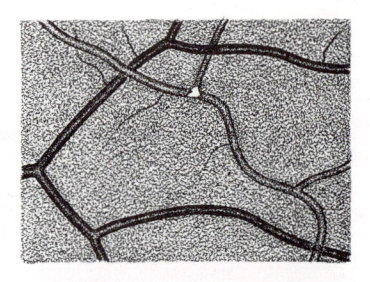

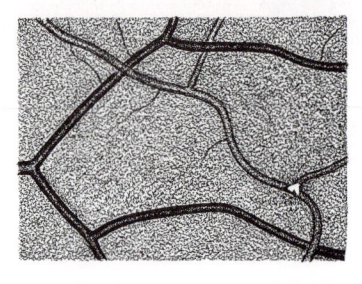

Fig 6-15 Upper Cholesterol embolus held up at an arterial bifurcation but not seriously impairing blood flow.

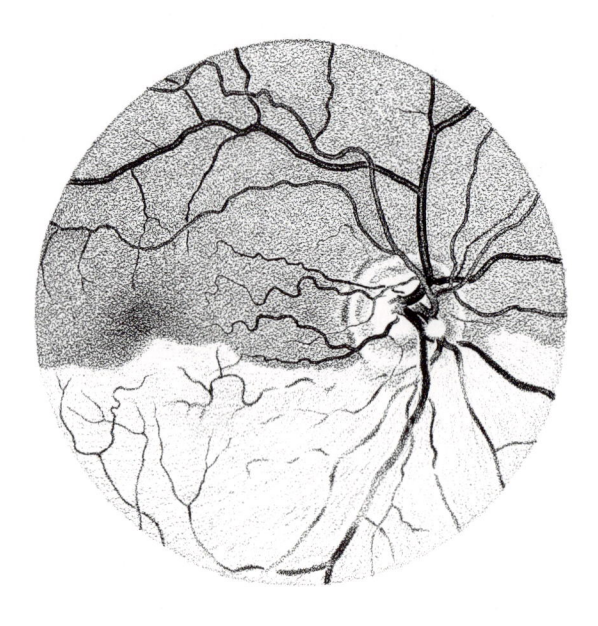

Lower One month later it had moved on to the next bifurcation.

Fig 6-16 Ischaemic infarct of the inferior retina caused by the impaction of a platelet embolus at the first bifurcation of the central retinal artery.

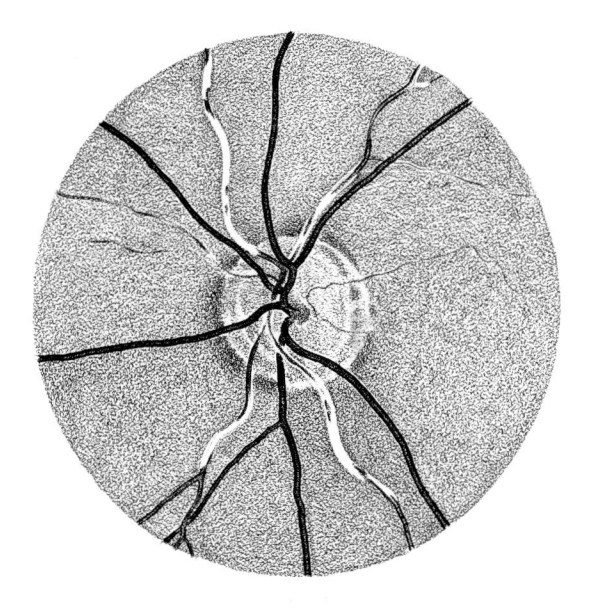

Fig 6-17 Sheathing of arteries in advanced retinal arteriolar sclerosis.

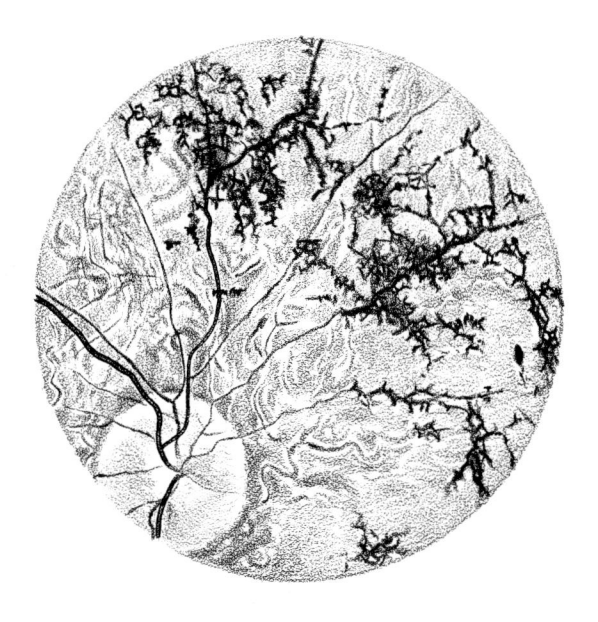

Fig 6-18 Generalized narrowing of retinal vessels in primary pigmentary degeneration of the retina (retinitis pigmentosa).

CHANGES DIFFICULT TO ASSESS AND OF DOUBTFUL SIGNIFICANCE

1 Generalized Narrowing

Clinical estimation of general arterial calibre is so uncertain that it should be disregarded unless attentuation of the arteries is strikingly obvious. The method commonly used is to compare the widths of companion arteries and veins, that is to estimate the AV ratio. Difficulties occur because of normal variations in the AV ratio, because there is commonly not an artery and vein which can be properly compared because of incomparable patterns of branching, and because there is much observer error in estimating relative vessel widths.

Generalized arterial narrowing, if quite obvious in a young person, is usually due to serve hypertension. It also occurs as a result of occlusion of the central retinal artery and of widespread retinal degeneration, e.g. pigmentary degeneration (Fig 6-18).

2 Altered Light Reflexes

Approximately the central third of normal arteries is overlain with a bright strip of reflected light, the light reflex. The cylindrical mirror surface from which the ophthalmoscope light is reflected is probably the interface between the blood and the vessel wall rather than the vessel wall itself.

Changes in the light reflex consist of widening of the reflex and loss of its distinct borders. These may be of such a degree as to more or less obscure the underlying blood. Traditional terms for this appearance are 'copper wire arteries' and, when the blood is completely obscured, 'silver wire arteries'. These terms should be discarded. The altered reflection probably results from changes in the refractive index of the vessel wall which becomes more refractile and less transparent.

Alteration of the light reflex is difficult to assess because of the subjective nature of the observation. Since increased light reflexes occur as a result of both ageing (involutional sclerosis) and hypertension (arteriolar sclerosis, replacement fibrosis) they are of little diagnostic value.

CHANGES WHICH CANNOT BE ASSESSED CLINICALLY

1 Increased or Decreased Tortuosity

The normal variation in tortuosity of the retinal arteries is so great that pathological changes in individuals can be detected only by repeated photographic observations.

Aterioles tend to become straighter with increasing age and more tortuous with increasing blood pressure, but these trends are slight and they are lost in the wide scatter of the normal range of tortuosity.

2 Actute-angled Branchings

In youth the branchings of the retinal arteries are wide-angled, but variation is great and assessment without resort to measurement is difficult. Some believe that with increasing age the angles between branches become smaller, but others believe the opposite — obviously a sign of no value.

In summary, look for irregularity of calibre, AV crossing changes, conspicuous generalized narrowing, and vessel opacities and ignore the other described changes.

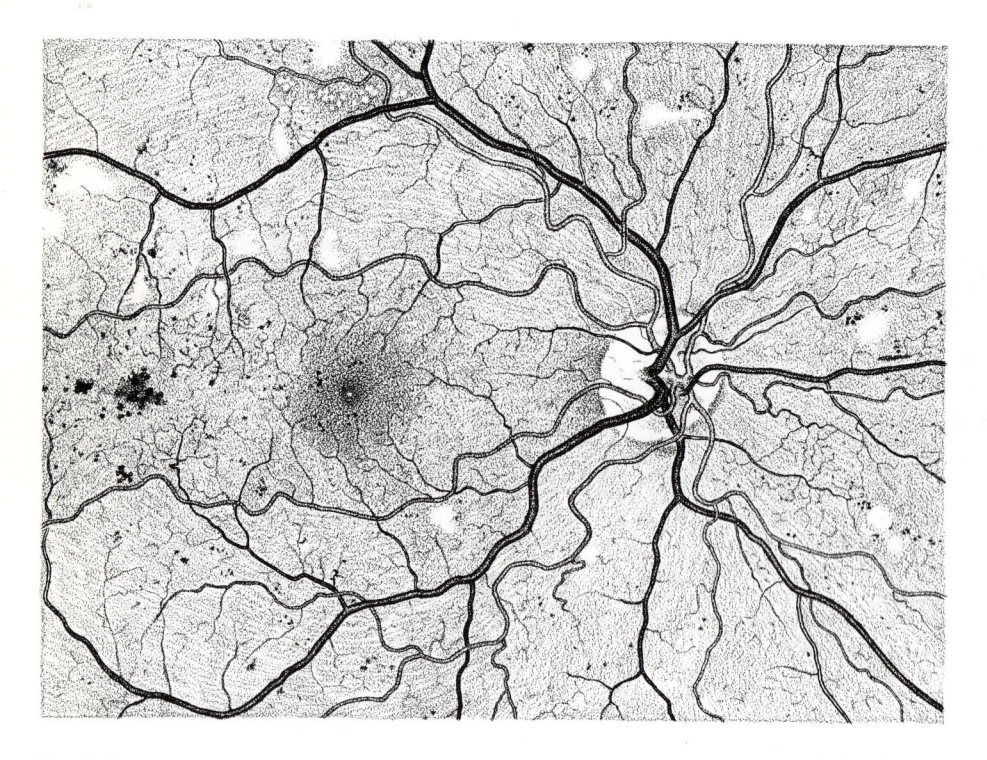

Fig 6-19 Patches of enlarged irregular capillaries, microaneurysysms, a few haemorrhages and soft exudates in the right eye of a 29 year old man diabetic for 21 years.

Capillary

Visibility of Capillaries

Individual normal capillaries are too small (5 μm diameter) to be seen with the ophthalmoscope. In some conditions, of which the commonest are diabetes and hypertension, capillaries may become abnormally dilated and therefore visible in localized areas of the fundus (Fig 6-19). These small vessels are often also irregular. Fluorescein angiography shows that they are commonly associated with closure of adjacent capillaries.

Microaneurysms

Aneurysmal dilatations of the retinal capillaries appear as small red dots varying in size from just visible to almost the width of a larger retinal artery (Fig 6-19). On ophthalmoscopic appearances alone they cannot be distinguished from some deep retinal haemorrhages.

They are characteristic of diabetic retinopathy, but they also occur in other ocular and general diseases, e.g. retinal vein occlusion, macroglobulinaemia.

Venous

Dilatation

As with assessment of general arterial calibre, clinical estimation of venous calibre is difficult. It is therefore best to disregard engorgement of the veins unless it is conspicuous. It occurs in a number of local and general conditions, e.g. retinal vein occlusions, papilloedema, polycythaemia. One unexpected cause is reduced pressure in the central retinal artery as a result of carotid artery insufficiency. In addition to dilatation and tortuosity of the retinal veins there may be blot haemorrhages and microaneurysms (carotid insufficiency retinopathy, venous stasis retinopathy) (Plate 11, p. 126).

Irregularity of Calibre

This usually occurs in association with other well-developed vascular changes in a variety of conditions, e.g. diabetic retinopathy, retinal vein occlusion.

Venous Collaterals

Dilatation of pre-existing vessels to by-pass areas of impediment to venous drainage occur not only in the retina (Fig 15-6) but also on the optic disc, e.g. in chronic open-angle glaucoma.

Neovascularization

Neovascularization can occur on the surface of the retina (intra-retinal) or in the vitreous in front of the retina or optic disc (pre-retinal). When they first appear intra-retinal new-formed vessels cannot be distinguished ophthalmoscopically from irregularly dilated capillaries but as they grow they form networks, loops, or arcades which are obviously new-formed (Plate 14, p. 127).

Pre-retinal new-formed vessels have broken through the internal limiting membrane and are drawn forwards as a result of shrinkage of the vitreous. They form vascular meshworks or long loops (Fig 6-20). Fibrous tissue proliferation always accompanies the vessels. At first filmy and hard to detect, it gradually becomes dense and conspicuous and eventually strangles the vessels. The fibrous tissue tends to shrink and

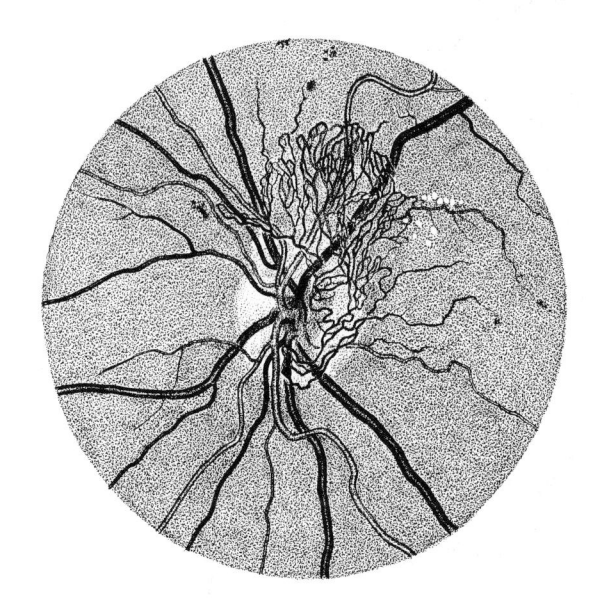

Fig 6-20 Preretinal neovascular meshwork arising from the left optic disc of a 30 year old diabetic woman.

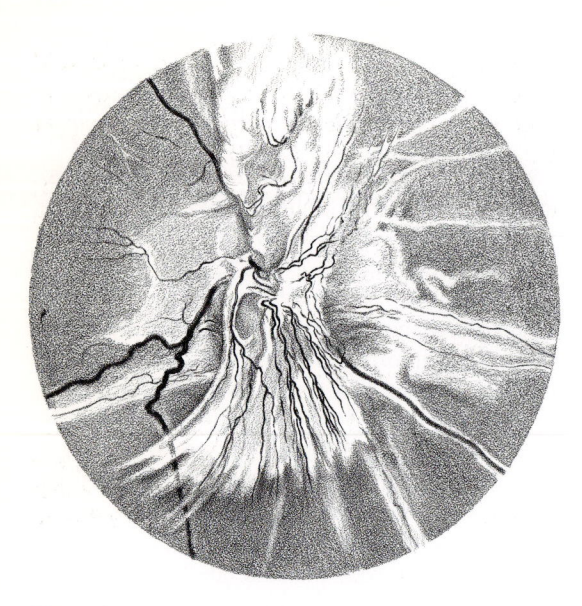

Fig 6-21 Retinitis proliferans obscuring the right optic disc and detaching the retina in a 47 year old diabetic woman.

by traction may cause detachment of the retina (Fig 6-21). The old term for this neovascular fibrosis is *retinitis proliferans* and it is still used even though there is no retinal inflammation.

New-formed vessels do not have the restricted permeability of normal retinal vessels and consequently plasma leaks from them into the tissues to cause oedema and hard exudates. They also behave as if they were abnormally fragile because spontaneous haemorrhages from them are common.

Retinal neovascularization occurs in a small proportion of eyes with diabetic retinopathy and also in other conditions, e.g. following retinal vein occlusion, retinal vasculitis (Eale's disease). Neovascularization from the periphery of the immature retina follows a period of arterial closure in response to neonatal oxygen levels that are too high in retinopathy of prematurity (formerly called retrolental fibroplasia).

Fundus Background

The *normal fundus background* is orange-red in colour because the ophthalmoscope light is reflected from the blood in the larger choroidal vessels and then modified by the overlying retinal pigment epithelium. This pigment acts both as a

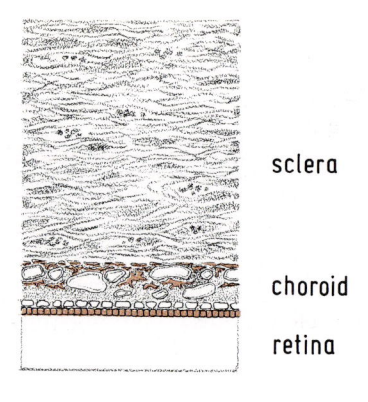

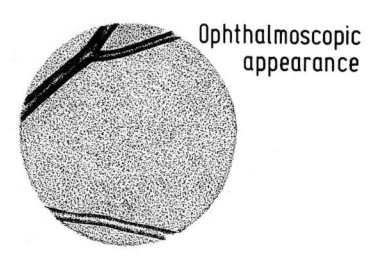

Fig 6-22 Structural basis for normal variations in the colour and pattern of the fundus background.

a Common, uniformly orange-red caucasian fundus.

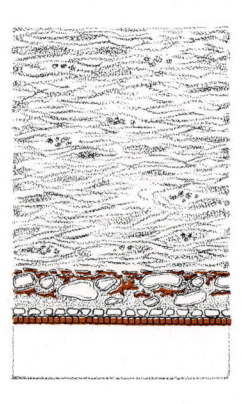

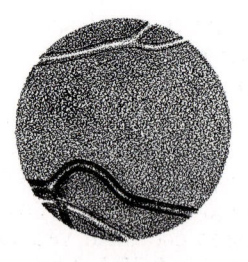

b Dusky negroid or polynesian fundus.

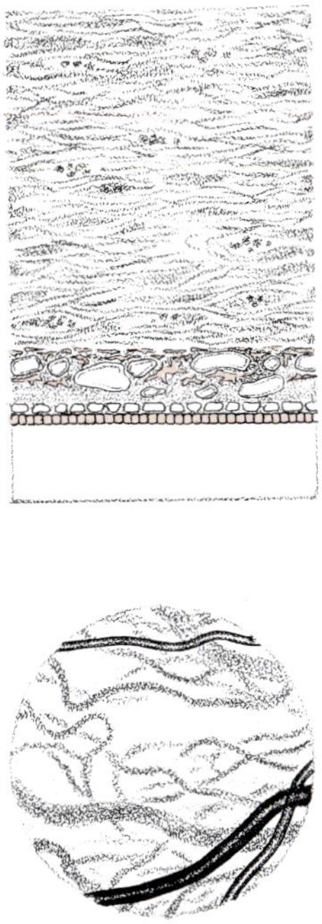

c Blonde fundus. 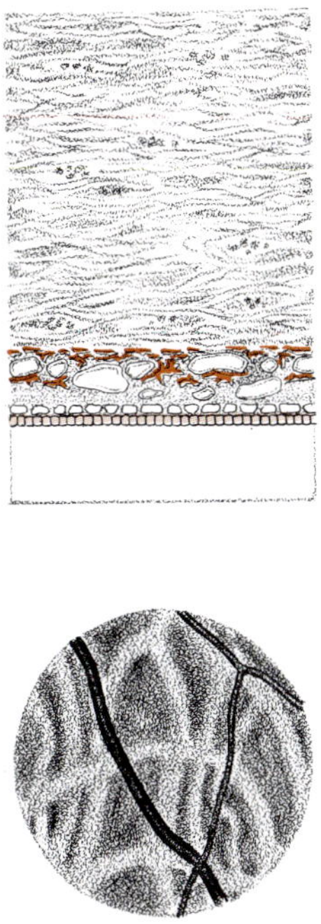   d Tessellated fundus.

diffusing screen which converts the discontinuous pattern of red vessels into a more or less uniformly coloured surface, and as a colour filter which changes the colour to an orange-red (Fig 6-22a). The retina internal to the pigment epithelium is necessarily transparent, except for the blood contained in the retinal arteries and veins, and therefore reflects little light.

As well as the pigment in the pigment epithelium, pigment also occurs in the choroid, especially in its outer part among the larger choroidal vessels. The densities of the pigment in these two situations are independent and they vary from individual to individual, with race, and with age. The shade of red and the pattern of the fundus background are determined by the densities of the pigment in the pigment epithelium and in the choroid.

Much pigment in the pigment epithelium gives rise to a dusky red, uniform background (Fig 6-22b). Little pigment in both the pigment epithelium and in the choroid gives rise to a light red background or one that is pale with discernible large choroidal vessels, the blonde type of fundus (Fig 6-22c). Little pigment in the pigment epithelium with much pigment in the choroid gives rise to the tessellated or tigroid fundus in which patches of choroidal pigment are seen more or less clearly outlined by the larger choroidal vessels (Fig 6-22d).

In the macular region there is heavier pigmentation of the pigment epithelium and this area is therefore slightly darker than the rest of the fundus. There is often some accumulation of retinal pigment at the margin of the optic disc, especially on its temporal side, where it is visible as an irregular line (pigment crescent).

Changes in the Fundus Background

Almost all of the alterations seen ophthalmoscopically in the fundus background are either pale (including white, grey, cream, or yellow), red, or black.

Pale Areas

Pale areas are produced either by loss of transparency of the retina which then reflects the light (Fig 6-23), or by exposure of the sclera through absence of the pigment epithelium and choroid (Fig 6-30; Plate 6, p. 123).

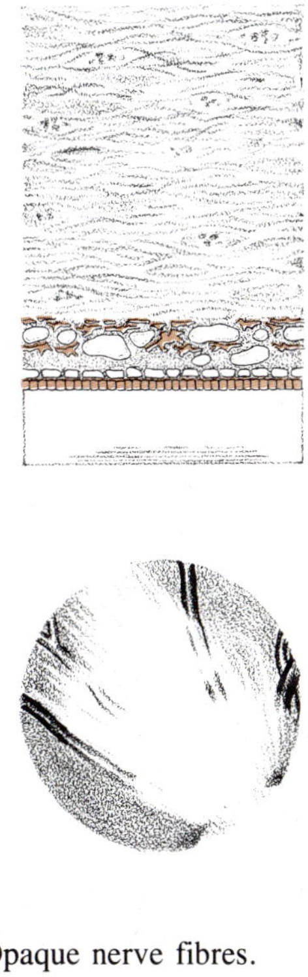

Fig 6-23 Opaque nerve fibres.

1 Opacities of the Retina

Various degrees of opacification of the retina result from
- congenital anomalies, e.g. opaque nerve fibres
- oedema, e.g. arterial occlusion, contusion of the globe
- inflammation, e.g. toxoplasmic choroidoretinitis
- retinal exudates
- retinal detachment
- retinal tumour

Opaque nerve fibres (myelinated nerve fibres) are the result of a developmental anomaly in which the myelin sheaths of the nerve fibres in some bundles do not stop at the lamina cribrosa but extend for varying distances into the retina where they opacify the inner layer (Plate 7, p. 124). Ophthalmoscopically the sectors affected are glistening faintly striated white patches with feathery edges which are usually continuous with the optic disc (Fig 6-23). There is a corresponding enlargement of the blind spot but no other interference with visual function.

What is usually called *retinal oedema* is in fact *cloudy swelling* of the inner retinal layers as a result of acute impairment of retinal arterial blood supply. It is seen most characteristically in central retinal artery or branch retinal artery occlusions (Plate 9, p. 125). The affected area of the fundus becomes cloudy and pallid or white (Fig 6-24). When the central part of the retina is involved the fovea, which contains no ganglion cells or nerve fibres and which is supplied by the choriocapillaris, retains its transparency and is seen as a small red disc in the surrounding pallor, traditionally called a 'cherry-red spot at the macula' (Fig 15-1). Occasionally mild cloudy swelling from transient retinal emboli is reversible, but usually the process signifies irreversible cell death. The opacity of the retina clears within two or three weeks to leave a misleadingly normal appearing fundus background.

Extracellular and therefore reversible retinal oedema may be superficial or deep. *Superficial retinal oedema* appears as a pale misty haze of the fundus near the optic disc and macula. The course of the nerve fibres close to the disc may be rendered more visible due to fluid separating bundles of fibres. It is seen most often in hypertensive retinopathy and with papilloedema. As the fluid absorbs during recovery fine hard exudates, oedema residues, appear which in the macular area take the form of a fan or a star. They last for many months before finally clearing completely and they cause no permanent impairment of retinal function.

Deep retinal oedema affects the deeper synaptic layer in a variety of conditions, for example retinal vein occlusion, diabetic retinopathy, following cataract extraction. It is not easy to recognize with an ophthalmoscope, the most useful sign being an increase in the glinting light reflexes from the surface of the retina which move with movement of the ophthalmoscope light over the fundus. It commonly affects the macular area and if prolonged it here collects in small cystic spaces (microcystic macular oedema) which can eventually coalesce to form a visible cyst at the macula. The appearance of microcystic macular oedema in fluorescence angiograms is characteristic. After transit of the fluorescein a radial star-like pattern slowly develops at the macula.

Inflammatory lesions tend to involve both choroid and retina although they may start as a choroiditis or as a retinitis. A common form of *choroidoretinitis* is the result of infestation with the protozoal organism, *Toxoplasma*. Active inflammation tends to recur adjacent to apparently quiescent scars at long intervals (Plate 6, p. 123). Another infestation, with a nematode of dogs, *toxocara canis*, is less common and causes a granulomatous lesion under the macular retina or beside the optic disc. Other rare known causes are tuberculosis (choroidal tubercles may be of great diagnostic help in miliary tuberculosis) and syphilis. In much of the lesion where there is an inflammatory cellular exudate the retina becomes densely opaque while around the edges inflammatory oedema makes the retina hazy (Fig 6-24). The ophthalmoscopic result is a white patch with indistinct margins. The inflammatory cells also enter the vitreous and the resulting vitreous haze further obscures the white areas. At the centre of the focus retina and choroid are destroyed so that when the active inflammation has subsided the sclera is exposed as a permanent visible white area which is commonly rimmed by accumulations of pigment. Inflammatory lesions thus illustrate the two ways in which pale fundus areas occur, loss of transparency in the active stage and exposure of the sclera when healed (Plate 6, p. 123).

The term *retinal exudate* is inapt but tradi-

OPHTHALMOSCOPIC CHANGES 143

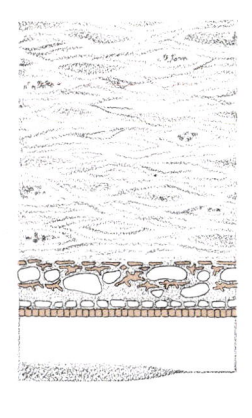

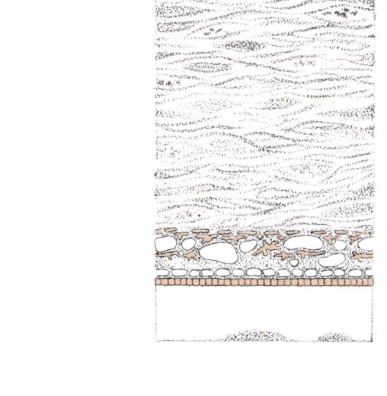

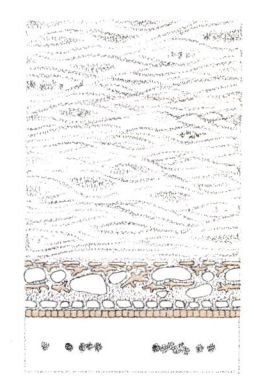

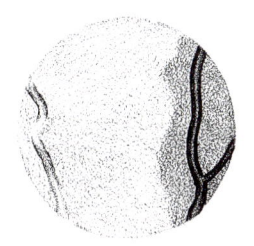

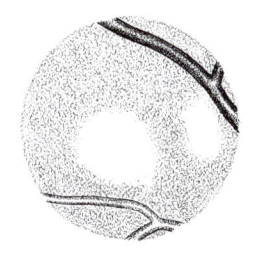

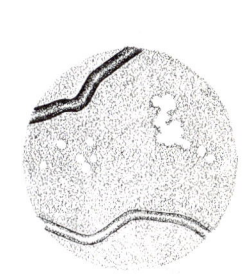

Fig 6-24 Retinal oedema or inflammation. **Fig 6-25** Soft exudates. **Fig 6-26** Hard exudates.

tional and fixed. Exudates are of two types synaesthetically called soft and hard.

Soft exudates, also called *cotton wool spots,* are ill-defined white or grey patches which occur superficially in the nerve fibre layer of the retina where the axons in a small area are swollen and opaque because normal axoplasmic flow has been locally held up by acute focal ischaemia (Fig 6-25). They are non-specific and occur in hypertension (if the diastolic BP is greater than 120mm Hg) and also in some retinal vein occlusions, disc oedema, diabetes, trauma, collagen diseases, e.g. disseminated lupus erythematosis, severe anaemia, and septicaemia. They become granular, grey, and fade within about two months leaving no visible trace. The soft exudates which occur in diabetic retinopathy are somewhat different in that they may be more faint and therefore less easily seen and they may persist for many months.

Hard exudates, also called fatty or waxy exudates, are sharply demarcated cream or yellow specks and spots which occur deep in the retina (Fig 6-26). They may be discrete or confluent. When confluent they may be in the form of incomplete or complete rings, patches, large plaques, or, at the macula, a fan or star (p. 15). They occur in many conditions in which there is chronic insufficiency of the deep retinal capillaries with probable hypoxia but not death of the retinal cells. They are composed of lipid debris either lying free or phagocytosed by microglia. At least in some conditions the fatty material is derived from leakage of plasma and consists of the larger molecules which are less readily reabsorbed by adjacent normal vessels. They are characteristic of diabetic retinopathy in which a ring distribution is often seen surrounding a focus of capillary abnormality from which leakage of plasma can be demonstrated by fluorescein angiography. Destruction of this central source by light coagulation leads to absorption of the surrounding exudate. Other conditions in which hard exudates occur are hypertensive retinopathy, retinal vein occlusion, disciform macular degeneration, and circinate retinopathy (a rare condition of older people in which an isolated inconspicuous vascular abnormality is surrounded by a 'fairy ring' of hard exudates).

Detachment of the retina refers to the separation of the neural retina from the pigment epithelium. In the most common form of detachment this occurs as a result of a hole or tear in the retina which allows fluid to accumulate between the two parts of the retina, thus recreating the space between the two layers of the embryonic optic cup. Detached retina becomes less transparent and the interposed fluid may be murky so that the red reflection from the underlying pigment epithelium and choroid is dulled and the retina is pale (Fig 6-27). Because the retinal vessels in the detached retina are retroilluminated they appear dark and, with the retina, they are often wrinkled and wavy because of the reduction in tension when they no longer have to follow the inner surface of the globe.

Tumours of the retina are rare, the one most frequently seen being a *retinoblastoma*. This is a solid mass which looks white (Fig 6-28). It occurs in babies and young children, is commonly bilateral and may be hereditary. It commonly presents as a pale mass behind the lens which is noticed by the parents as a white pupil, the 'cat's eye reflex'. Alternatively, as a consequence of the loss of sight, the infant may develop a squint and this is yet another reason why a child with a squint should receive specialist attention without delay.

2 Opacities of Bruch's Membrane — Colloid Bodies (Drusen)

Usually with age and commonly in degenerative and dystrophic conditions, small opaque hemispherical deposits from the pigment epithelium form on Bruch's membrane (p. 7). Commonly the pigment in the overlying epithelial cells is reduced and these *colloid bodies* are then seen as small round white or cream spots often with pigmented margins lying deep in the retina (Fig 6-29; Plate 8, p. 124). Distinction from hard exudates can be difficult; a colloid body glows when a fine spot of light from an ophthalmoscope is directed alongside it, an exudate does not. They do not reduce vision. Colloid bodies are often called *drusen*, but retinal drusen should not be confused with drusen of the optic disc (p. 164) which are different.

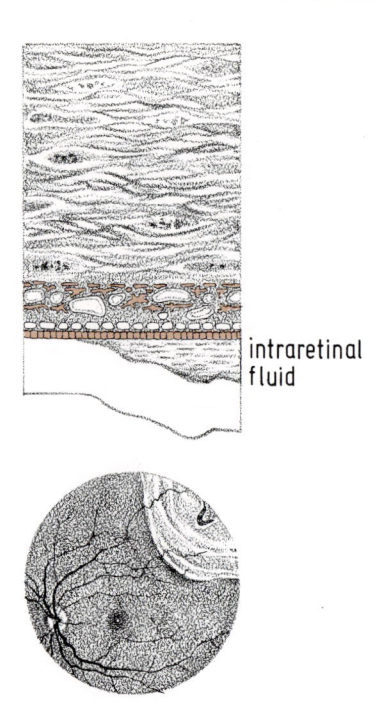

intraretinal fluid

Fig 6-27 Retinal detachment. Fundus drawing (to a different scale) of a ballooned peripheral detachment shows the horseshoe retinal tear which gave rise to it.

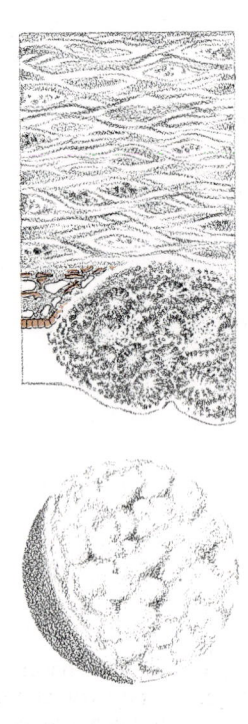

Fig 6-28 Retinoblastoma.

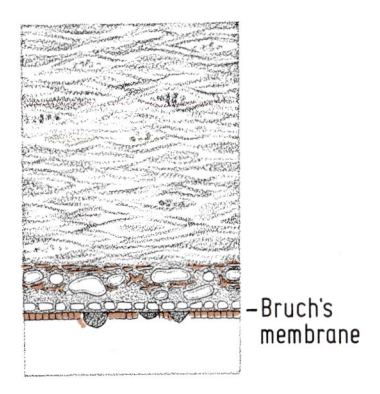

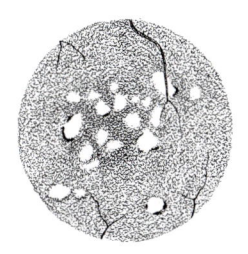

Fig 6-29 Colloid bodies.

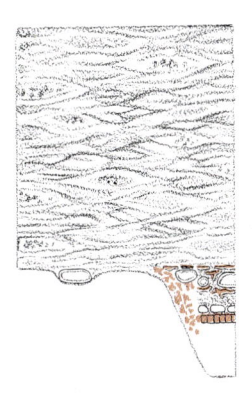

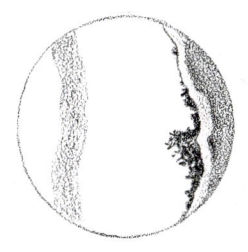

Fig 6-30 Post-inflammatory exposure of sclera with clumping of displaced pigment at the margin. A major choroidal vessel has survived the inflammatory destruction of tissue.

3 Exposure of Sclera

Loss of pigment epithelium and choroid to expose the white or cream sclera occurs as a result of congenital defects (coloboma), inflammation (Plate 6, p. 123), trauma, and a variety of degenerations. Sometimes the larger choroidal vessels escape destruction and often there is an irregular marginal fringe of pigment (Fig 6-30). A small crescent of sclera is commonly visible at the temporal margin of the optic disc (scleral crescent) and with age a ring of sclera encircling the disc may become visible (peripapillary atrophy). A more extensive myopic scleral crescent of peripapillary atrophy occurs pathologically in some highly myopic eyes (degenerative myopia) and this choroidoretinal atrophy may involve the macula in middle life.

Red Areas

Apart from microaneurysms, areas of neovascularization, retinal holes or tears and the rare angioid streaks, red areas on the fundus are due to haemorrhage. Extravascular blood can be in one or more of five anatomical situations.

i The appearance of a *vitreous haemorrhage* depends on whether the vitreous is a solid gel or whether, as a result of age or degeneration, part of the vitreous has become liquified. In the former case the blood is at first confined as linear or curled streaks and absorption is slower than in fluid vitreous where the blood is diffuse with denser blobs from the beginning. Vitreous haemorrhages clear slowly, the time ranging from a few weeks for a small haemorrhage in fluid vitreous to several years for a massive haemorrhage. With the ophthalmoscope the blood is red when illuminated directly, but it is more often seen as a black opacity silhouetted in the red reflex. Much blood eliminates the red reflex entirely. Recurrent vitreous haemorrhages are likely with retinal neovascularization from whatever cause. Other causes of bleeding into the vitreous are injury, and the formation of retinal holes — an old guide is to regard any unexplained vitreous haemorrhage as being associated with a retinal detachment until proved otherwise.

ii Blood escaping from a superficial retinal vessel may not rupture through the internal limiting membrane into the vitreous, but remain immediately *pre-retinal* between the retina and the vitreous (subhyaloid). In this situation the red

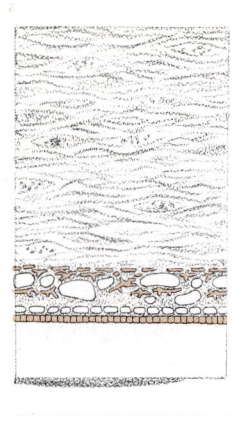

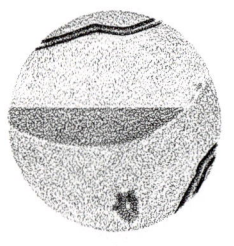

Fig 6-31 Preretinal haemorrhage and a mossy haemorrhage.

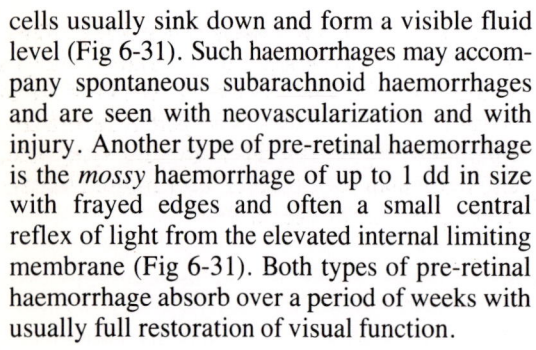

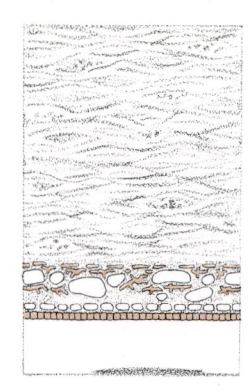

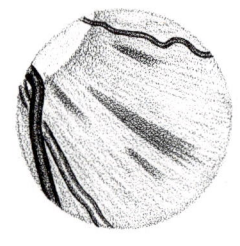

Fig 6-32 Superficial retinal haemorrhages.

cells usually sink down and form a visible fluid level (Fig 6-31). Such haemorrhages may accompany spontaneous subarachnoid haemorrhages and are seen with neovascularization and with injury. Another type of pre-retinal haemorrhage is the *mossy* haemorrhage of up to 1 dd in size with frayed edges and often a small central reflex of light from the elevated internal limiting membrane (Fig 6-31). Both types of pre-retinal haemorrhage absorb over a period of weeks with usually full restoration of visual function.

iii *Superficial retinal haemorrhages* are characteristically *linear* or *flame* shaped with their long axes directed towards the optic disc because the red cells lie between the nerve fibres (Fig 6-32). They absorb within a few weeks. They are characteristic of hypertensive retinopathy and are also seen in other conditions such as blood diseases and retinal vein occlusion.

iv In *deep retinal haemorrhages* the red cells within the retina are compacted by the tight structure of this tissue and these are characteristically round *dot and blot* haemorrhages (cf. hard exudates) (Fig 6-33). They occur especially when there is capillary or venous insufficiency, e.g. diabetic retinopathy, retinal vein occlusion.

v True *choroidal haemorrhages* are rare except as a result of traumatic rupture of the choroid. These dull red collections of blood lie deep to Bruch's membrane. What are commonly called choroidal haemorrhages are in fact in front of Bruch's membrane *deep to the pigment epithelium*. They occur in disciform macular degeneration, are a slate-grey colour, and have a rounded outline with commonly a partial red fringe of *subretinal haemorrhage,* that is blood which has seeped through the pigment epithelium to lie between it and the neural retina (Fig 6-34). They permanently destroy function in the overlying retina. The blood escapes from new-formed vessels which grow through breaks in Bruch's membrane from the choriocapillaris. Occasionally a patch of subretinal neovascularization detected by fluorescein angiography can be destroyed by careful photocoagulation before a haemorrhage occurs.

Retinal holes are breaks in the neural retina and

OPHTHALMOSCOPIC CHANGES

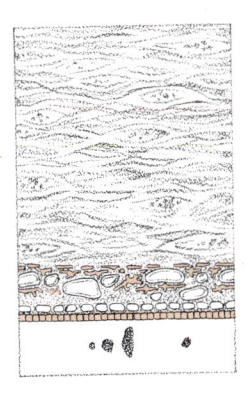

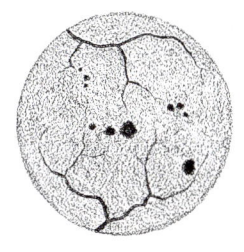

Fig 6-33 Deep retinal haemorrhages.

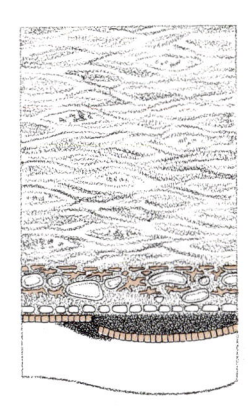

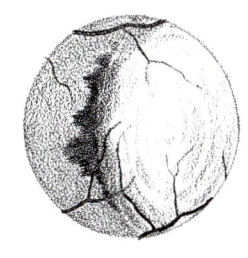

Fig 6-34 Choroidal haemorrhage with a margin of subretinal haemorrhage.

are the cause of primary retinal detachments. The great majority occur peripherally well anterior to the equator. They arise because of degenerative changes such as occur with age or in some cases of degenerative myopia, as a result of shrinkage of the vitreous in the presence of localized abnormal attachment of vitreous to retina (Fig 1-20), and following injury. The breaks are of various types such as a round hole, a crescentic U-shaped tear, or a dialysis (separation of the neural retina from the ora serrata around part of its circumference). Ophthalmoscopically, retinal breaks appear bright red because of the contrast between the unimpeded view of the pigment epithelium through them and the surrounding pale neural retina (Fig 6-27). They may be difficult to see but a detachment will not be cured unless they are found and closed by welding together retina, choroid, and sclera through inducing a controlled local choroidal inflammation by local heating or freezing.

Angioid streaks are rare, raggedly tapering red, brown, or grey striations looking something like cracks in dried mud which at first glance may be confused with blood vessels (Plate 15, p. 128). They are due to tears and degenerative changes in Bruch's membrane. In themselves they are of no significance but they may be part of generalized conditions, e.g. Grönblad-Strandberg syndrome, and more than half the eyes with angioid streaks develop macular degeneration.

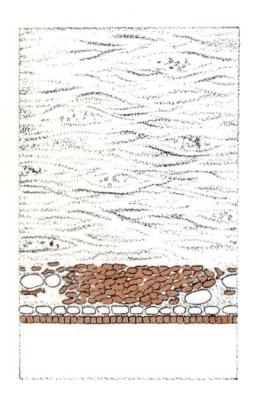

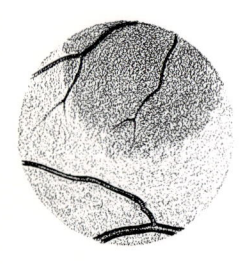

Fig 6-35 Choroidal naevus (benign melanoma).

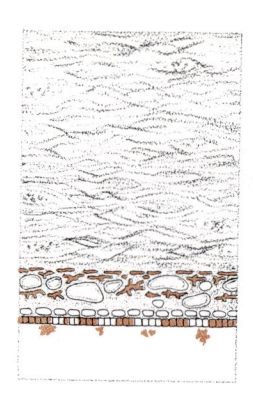

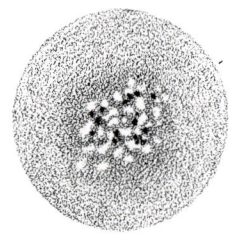

Fig 6-36 Pigmentary disturbance in macular degeneration.

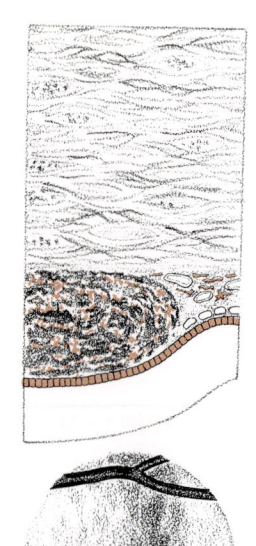

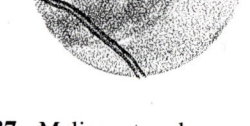

Fig 6-37 Malignant melanoma of the choroid.

Black Areas

The pigment of both the pigment epithelium and the choroid is commonly altered in amount and distribution. This occurs in the following circumstances.

Physiological

As well as the tessellated fundus background and the pigment crescent, localized patches of dense pigmentation of the pigment epithelium or of the choroid (naevus) occur as internal birth marks (Fig 6-35)

Post-inflammatory

In any severe disturbance of the retina and choroid the pigment granules are phagocytosed and commonly transported into clumps, especially at the margins of the affected area where they often remain permanently as black deposits (Fig 6-30; Plate 6, p. 123). With lesser or more diffuse disturbances, the uniform pigmentation is replaced by a non-uniform granular pigmentation, a pepper and salt appearance.

Degenerative Aggregation

In a number of degenerative conditions pigment granules are lost from the pigment epithelium and are deposited in the retina. In some conditions, e.g. senescent macular degeneration, the pigment is in small clumps so that a granular or stippled appearance of pale and dark specks is seen (Fig 6-36). In others, e.g. pigmentary degeneration of the retina, the pigment is deposited around the fine retinal blood vessels to produce the characteristic appearance of 'bone corpuscle pigmentation' (Fig 6-18).

Neoplastic

A malignant melanoma of the choroid is a primary melanotic tumour but while still subretinal it usually looks dark grey rather than black or brown (Fig 6-37). Great care and special investigations, e.g. fluorescence angiography, are necessary to avoid mistaking a haemorrhage beneath the pigment epithelium or a naevus for a malignant choroidal melanoma.

PART THREE

CLINICAL TOPICS

Chapter 7

RETINAL VASCULAR DISEASE

Pathophysiological mechanisms
    Capillary closure
    Endothelial incompetence

DIABETIC AND HYPERTENSIVE RETINOPATHIES

Diabetic retinal changes
    Fundus picture
    Fluorescein angiography
    Changes which destroy sight
    Detection and assessment
    Management
Hypertensive retinal changes
    Hypertensive vessel changes
    Hyptertensive retinopathy
    Associated retinal vascular abnormalities

RETINAL VASCULAR DISEASE

There are more than a dozen vascular retinopathies, some common and some rare, which can be recogised with an ophthalmoscope: diabetic, hypertensive, hyperviscosity, collagen disease and anaemic retinopathies; arterial occlusion, venous occlusion, retinal vasculitis, and so on. The beginner often finds it hard to distinguish these different conditions because they share the same component features such as irregularity of arteries, dilatation of veins, microaneurysms, haemorrhages, exudates, and neovascularization. These are the ophthalmoscopic pieces which make up the patterns of retinal vascular disease. With experience we learn to recognise the pattern.

Pathophysiological Basis of Vascular Retinopathies

It is easier to recognise the patterns if we know what the pieces mean, if we can translate ophthalmoscopic appearances into pathophysiological changes. When we do this we find that the underlying basis of most retinal vascular disease is reduced to only two fundamental mechanisms, underperfusion or closure of capillaries, and damage leading to incompetence of the capillary endothelium. In fluorescein angiograms non-perfused capillaries show up as small or large holes in the overall capillary network (Fig 7-5), while endothelial damage can be inferred if the dye diffuses out of the retinal vessels (p. 16) (Fig 7-6).

Where the retina is thicker in the neighbourhood of the optic disc and macula there are superficial capillaries in the nerve fibre layer as well as more deeply in the retina (Fig 1-17). Some conditions involve the capillaries of one layer more than those of the other. For example, hypertensive retinopathy tends to affect the superficial capillaries, diabetic retinopathy the deeper capillaries. We do not know why this happens, but the results of non-perfusion or damage are different in these two capillary layers.

Capillary Closure

When blood flow through the capillaries is reduced or stops the result depends on the area of retina involved and the speed with which it occurs. If capillary perfusion stops *abruptly* in a *large* area of the retina, or even in the whole retina, the retina becomes opaque with cloudy swelling and dies. Only occlusion of the retinal artery or one of its branches can cause this, so diffuse pallor means a retinal infarct.

If capillary perfusion is reduced *slowly and gradually* collateral vessels may have time to develop. This seems to happen mostly when the impediment is on the venous side of the retinal circulation. Therefore retinal collaterals are permanent evidence of present or past venous stasis.

When a small *focal* area of *deep* capillaries is not perfused there is no visible ophthalmoscopic change and only by seeing it in fluorescein angiograms have we learnt that this is a common feature of many retinopathies. However an abnormality which is visible may develop in adjacent capillaries, namely microaneurysms and these are therefore usually evidence of focal closure of deep retinal capillaries.

RETINAL RESPONSE TO VASCULAR DISEASE

	deep retinal capillaries	superficial retinal capillaries	optic disc capillaries
• capillary non-perfusion			pallid disc oedema
regional		retinal necrosis	
gradual regional		collateral vessels	
focal	microaneurysms	cotton wool spot	
widespread focal		neovascularization	
• endothelial damage		retinal oedema	disc oedema
	hard exudate		
	deep haemorrhage	superficial haemorrhage	

RETINAL VASCULAR DISEASE

The reaction to *focal* closure of *superficial* capillaries is quite different. Here the tiny infarct in the nerve fibre layer leads to local hold up of axoplasmic flow in the axons and the consequent opacity is seen as a cotton wool spot or soft exudate.

If capillary perfusion is defective in *numerous areas* but not bad enough to cause retinal necrosis, neovascularization is a likely response. New-formed vessels occur when the retina is 'sick but not dead'.

The arterial supply of the *optic disc* comes, not from the retinal artery, but from the ciliary arteries going to the choroid. This means that there can be non-perfusion of the optic disc capillaries with normal retinal circulation. When this happens the optic disc becomes pale and swollen, ischaemic optic neuropathy.

Endothelial Incompetence

Retinal oedema is not easy to detect with an ophthalmoscope but with angiography fluorescein leaking out of capillaries and persisting within the retina or optic disc is readily seen and this indicates oedema.

When plasma leaks from faulty capillaries into the *deeper* part of the retina the larger molecules, especially lipids, are not reabsorbed so well by adjacent normal vessels and they persist as visible *hard exudates*.

With more severe capillary damage *retinal haemorrhages* occur. Red cells from the *deeper* capillaries are confined by the tight structure of the retina and are seen as round dot and blot haemorrhages. Red cells from the *superficial* capillaries lie between the axons and are seen as linear haemorrhages following the course of the nerve fibres.

In the *optic disc* when the capillaries leak, oedema contributes to the loss of transparency which obscures the disc margin and adds to the swelling of the disc. If red cells escape they tend to be arranged in lines parallel to the axons.

The different patterns which these components make in the various systemic disorders is well illustrated by the two common conditions of diabetic retinopathy and hypertensive retinopathy.

RETINAL RESPONSE TO DIABETES

	deep retinal capillaries	superficial retinal capillaries	optic disc capillaries
• capillary non-perfusion regional gradual regional focal widespread focal	microaneurysms	cotton wool spot neovascularization	neovascularization
• endothelial damage	hard exudate deep haemorrhage	retinal oedema	

RETINAL RESPONSE TO HYPERTENSION

	deep retinal capillaries	superficial retinal capillaries	optic disc capillaries
• capillary non-perfusion regional gradual regional focal widespread focal		cotton wool spot	
• endothelial damage	hard exudate	retinal oedema superficial haemorrhage	disc oedema

DIABETIC RETINAL CHANGES

In countries with a high standard of living diabetes results in more blindness than any other systemic condition. Even so, only about one diabetic in forty is blind. On the other hand seventy per cent of diabetics have some degree of retinopathy by the time they die.

The occurrence of retinopathy is related to both the duration and the control of the diabetes. The average interval from the time of detection of the diabetes to serious visual handicap (vision less than 6/60) is 20 years for those with insulin dependent diabetes mellitus (IDDM) or juvenile onset diabetes, and 15 years for those with non-insulin dependent diabetes mellitus (NIDDM) or maturity onset diabetes. On balance the evidence suggests that good control delays the onset of retinopathy, especially in younger patients, but has less effect in retarding the progress of established retinopathy. The occurrence and progression of retinopathy are not related to the severity of the metabolic upset.

It is probable that the retinopathy is part of the generalized microangiopathy caused by the metabolic abnormality of diabetes and that the peculiarities of the retinal circulation determine the form that the angiopathy takes in the retina.

Fundus Picture

Diabetic retinal changes are sufficiently characteristic for most cases to be diagnosed with an ophthalmoscope. The basic picture consists of various combinations of microaneurysms, dot and blot haemorrhages, and hard exudates, with later changes in the retinal arteries and veins and, in some, neovascularization. But within this recognizable family likeness diabetic retinopathy varies greatly. In different individuals the component lesions in the fundus occur in different mixtures and progress at different rates to different endings. Progression is very variable. For long periods there may be no progression and occasionally there is regression of the lesions.

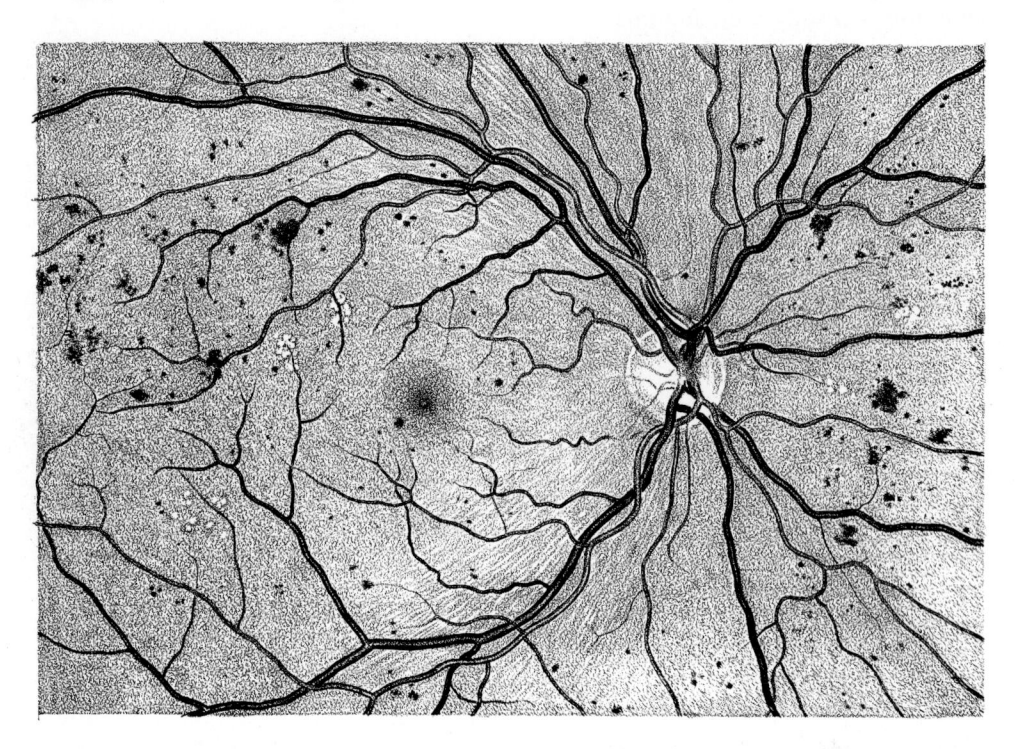

Fig 7-1 Non-proliferative diabetic retinopathy in the right eye of a 38 year old man diabetic for 20 years. There are many microaneurysms and dot and blot haemorrhages, but few hard exudates. The larger retinal vessels are normal.

DIABETIC RETINOPATHY

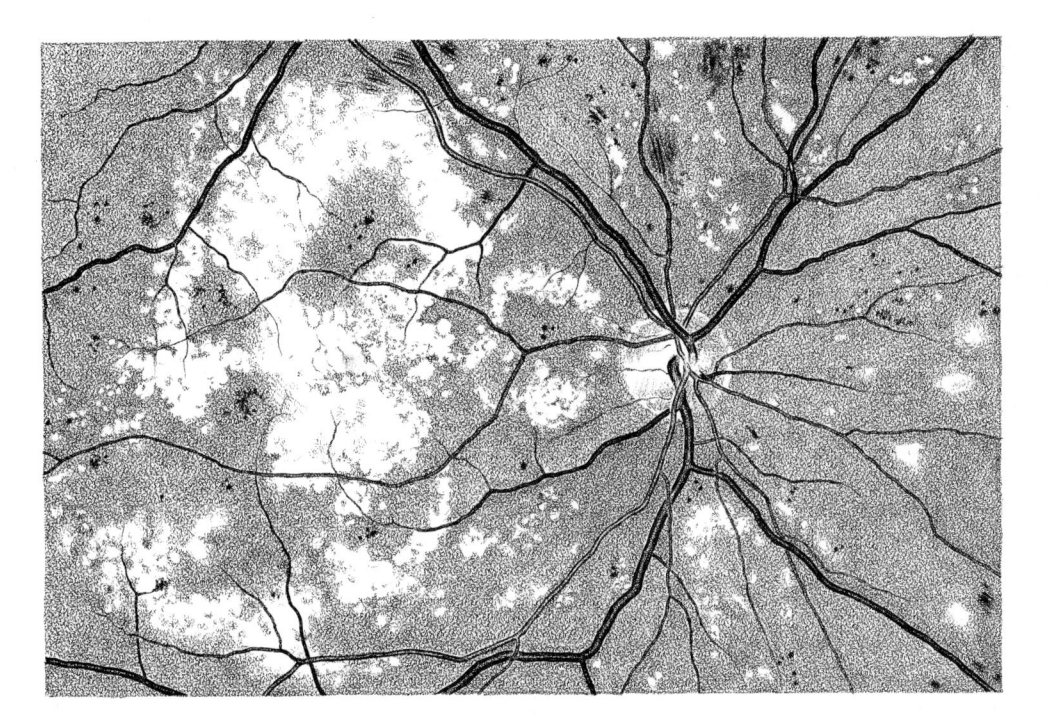

Fig 7-2 Non-proliferative diabetic retinopathy in which there are many hard exudates, some deep and superficial haemorrhages, and a few soft exudates. Some confluent hard exudates form rings or plaques. Right eye of 56 year old man not known to be diabetic until he presented with reduced vision and this diagnostic ophthalmoscopic appearance.

This variability makes evaluation of any treatment very difficult.

It is useful to subdivide diabetic retinopathy into non-proliferative and proliferative retinopathy. Very broadly there is the tendency for *non-proliferative retinopathy* to evolve into two types, either a 'wet', mainly haemorrhagic (Fig 7-1), or a 'dry', mainly exudative (Fig 7-2). The latter is more common in older patients with NIDDM.

Proliferative retinopathy is a separate entity in which there is neovascularization and its consequences (Fig 7-3; Plate 14, p. 127). It occurs in a small proportion of both long-standing juvenile-onset diabetics, who may have only slight non-proliferative retinopathy or rarely even no preceding retinopathy, and in older diabetics with established non-proliferative retinopathy.

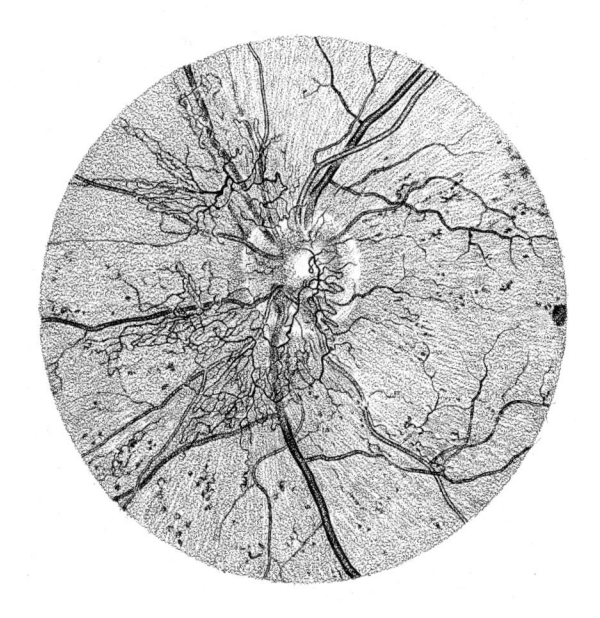

Fig 7-3 Proliferative diabetic retinopathy. A meshwork of new-formed vessels arises from the region of the optic disc in the left eye of 27 year old woman diabetic for 10 years.

CHANGES WHICH IN VARIOUS COMBINATIONS MAKE UP DIABETIC RETINOPATHY

- Microaneurysms
- Capillary dilatation and irregularity
- Dot and blot haemorrhages
- Hard exudates

- Soft exudates
- Retinal oedema
- Retinal atrophy
- Venous abnormalities
- Arterial abnormalities

- Neovascularization
  - intra-retinal
  - pre-retinal
- Pre-retinal and vitreous haemorrhages
- Fibrous proliferation
- Scarring
  - retinal detachment
  - retinal fibrosis

Microaneurysms are usually the earliest change which can be seen with the ophthalmoscope. It is easy to overlook them if an attempt is made to look at the fundus without previously dilating the subject's pupils. Microaneurysms are seen as small, round dots which may be either a pale arterial or a dark venous red colour (Fig 7-4; Plate 14, p. 127). They occur anywhere in the posterior part of the retina.

Capillary dilatation and irregularity is not so easy to see but is mentioned because it is one of the basic changes. Diabetic retinopathy starts in the retinal capillaries. Normal retinal capillaries are too small to be seen with the ophthalmoscope but it requires only a slight enlargement of these vessels for them to become visible. With a fully dilated pupil, a good ophthalmoscope, and preferably one with a green (red-free) filter, it is often possible to see some areas in the fundus of diabetics in which the capillaries are visible and are therefore dilated. They are often irregular also (Fig 7-4). Some refer to these intra-retinal microvascular abnormalities by their acronym, IRMA.

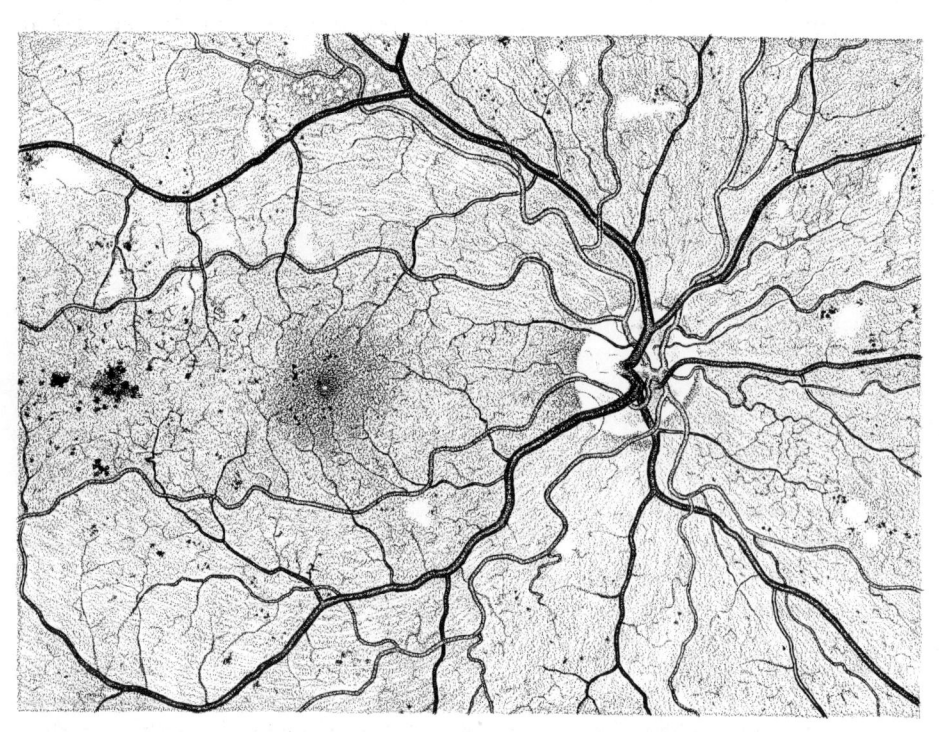

Fig 7-4 Patches of enlarged irregular capillaries, microaneurysms, a few haemorrhages, and soft exudates in the right eye of a 29 year old man diabetic for 21 years.

Dot and blot haemorrhages are deep in the retina and are characteristic of diabetic retinopathy. It is difficult to distinguish small ones from microaneurysms (Fig 7-4). They tend to be dark and are more irregular and last for a shorter time than microaneurysms.

Hard exudates are cream or yellow flecks which may be discrete or confluent. When confluent they may be in the form of incomplete rings, patches or large plaques (Figs 7-1, 7-2). Like dot and blot haemorrhages they are deep in the retina.

Soft exudates, or cotton wool spots, occur in a number of diabetics who are not hypertensive. They are commonly faint grey rather than white and last longer than soft exudates in other conditions (Fig 7-4).

Retinal oedema, especially macular oedema, is a fairly common cause of reduced vision in diabetics. Diabetic maculopathy is not easy to detect with ordinary ophthalmoscopy, does not show well in retinal photographs but is readily seen in fluorescein angiograms.

Retinal atrophy occurs as a result of ischaemia in some burnt out retinopathies.

Venous abnormalities are characteristic but appear late in the retinopathy. It is a long held opinion that dilatation of the veins is an early sign of diabetic retinopathy. However, this is so difficult to detect clinically that it should be disregarded. But there is no mistaking irregularity of calibre and some more rare bizarre loops and aneurysms which form on the retinal veins in the later stages of established retinopathy. Sheathing of the veins, which is due to opacification of their walls, is also a late change. The incidence of both branch and central retinal vein occlusions is higher in diabetics. Indeed when this occurs in any patient it is an indication for investigation of possible diabetes.

Arterial abnormalities which can be seen with the ophthalmoscope are not an early feature of diabetic retinopathy. This is one of the major differences between diabetic and hypertensive retinopathy. In the later stages of diabetic retinopathy irregularity of calibre, AV crossing changes, and sheathing usually appear.

Neovascularization may be either within the retina (intra-retinal) or in front of the retina in the vitreous (pre-retinal).

The new-formed small vessels in or on the retina when they first appear cannot be distinguished with the ophthalmoscope from irregularly dilated capillaries. As they grow they form loops and arcades which are obviously new-formed. These vessels have an abnormally increased permeability which allows plasma to leak into the tissues and is responsible for the occurrence of retinal oedema, exudates, and haemorrhages.

Pre-retinal new-formed vessels are drawn forwards as a result of shrinkage of the vitreous and form vascular network arcades or long loops. They arise most commonly from along the main retinal veins and from the optic disc (Figs 6-20, 7-3).

Pre-retinal and vitreous haemorrhages come from the new-formed vessels which are abnormally fragile.

Fibrous tissue proliferation always occurs around the new-formed vessels. At first filmy and hard to detect, it later becomes quite dense and eventually strangles the new-formed vessels which become atrophic (Fig 6-21).

Scarring of the fibrous tissue may result in traction bands across the retina, retinal detachment and disorganization, and choroidoretinal fibrosis and atrophy. An average time span from the appearance of new-formed vessels to the final, scarred, atrophic stage is about 5 years.

Fluorescein Angiography

Diabetic retinopathy is one of the most important indications for fluorescein angiography because this technique makes it possible to see retinal capillaries, and diabetic retinopathy is primarily a micro-angiopathy. It will demonstrate a change in function, in the form of an abnormal increase in permeability, as well as changes in structure of the retinal capillaries.

Focal areas of *capillary closure* show as small areas of darkness in the retinal capillary pattern. This is possibly the earliest lesion in diabetic retinopathy (Fig 7-5).

Capillary irregularity and dilatation are much more readily seen in fluorescein angiograms than they are with an ophthalmoscope. The capillary network appears coarser with dilated capillaries. They are often associated with microaneurysms. A patch of irregular capillaries with microaneurysms, is commonly found more or less centrally within a ring of hard exudates.

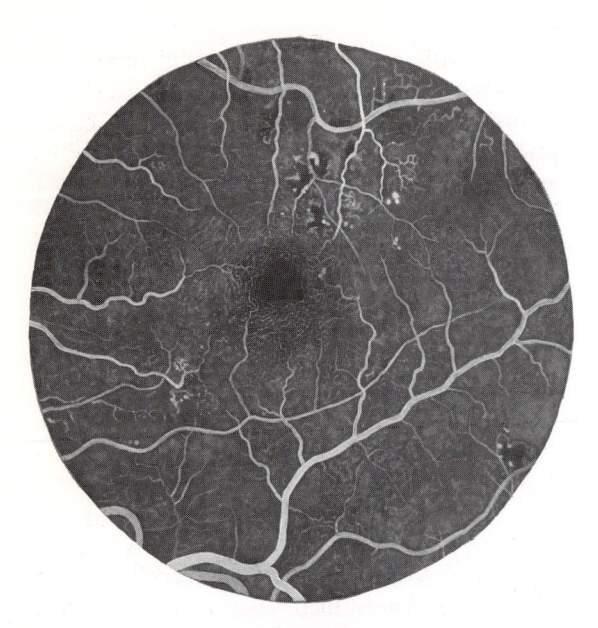

Fig 7-5 Foci of retinal capillary closure, irregular dilatation, and microaneurysms seen in a fluorescein angiogram of the left eye of a 65 year old man who was found to be diabetic when he presented with failing vision.

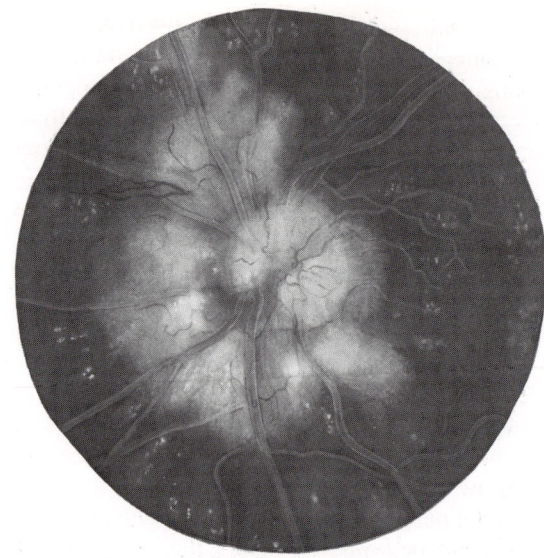

Fig 7-6 Fluorescein angiogram of the eye shown in Fig 7-3, taken some minutes after the injection of fluorescein, shows persisting diffuse fluorescence over and around the optic disc due to leakage of fluorescein from the new-formed vessels. The small fluorescent spots indicate foci of retinal capillary abnormality.

Microaneurysms appear as fluorescent dots anywhere in the area posterior to the equator of the eye (Fig 7-5). They are usually much more numerous than can be seen on ophthalmoscopy. (Colloid bodies also fluoresce, but these can be distinguished from microaneurysms because the former fluoresce much sooner after the injection of fluorescein than do the latter.) Most of the microaneurysms are about 15 to 50 μm in diameter, but some of the large ones can reach a diameter of about 100 μm.

Abnormal capillary permeability is responsible for hard exudates, the exudates being composed of the larger lipid molecules from the plasma which are not readily absorbed by adjacent normal vessels.

Leakage of fluorescein occurs from some microaneurysms, some dilated capillaries and all new-formed vessels (Fig 7-6).

When macular oedema occurs as a result of abnormal capillary permeability there is a slow, characteristic pattern of fluorescein accumulation at the macula which persists for some hours after the intravenous injection of fluorescein. This more certain evidence of oedema has shown it to be unexpectedly common in diabetic retinopathy.

New vessels are wider and more convoluted than are normal capillaries. They leak fluorescein profusely.

Haemorrhages do not fluoresce but, because they absorb the fluorescence from the capillaries, they appear as dark areas.

Hard exudates do not fluoresce and the capillaries can be seen fluorescing in front of them. As previously mentioned they are usually seen to be associated with abnormal leaking capillaries.

Changes Which Destroy Sight

Although loss of vision is the only thing that matters to the patient, function of the eye is not a good guide to the overall severity of the retinopathy. Whether poor vision occurs early or late in the disease is often an accident, in the sense that a lesion such as an exudate may happen to affect the macula rather than some other part of the retina, or that a pre-retinal haemorrhage breaks through into the vitreous to become a vitreous haemorrhage.

There are five principal causes of visual loss. The first three occur mainly in non-proliferative retinopathy and the last two occur mainly in proliferative retinopathy.

Hard exudates cause irreversible loss. Therefore the only treatment which could be effective would be one which prevented their occurrence.

Retinal oedema is at first reversible without any permanent loss of vision resulting. However, if oedema of the macula persists for longer than some months permanent loss of vision is inescapable.

Retinal atrophy is an irreversible end stage of burnt out retinopathy which results from closure of much of the fine vasculature of the retina.

Haemorrhages, if pre-retinal, absorb within a matter of some weeks, whereas vitreous haemorrhages take months and sometimes years to absorb. Pre-retinal and vitreous haemorrhages are likely to recur. They produce changes in the vitreous which cause it to shrink away from the retina.

Retinal detachment results from contraction of the fibrous component of proliferative retinopathy and usually progresses to ultimate total loss of vision.

Detection and Assessment

Because of the diverse natural history of diabetic retinopathy its onset and progression cannot be surely predicted. Treatment, when needed, should be given before the patient has any visual symptoms. It follows that diabetic retinopathy must be found and followed by regular examinations of diabetic patients' eyes.

As a guide for physicians who treat diabetics, it is suggested that, from five to eight years after diagnosis for those with IDDM and on diagnosis for those with NIDDM, at least once a year each patient's visual acuity should be recorded and his or her fundi examined with an ophthalmoscope through dilated pupils. In addition to this minimal assessment, some patients should have retinal photography at regular intervals. An alternative to routine ophthalmoscopy is to have standardized retinal photographic surveys taken with a red-free filter on black-and-white film. If desired an ophthalmologist can assess the photographs and advise which patients should be referred for ophthalmic examination and when each of the other patients should next be photographed. In any case, physicians and ophthalmologists obviously need to work together.

Management

Many regimes and treatments have been advocated for diabetic retinopathy but the evidence is strong only for the value of meticulous metabolic control and for photocoagulation. Randomized controlled trials of blood sugar levels are ethically not possible, but multicentre trials have confirmed the effectiveness of photocoagulation.

Good metabolic control delays by years the onset and probably the progression of retinopathy (Fig 7-7). The evidence has been conflicting, in part because of the difficulties in assessing the precision of blood sugar control. Some would claim that ideal control cannot be obtained with intermittent administration of insulin. Certainly for a number of patients the desired control can be achieved only with twice or thrice daily injections of insulin combined with an appropriate diet. Most patients control their blood sugar levels better when they directly test their own capillary blood glucose than when they have to estimate their insulin dosage from the more historical information provided by urine tests. Good control has its greatest effect and is therefore most important in the first years after diabetes is diagnosed.

Photocoagulation, in which a minute spot of high intensity light from a xenon arc or an argon laser is directed through an ophthalmoscopic or slit-lamp and contact lens system on to selected areas of the fundus, is used

to prevent and treat diabetic maculopathy by destroying the foci of vascular abnormality which are giving rise to macular oedema (provided they are not too close to the fovea);

to destroy the leaking vascular abnormality at

the centre of a large ring of hard exudate;

to destroy directly isolated patches of pre-retinal new vessels;

to indirectly cause regression of any new vessels which grow from the optic disc or of extensive pre-retinal neovascularization. This is achieved by what is called 'pattern bombing' or 'pan-retinal ablation' in which several hundred separate small burns are made in the fundus outside the area embraced by the optic disc and the upper and lower temporal vessel arcades. This destructive approach is based on the hypothesis that something which diffuses from inadequately perfused retina which is 'sick but not dead' is the stimulus for neovascularization.

Vitrectomy can help in selected cases of advanced diabetic retinopathy. In these procedures, performed with microsurgical instruments and an operating microscope, persistently opaque vitreous following vitreous haemorrhage or fibrous bands and membranes which pull on the retina are painstakingly cut and removed from the interior of the eye.

HYPERTENSIVE RETINAL CHANGES

The retinal changes seen with an ophthalmoscope in severe hypertension commonly form a pattern which is recognizable and therefore diagnostic. The nature and extent of the changes correlate with the duration and severity of the hypertension. Some of the changes are reversed by the reduction of the blood pressure to normal levels with treatment.

It follows that ophthalmoscopy has a role in hypertension and it may be of value in the following four ways. Hypertensive retinal changes may lead to the diagnosis of hypertension, past or present. They are of help in assessing the vascular damage caused by hypertension in a particular patient and thereby in estimating the patient's general prognosis and in deciding on the need for hypotensive treatment. They are a guide as to the adequacy of the treatment of a hypertensive patient. Additionally, ophthalmoscopy gives insights into the pathology of hypertension.

Hypertensive retinal changes may be confined to the retinal arteries — hypertensive vessel changes — or they may also involve the fundus background — hypertensive retinopathy.

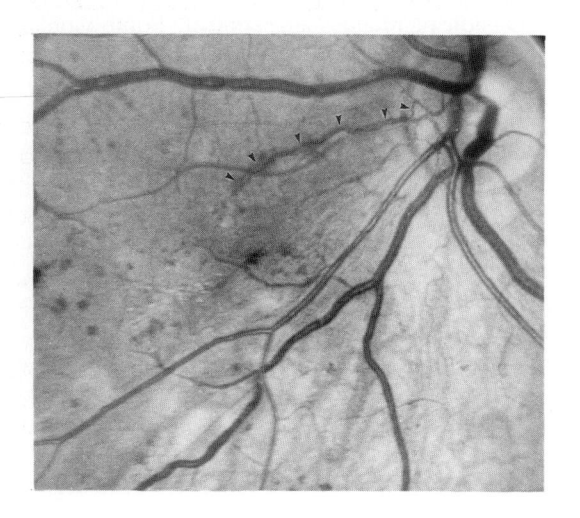

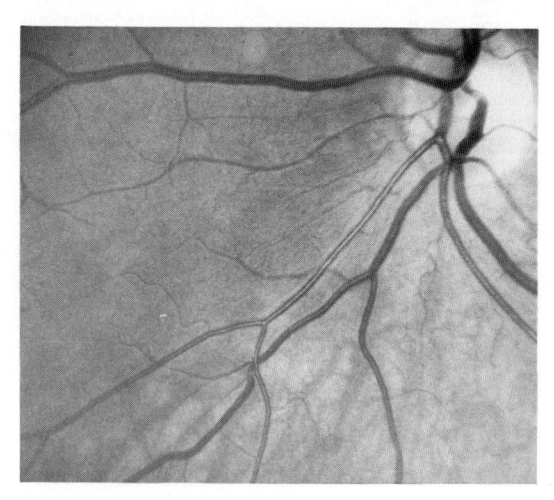

Fig 7-7 Red-free black and white photographs of an inferonasal part of the left fundus of a woman who had been diabetic since the age of three. The **left** photograph, taken when she was 23 and metabolic control was poor, show numerous microaneurysms and deep haemorrhages, a few flecks of hard exudate, beading irregularity of calibre of the main veins, and a leash of new-formed vessels (▲) arising from the optic disc. In the **right** photograph, taken two years later after metabolic control had been consistently good, there is an almost complete resolution of these abnormalities. A further ten years later the only evidence of diabetic retinopathy is a few scattered microaneurysms.

Hypertensive Vessel Changes

Many arterial abnormalities have been attributed to hypertension in the past 75 years. They include generalized and localized narrowing, AV crossing changes (venous nipping, concealment, deviation, and banking), alterations in the brightness of the arterial light reflex (copper wire and silver wire vessels), increased or reduced arterial tortuosity, and alterations in the angle of arterial branching. But some of these changes are difficult or impossible to assess clinically or they may occur as a result of ageing without hypertension. They are therefore of little clinical value and are best ignored (p. 137).

The vessel changes which can be assessed and which usually signify hypertensive damage are

definite irregularity of arterial calibre in more than two arteries,

definite AV crossing changes at more than two crossings,

and obvious generalized narrowing of arteries in a young person.

Segmental arterial narrowing when marked signifies that the diastolic blood pressure is or has been greater than 120mm Hg. Generalized AV crossing changes probably signify moderate hypertension of long duration, e.g. 10 years plus (Fig 7-8).

It should be emphasized that, while segmental narrowing and generalized AV crossing changes signify present or previous hypertension, their absence is of no significance. Many hypertensive patients do not develop these changes. Possibly as many as two-thirds of hypertensive patients (BP greater than 160/100mm Hg) do not develop irregularity of calibre and more than a half do not show AV crossing changes.

The generalized narrowing of arteries in young patients with abruptly increased blood pressure, e.g. renal disease, toxaemia of pregnancy, is reversible if the blood pressure is therapeutically returned to normal. In the majority of cases localized narrowing and AV crossing changes are permanent and not influenced by treatment. However a few photographically documented examples of dilatation of narrowed segments following treatment have been seen (Fig 7-9). It is probable that in older people hypertension results in dilatation of the larger and constriction of the smaller retinal vessels. This is based on photographic evidence of the reverse changes in calibre having occurred with lowering of the pressure.

The Keith, Wagener and Barker prognostic classification of hypertensive retinal changes should be discarded because their group I is undiagnosible, and groups I and II do not distinguish hypertensive and involutional vessel changes. Further, a few haemorrhages or a few hard exudates in older people may not mean dangerous hypertension (group III). On the other hand, it is still true that soft exudates are of serious significance and that papilloedema, or macular oedema causing reduced vision, are of sinister significance (group IV).

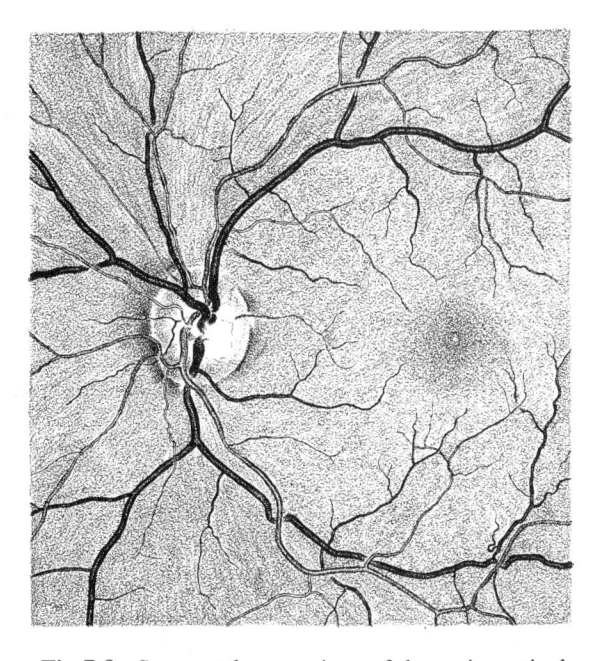

Fig 7-8 Segmental narrowings of the major retinal arteries and narrowing of some terminal branches in the left retina of a 49 year old man with treated hypertension. At two inferotemporal AV crossings there is deviation of the vein and at two superior AV crossings there is concealment of the vein.

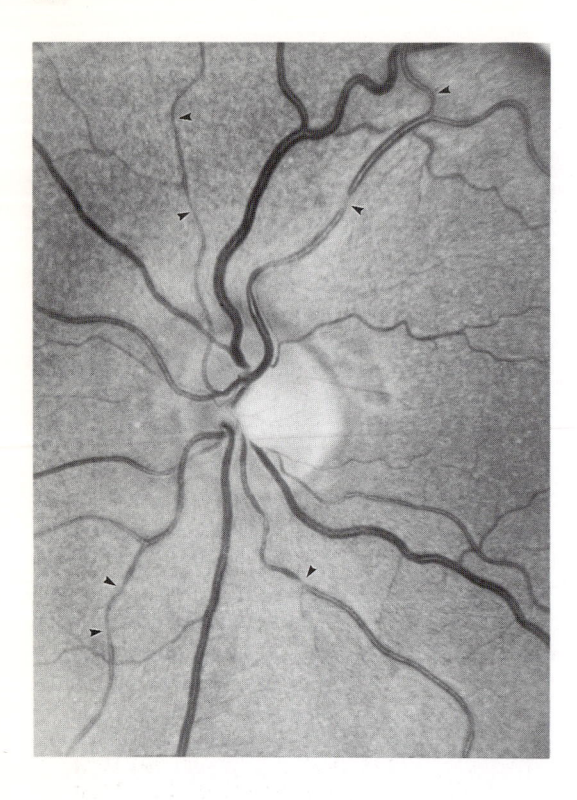

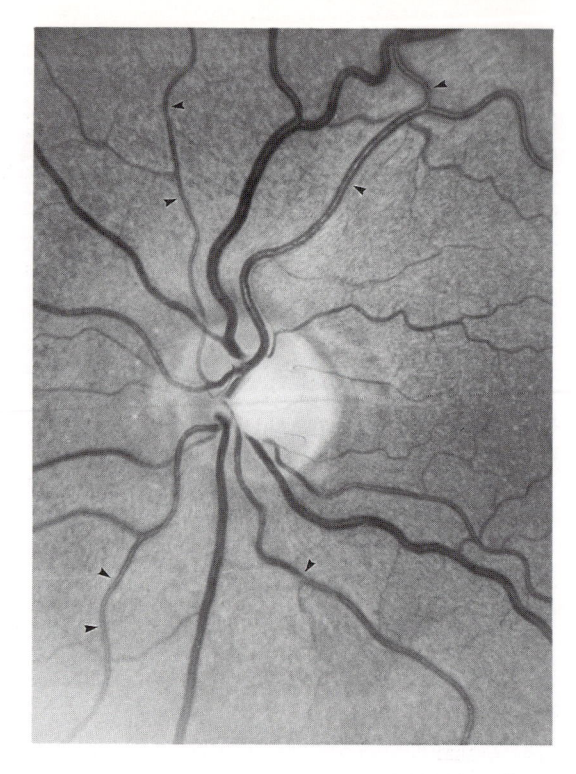

Fig 7-9 The **left** red-free black and white retinal photograph was taken when a 51 year old woman was discovered to have high blood pressure. The retinal arteries are locally narrowed in many places (▲). In the **right** photograph taken five years later after adequate treatment of her hypertension there is very little irregularity of arterial calibre.

Hypertensive Retinopathy

The changes in the fundus background and optic disc which constitute hypertensive retinopathy are haemorrhages, soft exudates, hard exudates, and, in the most severe form of retinopathy, papill-oedema and retinal oedema (Fig 7-10; Plate 13, p. 127). Retinopathy is evidence of accelerated hypertension and is therefore seen in middle rather than old age.

Haemorrhages, which are characteristically superficial, usually signify hypertensive damage which requires treatment, but in older people with systolic hypertension only and prominent vessel changes a few haemorrhages do not necessarily mean that the hypertension is severe enough to require treatment. With adequate treatment of the hypertension haemorrhages clear within three months (Fig 7-11).

Cotton wool spots are always of serious significance. With correct management they disappear in one to three months and do not recur.

Hard exudates in hypertensive retinopathy are oedema residues and may increase for a few weeks as retinal oedema subsides with treatment. They are discrete white flecks which occur between disc and macula (where they may form a macular fan), in the radial spoke-like pattern of a macular star, and nasal to the optic disc (Fig 7-12). On the other hand a few hard exudates and no other changes in an older patient may not mean dangerous hypertension. Surprisingly and in contrast to diabetic hard exudates at the macula,

HYPERTENSIVE RETINOPATHY

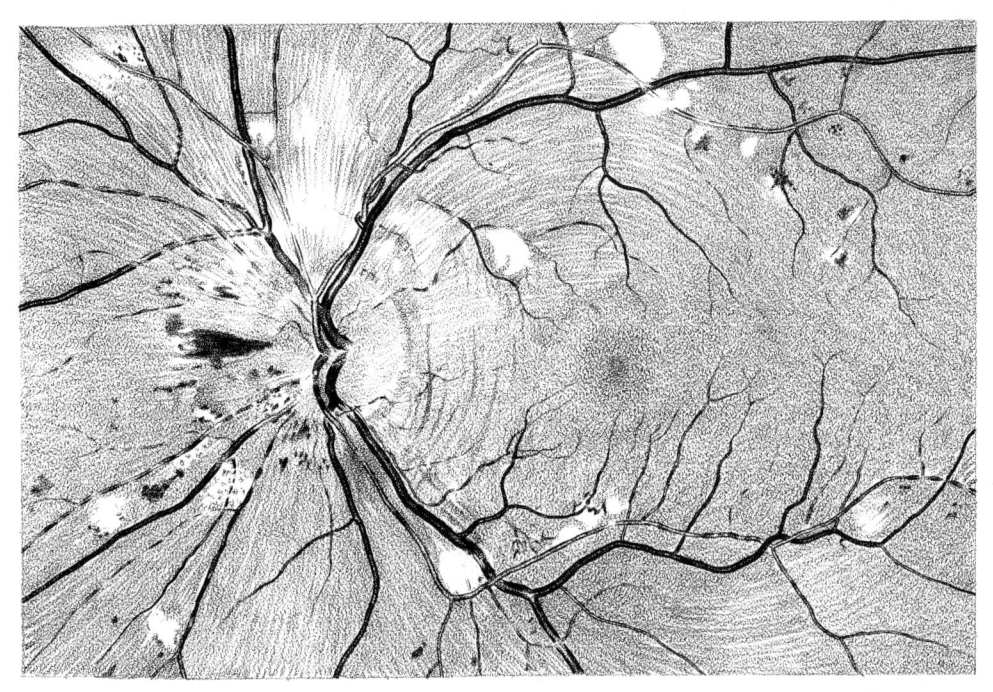

Fig 7-10 Severe hypertensive retinopathy in a 45 year old man who presented because of blurred vision. The retinal vessels are obscured in places by retinal oedema and by soft exudates. There are also focal narrowings of the arteries. The inferior temporal vein is slightly displaced by a large soft exudate. Most of the scattered haemorrhages are superficial. There is disc oedema; the swollen disc has wrinkled the retina on its temporal side into visible concentric lines.

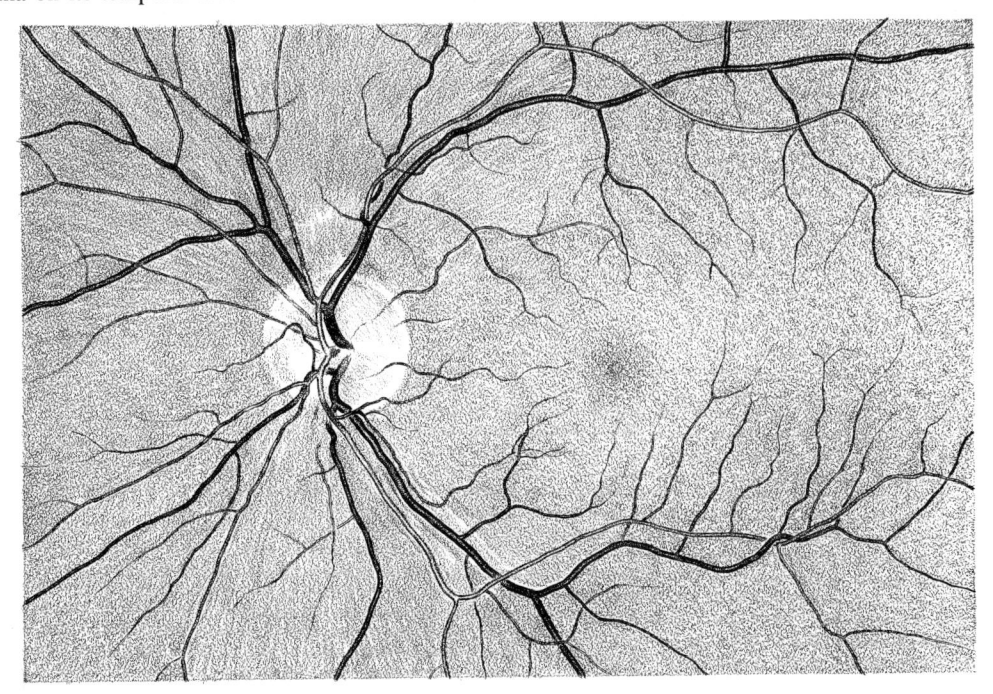

Fig 7-11 Complete resolution of the retinopathy pictured in Fig 7-10 after hypotensive treatment. In this patient there is unusually little residual irregularity of calibre of the retinal arteries.

a macular fan or star does not permanently damage central vision. With effective treatment they take from six to twelve months to disappear.

Oedema of the optic disc or of the retina or of both has the most sinister general significance. When due to hypertension it is associated with hypertensive vessel changes. With adequate treatment the papilloedema resolves within one to three months. With inadequate treatment it may result in permanent loss of vision.

Associated Retinal Vascular Abnormalities
Central retinal vein and branch vein occlusions are more common in eyes whose vessels have been damaged by hypertension (p. 217). About two-thirds of the patients who suffer a retinal venous occlusion are hypertensive. Retinal artery occlusions also occur with greater frequency in hypertensive than in normotensive people (p. 216).

It is these associated retinal disasters which constitute the major threat to vision in hypertension. Loss of vision due to macular oedema in a severe retinopathy may lead to the discovery of hypertension, but if treatment is adequate permanent loss of sight from hypertensive retinopathy should not occur. The major role of ophthalmoscopy in hypertension is not so much to save sight as to contribute an essential ingredient to the management of the patient's general condition.

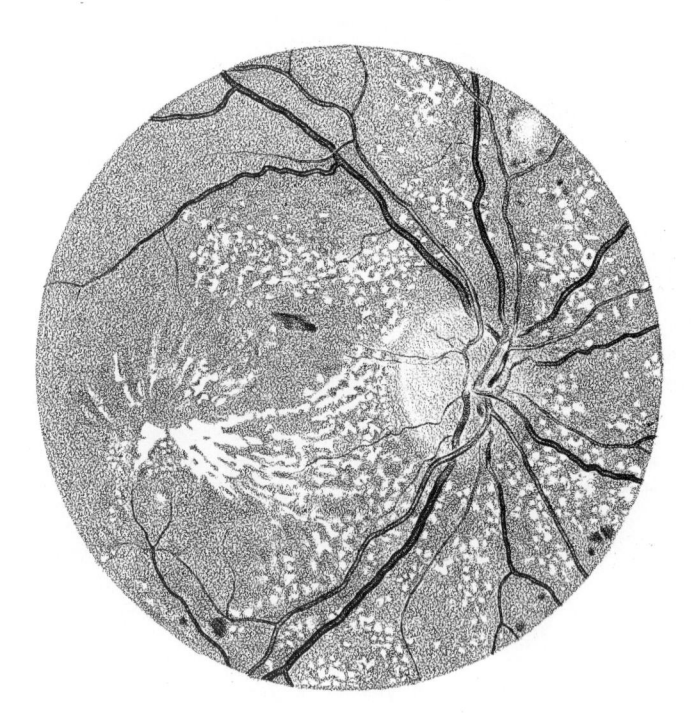

Fig 7-12 Hard exudates forming a macular star in a patient with long-standing untreated hypertension.

Chapter 8

OPTIC DISC OEDEMA AND OPTIC ATROPHY

Optic disc oedema
  Papilloedema, papillitis, and
    pseudopapilloedema
  Ophthalmoscopic features
  Causes
  Pathogenesis
  Fluorescein angiography

Optic atrophy
  Colour of optic disc
  Ophthalmoscopic features
  Visual function impairment
  Causes

OPTIC DISC OEDEMA

The words papilloedema and disc oedema have come to be used in different ways by different people and so it is necessary to define one's usage of these terms.

Oedema of the optic disc or *disc oedema* is a swelling of the disc associated with an abnormal accumulation of fluid. These synonymous terms embrace all types of pathological swelling of the optic disc.

Papilloedema includes all forms of disc oedema other than papillitis, that is it is applied to non-inflammatory swellings of the disc. The literal meaning of papilloedema is disc oedema, the component 'papill-' being derived from the old anatomical term for the optic disc of optic papilla. An occasionally used term for oedema due to raised intracranial pressure is plerocephalic papilloedema.

Papillitis is disc oedema due to optic neuritis. The ophthalmoscopic appearances of papilloedema and papillitis are the same; the distinction has to be made on the invariable loss of function in papillitis.

Pseudopapilloedema is a non-pathological elevation of the optic disc due to variations of normal anatomy or to buried drusen (Fig 8-1; Plate 5, p. 123). *Drusen* are glistening rounded tapioca-like bodies composed of concentric layers of hyaline material which occasionally form within the optic disc (Plate 5, p. 123). In children they are covered by disc tissue and are therefore not easily seen, but with time they show through the surface of the disc. The cause is not known; they may be familial and they interfere very little with function (cf. retinal drusen, p. 144).

(Some clinicians use the word papilloedema only for disc swelling due to raised intracranial pressure and for all forms of disc swelling other than papilloedema and papillitis they use the term disc oedema.)

Ophthalmoscopic Features

Fully developed papilloedema is easily recognized (Fig 8-2). The ophthalmoscopic picture is that of a disc enlarged both in height and in area with an absent or diminished cup, indistinct margins due to loss of translucency of the swollen disc tissue, and either hyperaemia (dilated retinal veins, visible disc capillaries, haemorrhages) or,

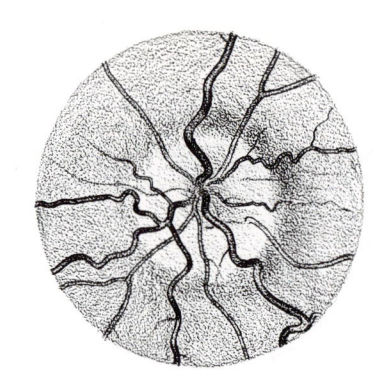

Fig 8-1 Pseudopapilloedema. The disc margin is obscured. A two dimensional drawing cannot show that the disc projects forwards; on altering the angle of view with an ophthalmoscope there would be parallactic movement of the elevated disc relative to the surrounding retina.

occasionally, pallor. On the other hand the differentiation of early papilloedema from pseudopapilloedema can be very difficult and may be impossible on ophthalmoscopic appearances alone.

The three principal changes of early papilloedema due to raised intracranial pressure are abnormal elevation, loss of translucency and, in a majority, hyperaemia of the optic disc (Fig 8-3).

One disc is commonly affected in advance of the other and therefore comparison of the two discs, which usually are similar in appearance, can be most helpful.

The *elevation* starts at the upper or lower poles of the disc, it may be slight and detectable only by eliciting parallactic movement, it spreads outwards into the surrounding retina before inwards into the physiological cup, and it may eventually have steep rather than sloping sides. Loss of the physiological cup is not necessarily an early change in papilloedema because the original size of the cup influences the time it takes to become filled in.

DISC OEDEMA

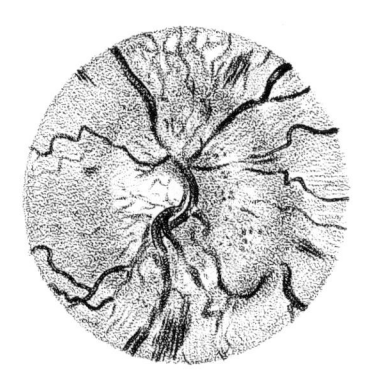

Fig 8-2 Papilloedema from raised intracranial pressure. The disc is swollen forwards and also outwards into the surrounding retina. The disc margin is completely hidden and in places retinal vessels are concealed, because oedema has impaired the translucency of the disc tissues. The retinal veins are congested and there are a few haemorrhages.

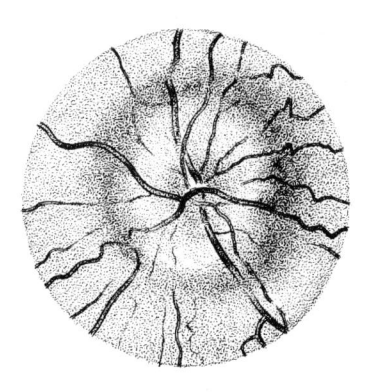

Fig 8-3 Early papilloedema. The vessels crossing the disc are obscured in places due to the loss of translucency of the prelaminar tissue in which they lie.

The *loss of translucency* of the prelaminar tissue of the disc has three effects. It more or less obscures the disc margin, it may make the disc look paler, and with high-magnification binocular instruments it makes visible the thin layer of nerve tissue which lies in front of portions of the major vessels (Plate 3, p. 122). Because partly obscured disc margins are common in normal eyes and the colour of discs varies greatly these two signs are not very helpful. But a buried appearance of portions of the vessels as they cross the disc is useful evidence of oedema.

Hyperaemia of the deeper capillaries may impart a general redness to the disc, but this is by no means invariably present because a mildly oedematous disc may be pale as a result of the reduced translucency masking the underlying hyperaemia. Hyperaemia of the surface radial papillary network may render these vessels individually visible. Visibility of the deeper vessels in the disc due to their tortuous dilatation, and engorgement of the larger retinal veins are not usually present when papilloedema begins. In general the severity of the vascular changes depends on the rate of onset of the papilloedema. When the onset is abrupt superficial haemorrhages may be present from the start but they usually appear later. Soft exudates on the disc and surrounding retina are also a late sign.

Pulsation of the retinal *veins* just before they leave the interior of the eye is a common normal appearance. It does not happen when the intracranial pressure is higher than about 200mm CSF and therefore when there is spontaneous pulsation of the retinal veins on the disc it is unlikely that there is papilloedema due to raised intracranial pressure (p. 15). Absence of venous pulsation is of no significance.

There are usually no *symptoms* directly attributable to papilloedema. Some patients experience transient obscurations of their vision especially on turning their head or eyes. In the first weeks the only functional change is enlargement of the blind spot. After some months of unrelieved papilloedema, secondary optic atrophy occurs and, if allowed to, this will eventually result in irreversible blindness. In papillitis visual function is always impaired, the greatest impact usually being on central vision.

Causes of Disc Oedema

In order of importance and frequency the causes of disc oedema are

Raised intracranial pressure
  Tumours
  Inflammation of brain and/or meninges — abscess, meningitis, encephalitis
  Haemorrhage — extradural, subarachnoid
  Benign intracranial hypertension
    dural sinus thrombosis
    in obese young women
    iron deficiency, low serum iron with or without anaemia
    hypoparathyroidism
    adrenal insufficiency, after systemic steroids in children
    after tetracyclines in children
    vitamin A intoxication
  Deficient cranial capacity, e.g. oxycephaly
Vascular hypertension
Optic neuritis
  Papillitis
  Retrobulbar neuritis
Ischaemic optic neuropathy
  Giant cell arteritis
  Atherosclerosis
Retinal vasculitis
Ciliary vasculitis, uveitis
Orbital lesions
  Thyroid disease
  Tumours and pseudotumours
  Optic nerve tumours
Miscellaneous
  Vascular disorders
    cavernous sinus thrombosis
    macroglobulinaemia
    polycythaemia
    following blood loss
  Chronic pulmonary insufficiency, Pickwickian syndrome
  Low intraocular pressure

About two-thirds of patients with cerebral *tumours* ultimately develop papilloedema. Disc oedema is earlier and more severe in posterior fossa tumours.

When due to *hypertension* papilloedema is associated with hypertensive vascular changes and usually other features of hypertensive retinopathy.

Optic neuritis is an inflammatory lesion of the optic nerve in which there are areas of nerve fibre demyelination surrounded by oedema. It is usually unilateral and presents as a sudden loss of vision. The extent of visual field loss ranges from a small central scotoma to bare perception of light. There is often pain on movement of the eye and tenderness on applying gentle pressure over the superior rectus tendon. The pupil reacts less well to direct light than to the same light shone into the other eye. This result of impairment of the afferent pupillary light reflex pathway is most readily detected by the swinging flashlight test (p. 106).

When optic neuritis involves the optic disc it is *papillitis* whereas involvement of the optic nerve behind the globe is called *retrobulbar neuritis*. In papillitis there is an active inflammatory oedema of the disc but the swelling is usually less than occurs in papilloedema (Plate 4, p. 122). In retrobulbar neuritis, if the patch of inflammation is close to the globe there is passive oedema of the disc, but when it is further posterior than the site of entry of the retinal vessels into the nerve there is no change in the disc, which looks normal. The situation is summed up by the old saying that in retrobulbar neuritis neither the patient nor the doctor sees anything.

Multiple sclerosis is the cause of about one-third of all cases of optic neuritis. In about one-fifth of patients with multiple sclerosis optic neuritis is the presenting symptom. Often optic neuritis is the only manifestation of multiple sclerosis; in the long-term probably about one-third of patients with optic neuritis will develop other manifestations of multiple sclerosis. Recovery of function within some weeks is usual in this type of optic neuritis. Optic atrophy may be a permanent legacy. Recurrences occur.

Other causes of optic neuritis include neuromyelitis optica (Devic's disease, in which, usually in children, there is a myelitis with bilateral optic neuritis from which good recovery can occur), encephalitis associated with measles, mumps, etc., and Leber's hereditary optic neuritis. This latter condition is a rare sex-linked (females transmit, males affected) hereditary condition with rapid onset about the age of 20 which results in permanent loss of central vision and optic atrophy.

Rarer causes are inflammation locally adjacent to the optic nerve in the orbit or nasal sinuses, diabetes, pernicious anaemia, and vitamin B deficiency.

Ischaemic optic neuropathy presents as a sudden loss of sight and manifests as a pallid disc oedema, perhaps with a few haemorrhages (Plate 12, p. 126). It results from impairment of blood flow in the posterior ciliary arteries which supply the optic disc due to giant cell arteritis or to atherosclerosis. Giant cell arteritis which affects old people is important because, although it is often bilateral, one eye is usually affected before the other and if recognized this gives time to prevent involvement of the second eye by urgent treatment with systemic corticosteroids. Loss of vision is commonly total and once it has occurred treatment is usually unavailing. Giant cell arteritis classically causes anorexia, loss of weight, head pains, and a painful, tender, firm, tortuous thickening of the superficial temporal arteries (hence the old name of temporal arteritis), but many patients do not have these symptoms or signs. The majority do have an elevated ESR and this, with an unexplained sudden uniocular vision loss, is sufficient grounds for starting treatment.

In *retinal vasculitis* there is an inflammation of the retinal veins which as well as a usually mild disc oedema causes engorgement of the affected veins and haemorrhages in their drainage territory. *Ciliary vasculitis* is a uveitis which happens to occur close to the disc. This is traditionally called juxtapapillary choroiditis (Fig 8-4). The appearance can superficially resemble papilloedema due to raised intracranial pressure, but the associated signs of a choroiditis and interference with visual function enable the distinction to be made.

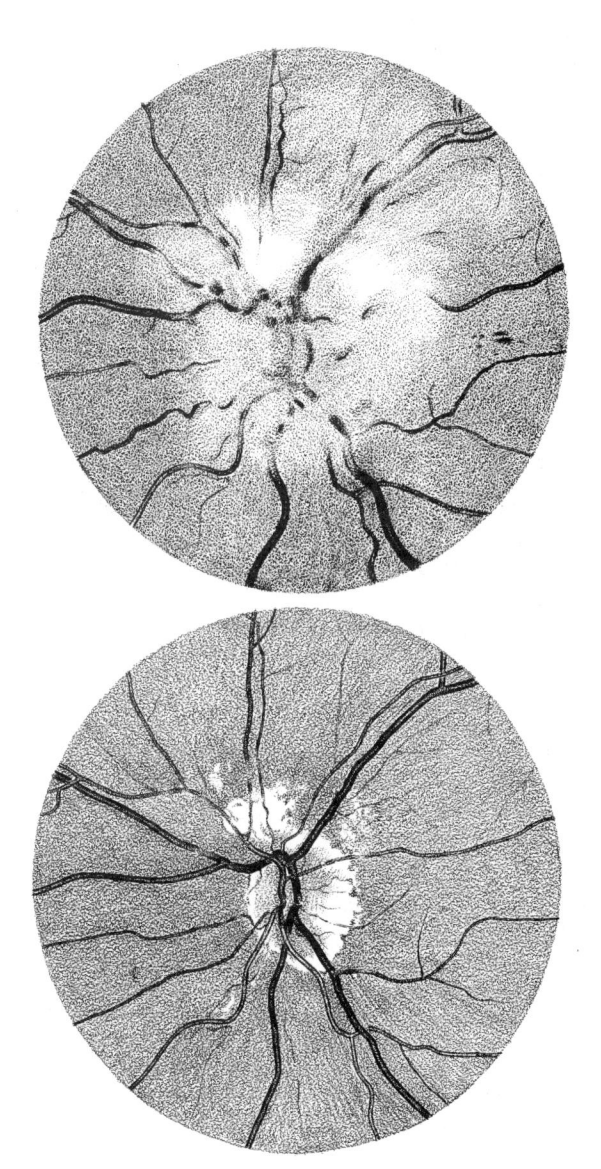

Fig 8-4 Upper Juxtapapillary choroiditis. Oedema of the disc caused by an adjacent focus of uveal inflammation.

Lower After the inflammation has subsided and the oedema has resolved the white patch of exposed sclera above the disc indicates where the inflammation was most severe and destroyed retina and choroid.

Pathogenesis

The pathophysiology of papilloedema due to raised intracranial pressure is not fully understood. The intracranial subarachnoid space normally extends within the dural sheath of the optic nerve to its distal end at the eye. The normal pressure relationship on either side of the lamina cribrosa is therefore an intraocular pressure of 15mm Hg and a CSF pressure of between 6 and 9mm Hg. A reversal of this difference, either by an increase in CSF pressure above about 15mm Hg or by a decrease in the intraocular pressure below a few mm Hg, can give rise to papilloedema. Surgical opening of the nerve sheath behind the globe leads to the resolution of established papilloedema due to raised intracranial pressure.

As the central retinal vein crosses the subarachnoid space it is exposed to the pressure within the nerve sheath and as this pressure increases so must the intravenous pressure also increase for blood flow to be maintained (Fig 1-16). This increase in retinal venous pressure above intraocular pressure is responsible for the loss of venous pulsation on the disc but not for the swelling of the disc as some once thought.

There is evidence that the raised CSF pressure within the optic nerve sheath by compressing the optic nerve blocks both fast and slow orthograde axoplasmic flow in the axons. These then individually swell where they are not supported by fibrous tissue, i.e. anterior to the lamina cribrosa, and collectively they cause swelling of the optic disc and peripapillary retina. In turn, the swollen nerve fibres compress the venules of the optic disc which dilate and leak fluid. At this stage there is true oedema with increased extracellular fluid. Flow in the central retinal vein is further impeded and the retinal veins are visibly engorged. Axons continue to conduct nerve impulses for a few months after the onset of stasis of axoplasmic flow. This is why optic nerve function is normal during this time.

This mechanism explains why papilloedema does not occur in an atrophic disc in which there is little or no axoplasmic flow to be obstructed. It also explains why fluorescein angiography may not help in making the differential diagnosis between early papilloedema and pseudopapilloedema.

Fluorescein Angiography

In fluorescein angiograms normal optic discs show an early faint fluorescence of the centre and a later venous phase fluorescence of the margins (Fig 8-5a). There is some normal leakage of fluorescein from optic disc capillaries because these are largely derived from the ciliary arteries and so there is a variable persisting fluorescence of normal optic discs after the transit of the injected fluorescein. But this is faint and confined to the optic disc.

In papilloedema the dilated capillaries show up during passage of the fluorescein and there is increased escape of fluorescein from the disc vessels (Fig 8-5b). This results in fluorescence spreading beyond the disc margin and in an increase in the intensity of the fluorescence for 15 to 30 minutes after the injection.

However in the initial stage of papilloedema, before the permeability of the disc capillaries is increased secondarily to compression of the venules by the swollen axons, there is no leakage of fluorescein and the angiogram is normal. In other words, a normal angiogram does not exclude disc oedema. This greatly lessens the value of angiography in just those cases in which the differential diagnosis is difficult.

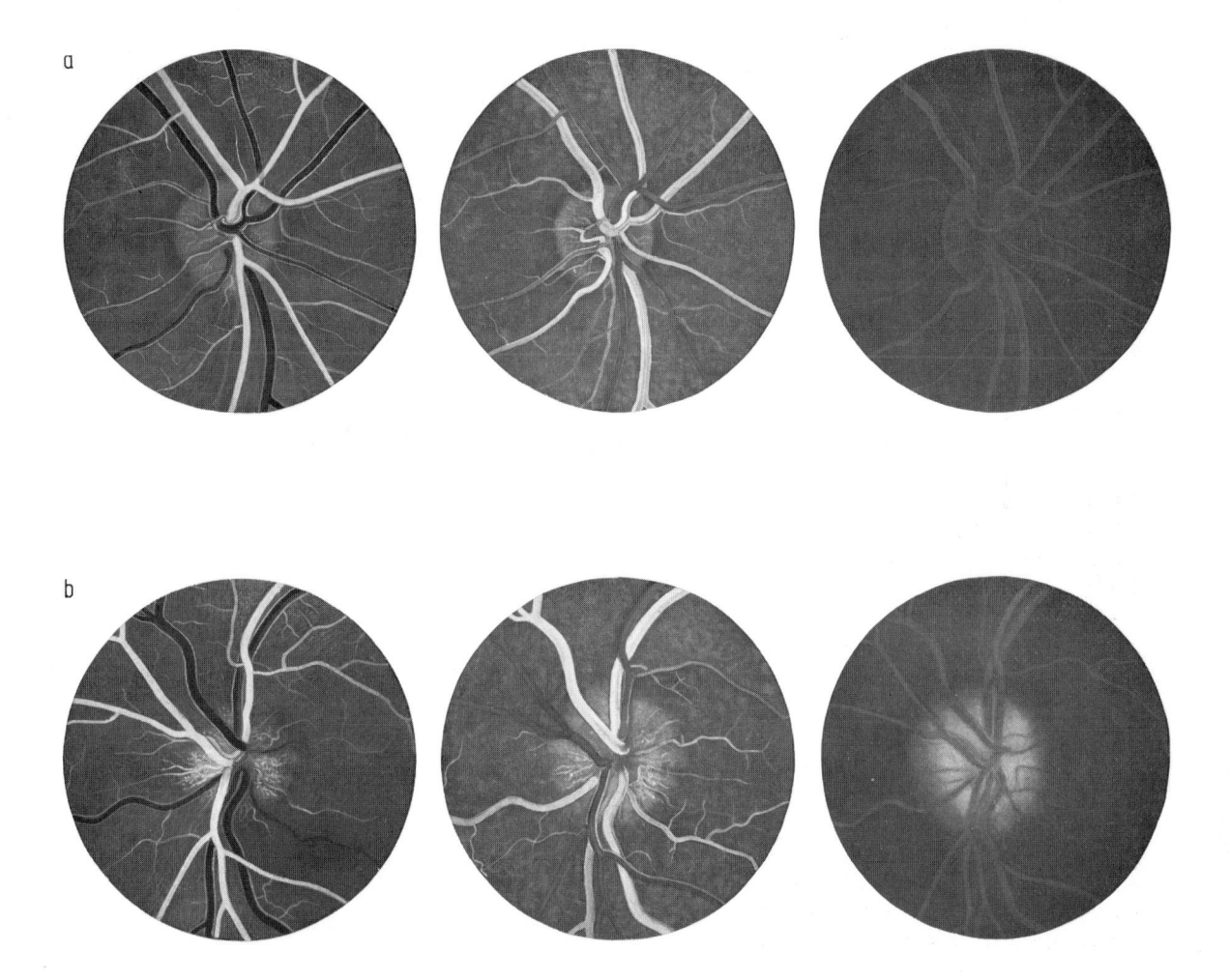

Fig 8-5 Fluorescein angiograms from a patient with unilateral early papilloedema.

    a Arterial, arteriovenous and late phases of the normal right disc.

    b Arterial, arteriovenous and late phases of the oedematous left disc.

In the arterial phase, the increased vascularity of the left disc is already apparent. In the arteriovenous phase, the fluorescence of the normal disc is fading, but that of the abnormal disc is increasing. In the late phase, fluorescein, which has leaked from the capillaries of the oedematous disc and spread into the adjacent retina, continues to fluoresce. There is faint fluorescence of the normal disc and recirculating diluted fluorescein dimly outlines the retinal vessels in both eyes.

OPTIC ATROPHY

Optic atrophy is a pathological partial or complete loss of nerve fibres and their myelin sheaths in the optic nerve with associated impairment of visual function. An ophthalmoscopic definition is pathological pallor of the optic disc.

The Colour of the Optic Disc
The colour of a disc is judged by the colour of the rim of nerve tissue peripheral to any cup which may be present and central to any scleral ring or crescent which may adjoin the disc.

The normal yellowish red colour varies from person to person. It is lighter than and lacks the dusky shade of the surrounding retina because there is no pigment comparable to the retinal pigment epithelium. Commonly the temporal part of a disc is paler than the nasal part. The optic disc is pale in infants.

Three layers contribute to the colour of the disc. They are (1) the opaque lamina cribrosa, (2) the translucent prelaminar layer of nerve fibres, with an ophthalmoscopically invisible plexus of capillaries among the nerve fibres, and (3) a radial network of capillaries on the surface. The prelaminar layer is a stiff red-tinged jelly overlying the lamina cribrosa and, where this layer is thinner, as over the floor of the physiological cup, the white lamina shows through as a paler area.

Pathological pallor is due to thinning of the nerve fibre layer, with reduction of its capillaries, or to opacification of this layer.

Ophthalmoscopic Features
The one constant feature is pallor of the optic disc (Fig 8-6). This may not parallel the severity of the atrophy. It may be limited to part only of the disc, for example, temporal pallor following optic neuritis. But remember that physiological temporal pallor is common.

A subtle pallor of one disc may be detected only by comparing the two discs which, unless there is a large difference in refractive errors, when normal almost always look the same. In infants one can be sure of optic atrophy only when pallor of the disc is marked.

When there is no other change in the appearance of the disc (primary optic atrophy) the disc margin is sharply defined.

If there is pathological cupping with the pallor it is glaucomatous optic atrophy. This is the commonest cause of optic atrophy.

When there is blurring of the disc margins with the pallor (secondary optic atrophy) this is the result of gliosis on the surface of the disc and adjacent retina which may follow prolonged disc oedema.

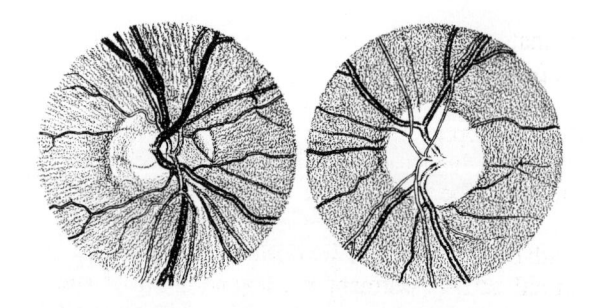

Fig 8-6 Optic discs of a patient with traumatic left optic atrophy. In the right eye the streaky pattern of nerve fibres converging on the normal optic disc can be detected. The left optic disc is white and flat, and the nerve fibre pattern is not seen in the surrounding retina.

Visual Function Impairment
There is always some loss of vision but this may be detected only by careful testing of the visual field.

Reduced central vision and a central scotoma occurs in optic neuritis and in toxic lesions, for example tobacco amblyopia. Reduced colour vision can be tested for with Ishihara or similar pseudo-isochromatic plates and this test of visual function is useful for comparing the two eyes when there is suspicious pallor of one disc.

Peripheral field defects occur in a variety of forms. An arcuate scotoma is characteristic of glaucoma, a ring scotoma of pigmentary retinal degeneration, a temporal field loss of a chiasmal lesion, and a peripheral contraction of neurosyphilis.

Causes of Optic Atrophy
Since the optic nerve fibres originate from the retinal ganglion cells and synapse in the lateral geniculate body any infrageniculate lesion of the visual pathway can cause optic atrophy. It is most practical to classify causes of optic atrophy on

an anatomical basis and consider the pathway in six parts, namely retina, optic disc, optic nerve in the orbit, optic nerve in the optic canal, chiasma, optic tract. The atrophy is ascending when it is due to a retinal lesion and descending when it is due to a lesion in one of the other sites.

Examples of *retinal* lesions which can cause death of ganglion cells are occlusion of the central retinal artery, pigmentary degeneration of the retina, extensive choroido-retinitis, and poisoning with lead, methyl alcohol, quinine, and tobacco.

The *optic disc* is the part of the eye most vulnerable to the raised intraocular pressure of primary, secondary, or congenital glaucoma which, if untreated, will result in optic atrophy. Long-continued papilloedema will eventually cause secondary optic atrophy and atrophy is usual after papillitis and ischaemic optic neuropathy.

The optic nerve can be affected in the *orbit* by various inflammatory lesions such as multiple sclerosis, Leber's disease, and syphilis, and lesions of uncertain mechanism such as diabetes, vitamin B deficiency, and pernicious anaemia, by compression from orbital tumours and pseudotumours and in thyroid exophthalmos, by trauma, and by intrinsic tumours such as an optic nerve glioma.

The *intracanalicular* part of the nerve can be compressed by bone disease, such as Paget's disease or craniostenosis, or following injury and fracture.

The *chiasma* with the intracranial part of the nerve is vulnerable to compression and/or stretching from a pituitary tumour, a craniopharyngioma, a meningioma, an intracranial aneurysm, or tuberculous meningitis, to rupture from injury, to stretching in congenital hydrocephalus, and to gliomatous infiltration.

The *suprachiasmal* optic tract is sometimes affected by a tumour of the basal ganglia or of the temporal lobe or by an adjacent cerebral abscess.

Chapter 9

GLAUCOMA

Definition and classification
Physiology of the intraocular pressure
Abnormally increased intraocular pressure
Angle closure glaucoma
   Sub-acute
   Acute
Open angle glaucoma
Congenital glaucoma

Definition and Classification

The word glaucoma is used for a group of ocular diseases with the common features of abnormally elevated intraocular pressure (IOP) and ultimate loss of vision if untreated. The conditions which share this label are diverse as is shown by the following simplified *clinical classification*.

   Primary glaucoma
      Angle closure (congestive)
         Sub-acute or chronic
         Acute
      Open angle (chronic simple)
   Secondary glaucoma
   Congenital glaucoma (buphthalmos)
   Low tension glaucoma
   Ocular hypertension

In *primary glaucoma* the abnormality of the eye which causes the increased IOP is not clinically obvious. In *secondary glaucoma* the IOP is secondary to recognizable local causes such as iritis, injury, occlusion of the central retinal vein, or the use of steroid eye-drops (p. 206; Plate 2, p. 121). The two principal types of primary glaucoma, angle closure and open angle, are quite dissimilar conditions with different aetiologies, symptoms, signs, and treatments. Open angle glaucoma is about ten times as common as angle closure glaucoma.

Glaucoma which occurs during the first three years of life is classified as *congenital glaucoma*.

The paradoxical label of *low tension glaucoma* is given to the condition in which there are the features of open angle glaucoma, such as pathological cupping of the optic disc and visual field loss, without an abnormally elevated IOP ever being detected. It is as if the eye had slowly succumbed to what are for most eyes normal levels of pressure.

The term *ocular hypertension* is applied to those eyes in which the IOP is elevated (commonly when it is consistently higher than 21mm Hg) but in which there is no other evidence of glaucoma such as pathological cupping of the optic disc or a glaucomatous field defect. This must always be a temporary diagnosis because some will be early cases of chronic glaucoma, but this will not become apparent until later when loss of vision can be detected.

Glaucoma is important because it is common, with a *prevalence* in the population over the age of 40 years of 1%, and because it destroys sight. Primary glaucoma is very rare in some races, e.g. Polynesians, but the reasons for this genetic difference are unknown.

Physiology of the IOP

The intraocular pressure is normally maintained by a controlled balance between the formation of aqueous within the eye and the drainage of aqueous from the eye. The aqueous is largely formed as a secretion of the ciliary processes and flows from the posterior chamber through the pupil into the anterior chamber (Fig 9-1). It leaves the interior of the eye through the trabecular meshwork in the angle of the anterior chamber to enter the canal of Schlemm and from this it seeps by way of a plexus of fine veins (collector channels) through the sclera into the episcleral veins. About 2.0 microlitres of aqueous, i.e. about one-tenth of the total volume of aqueous, flow from the eye per minute.

When estimated clinically the IOP is often called the ocular *tension* and this is determined by *tonometry* (p. 107). Indentation tonometers of the Schiotz type measure the indentation of the cornea produced by a given force. The scale reading on the instrument may be translated into mm Hg by reading from a conversion table. In applanation tonometry the force required to flatten a pre-determined area of the cornea is measured. This method is more accurate because it eliminates errors due to differences in the resistance to distension of the walls of different eyes (scleral rigidity).

The *normal range of IOP* can be expressed as a mean and standard deviation. It is 15 ± 3 mm Hg. In practice an IOP greater than 24mm Hg is regarded as being pathological, while pressures of 22, 23 and 24mm Hg are regarded as being suspicious of glaucoma and requiring further investigation.

As with most physiological functions there is a diurnal variation in the IOP; normally this does not exceed 5mm Hg. The difference between the pressures of an individual's pair of eyes is not normally greater than 4mm Hg. Both of these values may be exceeded in the early stages of glaucoma.

GLAUCOMA

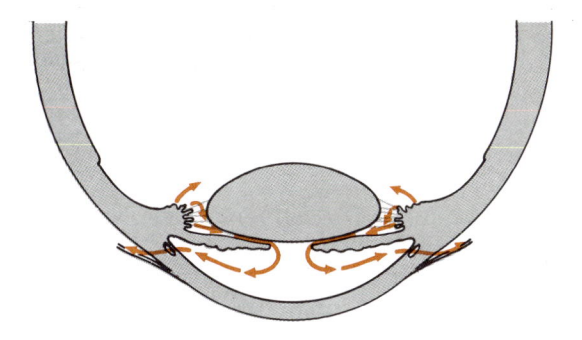

Fig 9-1 Circulation of the aqueous humour.

Abnormally Increased IOP

In common with other physiological measurements, e.g. blood pressure, it is inappropriate to think of an absolute upper limit of normal for the IOP. A pressure can be judged to have been abnormal with certainty only if it is associated with loss of visual function, in either the short or long term. The level of pressure at which an eye suffers damage is not the same for all eyes. For example, some eyes withstand pressures of up to 30mm Hg for many years without showing any structural or functional change and there are other eyes which develop pathological cupping of the optic disc and loss of visual field with pressures which are never higher than two standard deviations above the mean. In general, however, the higher the IOP or the older the person the more likely is loss of visual function. Unfortunately we do not yet have good methods of measuring for the individual how well a particular eye will tolerate a particular pressure. We are not able to detect clinically the difference between 'ocular hypertensives' whose eyes suffer no damage from elevated pressures and those patients with 'low tension glaucoma' whose eyes lose vision at pressures which cause no damage to most eyes.

A *pathological increase in IOP* can result from (1) increased production of aqueous, (2) alteration in the composition of the aqueous, or (3) obstruction to the outflow of aqueous. There is little evidence that (1) and (2) commonly cause elevation of IOP.

Obstruction to outflow can occur (1) at the pupil, (2) at the angle of the anterior chamber, or (3) in the drainage channels in the wall of the globe.

1 Occlusion of the pupil, e.g. by a total circumferential posterior synechia, results in iris bombé (a forward ballooning of the iris between pupil and periphery) and acute secondary glaucoma with a very high IOP (Fig 9-2).

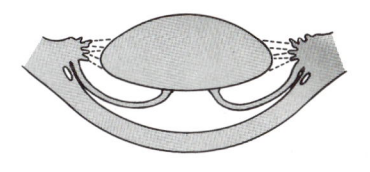

Fig 9-2 Iris bombé. Inflammatory adhesion of the pupillary margin of the iris to the lens blocks the flow of aqueous into the anterior chamber.

2 The angle of the anterior chamber may be occluded by the periphery of the iris becoming displaced forwards so that it touches the overlying cornea and covers the trabecular region (Fig 9-3c). This is called *angle closure* and it can occur only in eyes which have a narrow angle. In this inherited variation in anatomical configuration there is only a slit-like space between the anterior surface of the periphery of the iris and the overlying cornea (Fig 9-3b). It is associated with a shallow anterior chamber.

The angle of the anterior chamber may also be blocked by adhesions of the peripheral iris to the posterior surface of the cornea (peripheral anterior synechiae), e.g. as the result of iritis, following repeated episodes of primary angle closure, and following injury.

3 Pathological changes in the trabecular meshwork, canal of Schlemm, or exit venous plexus can obstruct the flow of aqueous. In these cases the *angle* is not closed but remains 'open' (Fig 9-3a).

The angle of the anterior chamber can be directly visualized by a procedure called *gonioscopy* (p. 21). A special contact lens is placed on the cornea and it refracts light so that the normally

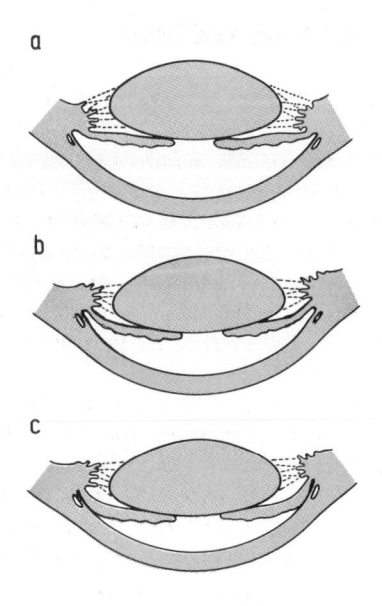

Fig 9-3 Configuration of the anterior chamber.

a The common, open (wide) angle.

b The uncommon, narrow angle.

c Angle closure in an eye with a narrow angle.

hidden angle comes into view. In this way one can distinguish narrow or closed angles from open angles. It is the basis for the classification of the primary glaucomas into angle closure and open angle types.

ANGLE CLOSURE GLAUCOMA

This type of glaucoma occurs typically in predisposed narrow-angle eyes which usually have shallow anterior chambers. Angle closure glaucoma is episodic and between attacks the affected eye is normal. Abrupt and usually large rises in IOP occur which produce pain, fogginess of vision, and rainbow-coloured haloes round lights. Sooner or later an episode of raised pressure does not spontaneously resolve and the classical acute congestive glaucoma results.

In most cases the forward movement of the peripheral iris which closes the angle is due to a partial block to the flow of aqueous through the pupil into the anterior chamber *(pupillary block)*. This results in an increase in the aqueous pressure in the posterior chamber and it is this difference in pressure between the anterior and posterior chambers which balloons the periphery of the iris so that it obliterates the already narrow angle. Pupillary block is most likely to occur when the pupil is partly dilated. Dilatation of the pupil with emotion or in a theatre may precipitate an attack of angle closure. Dilatation of the pupil with mydriatics for ophthalmoscopy may similarly bunch the periphery of the iris into a narrow angle sufficiently to block the exit of aqueous. This is sometimes used as a provocative test for angle closure glaucoma.

Sub-acute Angle Closure Glaucoma

Sub-acute attacks result from angle closure which is less than total. Oedema of the corneal epithelium causes diffraction of light and this is seen as rainbow-coloured haloes around lights. This symptom always warrants referral for ophthalmic investigation. Some mistiness of vision and discomfort in the eye usually accompany an attack.

Attacks can be prevented either by regular use of miotics to prevent dilatation of the pupil or by a peripheral iridectomy or laser iridotomy which, by preventing pupillary block, is curative (Fig 9-4).

Acute Angle Closure Glaucoma

The *symptoms* of acute angle closure glaucoma are
  sudden profound reduction of vision,
  severe pain in and around the eye, and
  often nausea and vomiting.
The *signs* are
  reduced visual acuity,
  a red eye,
  corneal haze and loss of lustre (oedema),
  a shallow anterior chamber,
  a moderately dilated, ovoid, fixed pupil, and
  greatly increased ocular tension.
The *differential diagnosis* is that of 'the acute red eye' and includes iritis, conjunctivitis, keratitis, and scleritis (p. 204).

Total and permanent loss of vision can occur in 12 hours, and *treatment is therefore urgent.* The aims are to unblock the angle, to reduce the volume of aqueous secreted and to abstract water from the eye. Miotic drops used intensively, e.g. pilocarpine 4% eye drops every 15 minutes for two hours, may achieve the first objective. If the drops succeed in causing the pupil to constrict the angle will be opened. If the attack has lasted

GLAUCOMA

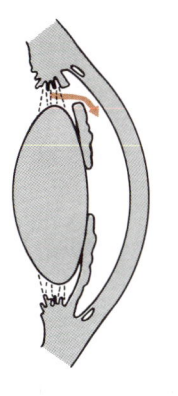

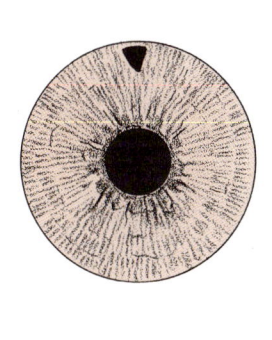

Fig 9-4 Peripheral iridectomy in vertical section and anterior view. Aqueous can bypass the pupil by flowing through the surgical hole in the iris from the posterior chamber to the anterior chamber.

too long, e.g. 10 hours, due to damage to the ciliary nerves, the pupil does not respond.

Acetazolamide (Diamox) 500 mgm i.v. and then 250 mgm by mouth 4 hourly inhibits the secretion of aqueous and thereby often lowers the IOP sufficiently for the miotic drops to be effective.

The third objective is attained by giving glycerine by mouth (150ml of 50% flavoured glycerine). By increasing the hypertonicity of the blood, fluid is abstracted from the eye. Intravenous urea or mannitol act similarly and are even more effective.

If there is no response after six hours of medical treatment, surgical treatment must be undertaken. An iridectomy is the classical operation.

If medical treatment reduces pressure to normal and when the eye has fully recovered it is usually wise to do a peripheral iridectomy or laser iridotomy with either an argon or YAG (p. 193) laser to prevent a future attack. Most authorities recommend prophylactic peripheral iridectomy or iridotomy on the other eye.

OPEN ANGLE GLAUCOMA

Open angle glaucoma is a bilateral, insidious, slowly progressive disease which causes no symptoms until considerable visual impairment has occurred, often too late for useful vision to be salvaged. Early treatment prevents or delays visual loss in nearly all cases. It is therefore obvious that early diagnosis is imperative and this can only be achieved by routine medical examination of the eyes of all people over the age of say 50 years.

The aetiology is not fully understood. It is thought that there is a pathological increase in the resistance to aqueous outflow due to changes in the trabecular meshwork. It probably takes about ten years for the resulting modest increase in IOP to cause detectable damage to the optic nerve.

The most likely site of damage to the ganglion cells which leads to their degeneration is where their axons pass through the optic disc. An old belief is that some associated impairment of the blood supply to the optic disc makes it more susceptible to the effects of the raised pressure, and this vascular abnormality has been thought to be a major factor in low tension glaucoma. An alternative view for which there is some recent evidence is that a mechanical weakness of some components of the lamina cribrosa allows kinking and compression of some axons as they pass through the lamina.

Genetic factors play a large part and therefore examination of relatives of affected individuals is indicated.

Symptoms and Signs

There are no *symptoms* at all in the early stages and the patient usually notices no abnormality until much of the peripheral visual field has been destroyed. Untreated, the final outcome is total blindness.

There are three *signs* of chronic open angle glaucoma. Ophthalmoscopically there is pathological *cupping* of the optic disc in which the cup becomes wider and maybe deeper and the remaining rim of disc tissue becomes atrophic (Fig 9-5; Plate 1, p. 121). It can be difficult to differentiate early glaucomatous cupping from a large physiological cup (p. 130). Tiny splinter haemorrhages are common on the margins of discs which are or will become glaucomatous.

Except in low tension glaucoma, *ocular tension is increased.* This may not be great, e.g. to 30mm Hg, and will not therefore usually be detected by palpation. The ocular tension commonly varies greatly and in the early stages is often normal at some time during the day. One normal pressure measurement therefore does not exclude chronic glaucoma. To be reasonably sure that the ocular tension is at all times normal it is necessary to perform tonometry either every four hours for 48 hours, or at varying times of the day on a number of occasions over a period of a week or so. Only after doing this can a diagnosis of low tension glaucoma be made in those eyes with cupping and field loss and apparently normal pressure. More often phases of elevated pressure are discovered and the diagnosis of true glaucoma confirmed.

Visual *field changes* are evidence of impaired visual function (Fig 9-6). Initially these are always peripheral and therefore central vision, i.e. visual acuity, is not affected. Nerve fibre bundle defects are characteristic (arcuate scotomata) (p. 12). In addition to their importance in diagnosis, visual field studies are the best criterion of effectiveness of treatment.

Gonioscopy reveals an open angle.

Although the disease is nearly always bilateral, one eye is frequently involved earlier and more severely than its fellow eye. Because of this the diagnosis is often made at an early and therefore more hopeful stage in the second eye.

Treatment

The aim of treatment of open angle glaucoma is to maintain a 'normal' intraocular pressure at all times and if this end is achieved the results are good.

On the other hand, because treatment is trying for the patient, it is important to be sure of the diagnosis of glaucoma before starting treatment. It is not usually necessary to treat *ocular hypertension* unless the pressures are higher than about 30mm Hg. However, because we are unable to predict which patients with ocular hypertension will eventually develop glaucoma, it is necessary to keep all such patients under observation indefinitely.

Treatment can be both medical and surgical. *Medical* treatment aims at increasing the facility

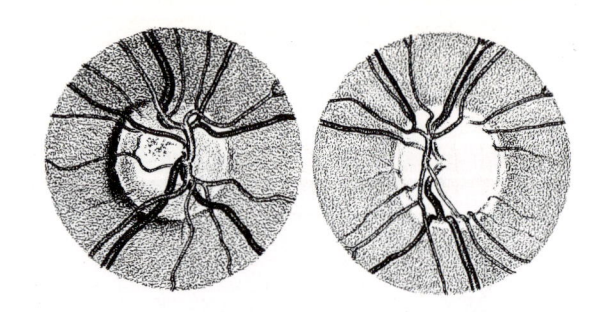

Fig 9-5 The two optic discs of a patient with open angle glaucoma which has not yet damaged the right optic disc. The left optic disc is grossly cupped and atrophic.

of outflow and suppressing the secretion of aqueous.

Regular use of miotic eye drops controls but does not cure and must therefore be constant, consistent, and continuing. In angle closure glaucoma miotics act by freeing the angle of the anterior chamber from iris block. In open angle glaucoma miotics probably act by opening the microscopic spaces in the trabecular meshwork through contraction of the ciliary muscle pulling on the scleral spur. They also have an ill-understood effect on the intraocular blood vessels which improves the outflow facility.

The drug of choice is pilocarpine, 1% to 4% eye drops, used twice to five times daily. Other miotics are physostigmine (eserine) ¼ or ½% and echothiophate (phospholine) 0.125%.

Acetazolamide (and some other carbonic anhydrase inhibitors) reduces the secretion of aqueous (up to 60%). It can be used 250mgm once to thrice daily for lengthy periods to supplement miotic therapy.

Adrenalin (epinephrine) 2% eye drops, or dipivalyl adrenalin (dipivefrin) 0.1% eye drops, which is converted to adrenalin after absorption through the corneal epithelium, inhibits aqueous secretion. Because it dilates the pupil even when used together with miotics it is dangerous in angle closure glaucoma.

Beta-adrenergic blocking drugs, e.g. timolol maleate 0.25% or 0.5% eye drops, also suppress aqueous secretion but do not affect the pupil or accommodation. However timolol used only as eye drops twice daily can cause serious systemic effects such as asthma.

In general the least aggressive medical therapy

GLAUCOMA

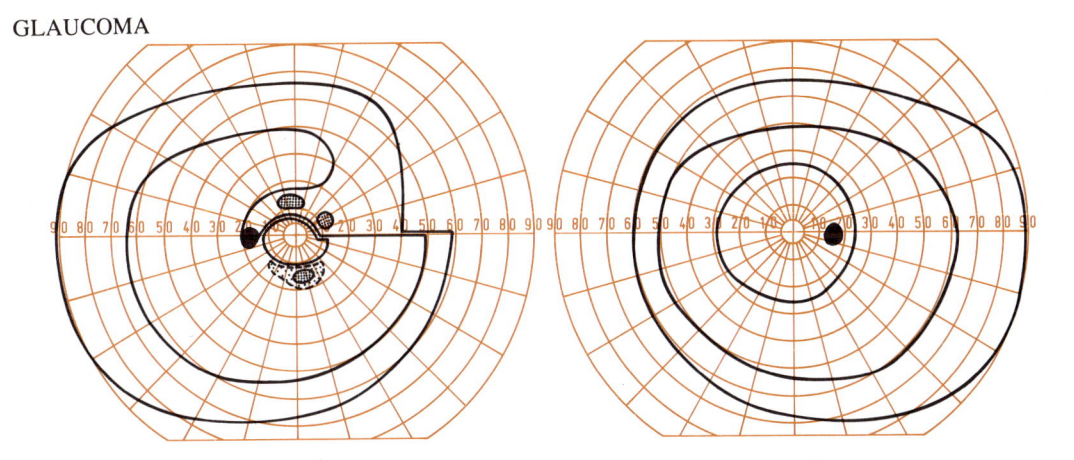

Fig 9-6 Visual fields of a patient with chronic open angle glaucoma recorded with a Goldmann perimeter. The continuous lines are the isopters which denote the thresholds to three stimuli of different sizes or brightnesses. At this stage the right visual field is normal.

In the left visual field when the maximum stimulus is used there is an upper 'nasal step', two paracentral scotomata within the upper arcuate area and one scotoma within the lower arcuate area. To the intermediate stimulus there is an upper arcuate defect which has 'broken through to the periphery' and the inferior scotoma is larger. To the least intense stimulus the whole field is reduced in size but central vision would be normal.

which will control tension throughout the 24 hours and which prevents further visual field loss is used. Adequacy of control is assessed by periodic tonometry measurements at varying times of the day and by periodic, e.g. 2-, 3-, or 6-monthly, visual field studies.

Only when medical treatment fails is *surgery* resorted to. The standard operations are called drainage or filtering operations, e.g. trephine, trabeculectomy (Fig 9-7). These create a fistula in the corneoscleral wall through which aqueous can escape into the subconjunctival space and thence through the conjunctiva to mix with the tears.

In recalcitrant cases a fine tube from the angle of the anterior chamber is used to drain aqueous posteriorly to the external surface of a 13mm diameter plastic plate which rests on the globe inside Tenon's capsule (a Molteno drain). The plate maintains a sufficient surface area of tissue to absorb the drained aqueous and the permeability of the surface is preserved by controlling fibrous scarring after the operation with a combination of local and systemic anti-inflammatory agents.

Laser trabeculoplasty, in which with a gonioscopic lens the argon laser is used to cause a row of small mild burns along the trabecular meshwork reduces the intraocular pressure in some patients but the effect is not always maintained.

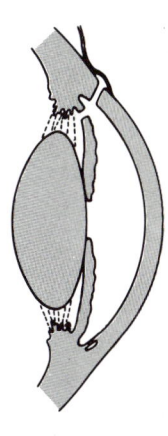

Fig 9-7 Filtering operation in vertical section. The small hole in the corneo-sclera is covered externally by conjunctiva. A peripheral iridectomy is done to prevent the underlying iris from blocking the internal opening of the fistula.

CONGENITAL GLAUCOMA

The word buphthalmos, which is also used for congenital glaucoma, literally means ox eye and refers to the enlargement of the eye which occurs. The condition is due to maldevelopment of the angle of the anterior chamber. It is rare, but early diagnosis is crucial if sight is to be preserved.

The earliest and most constant symptom is photophobia which makes affected infants almost close their eyes in ordinary daylight and consequently wear a worried frown. The infant eye can enlarge with increased IOP (like the infant skull in hydrocephalus) and the corneal diameter increases beyond 11.0mm. The 'beautiful big eyes' of the baby are often remarked on. The cornea is hazy and the anterior chamber is deep.

Although miotics are of slight help, treatment is surgical and in the early stages is commonly (60-80%) effective. The appropriate operation is goniotomy in which aqueous drainage is established by incising the abnormal tissue which covers the trabecular region. In the late stages or when goniotomy fails a Molteno drainage operation is required (p. 179).

Chapter 10

SQUINT AND AMBLYOPIA

Squint in children
  Causes
  Sensory changes
  Common squints of children
  Simple tests
  Treatment
  Definitions
Amblyopia
  Detection
  Treatment

SQUINT IN CHILDREN

A squint or strabismus is a failure of the two eyes to look at the same thing. When this happens binocular vision is not possible.

Causes

Binocular vision can occur only if there is precise co-ordination of the movements of the two eyes for all directions and distances of gaze. It also requires clear images from both eyes and their fusion into a single mental percept. The ability to see singly and in 3D is normally acquired during the first years of life; it cannot be acquired later. Development of binocular vision in an infant can be arrested or perverted by any imperfection of the motor, sensory, or central components. An initial defect in one of these components is therefore likely to result in defects in the other two. A squint, which is a motor abnormality, can thus be due to a primary nerve or muscle defect or, more commonly, it is secondary to a sensory or a central defect. However it is caused, a squint is always more than an altered appearance.

Although the causes of many squints are not fully understood, in the majority of squinting children there is an hereditary factor and in others the responsible defect can be recognized. Examples are: an ocular abnormality which prevents good central vision (unilateral congenital cataract, retinoblastoma, a macular lesion, etc.), paresis of a lateral rectus muscle (birth injury, maldevelopment), the brain damage of cerebral palsy, and large refractive errors.

Refractive errors are important because they can be easily corrected with glasses. They may act in two ways, directly by preventing clear vision and indirectly through the normal association of convergence and accommodation. There is a linkage between these two mechanisms so that for near vision the two occur together and normally it is impossible to converge without accommodating and conversely to accommodate without converging. When a child is hypermetropic, to see clearly he or she has to accommodate more than is normally required both for distant and for near vision. As a result of the linkage of convergence with accommodation, this excess accommodation gives rise to excessive convergence and, if the binocular fusion mechanisms are not strong, a convergent squint results. Spectacles which correct the hypermetropia eliminate the need for the excess accommodation and so the associated over-convergence does not occur. In many children this type of squint, an *accommodative squint,* is cured simply by wearing of proper spectacles. This relationship between accommodation and convergence also explains the occurrence of a divergent squint in a few children who are myopic.

Sensory Changes in Squints

If the binocular sensory mechanisms are normal, any squint must result in double vision and this occurs at the onset of most squints. However, an infant is able to suppress the images arising from one eye and, by this inhibition, prevent them from reaching consciousness. Double vision is thereby overcome. The younger the infant, the more readily does suppression occur.

Suppression is a faculative inhibition of vision which occurs only while it is useful. In squints in which either eye is used as the fixing eye (alternating squints) suppression switches from eye to eye as each becomes the squinting eye. If this alternating suppression is allowed to continue during the years of infancy it becomes permanent and simultaneous vision with the two eyes is never possible.

In many squinting children it is always the same eye which turns (unilateral or monocular squint) and in these children the vision of the squinting eye fails to develop normally. This permanent defect is called *amblyopia.* Untreated, it lasts for life, even if the sight of the other eye is lost. The younger the child the more quickly does amblyopia occur and the more firmly it is established. Amblyopia does not occur after the age of about seven years.

A number of other abnormalities may develop as a consequence of a squint. These include eccentric fixation, in which the squinting eye, even when used alone, does not look directly at an object with the result that the image falls on some part of the retina other than the fovea, and abnormal retinal correspondence, in which a degraded type of binocular vision becomes established.

Because of these ensuing sensory changes, the prompt investigation and treatment of a squinting child is always mandatory. After the

age of six months no infant with a squint is too young to be referred for ophthalmological examination. **No squint should be ignored. Children do not grow out of squints.**

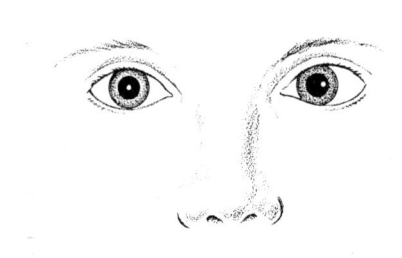

Fig 10-1 Left convergent squint.

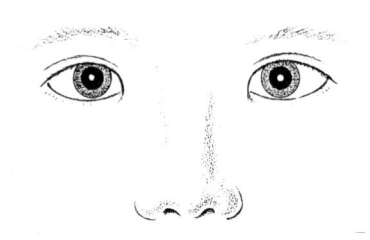

Fig 10-2 Wide nasal bridge and epicanthic folds as commonly seen in babies and infants. The central corneal light reflexes show that the convergent appearance is illusory.

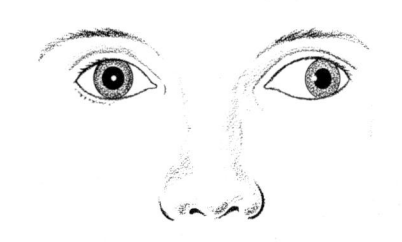

Fig 10-3 Left divergent squint.

Common Squints of Children

Convergent squints are the most common (Fig 10-1). Some appear soon after birth and are not associated with refractive errors. Others appear in the second or third year, may be intermittently present at first, and are associated with hypermetropia.

Pseudo-squints are common (Fig 10-2). This is the illusory appearance of a convergent squint which occurs because a wide nasal bridge and/or epicanthic folds hide the sclera of the medial part of the eyes. On looking slightly to the side the adducting eye appears to turn in excessively because the inner white sclera disappears. This apparent squint is usually lost as the bony nasal bridge develops. Pseudo-squints are in part responsible for the folklore that some squints disappear with growth.

Divergent squints often occur only when the child looks at distant objects or daydreams (Fig 10-3). Shutting one eye in bright light often heralds a divergent squint.

A paresis of one of the vertically acting eye muscles gives rise to a *vertical squint;* the deviation is often small and the squint therefore inconspicuous. Some children adopt a compensatory abnormal head posture (ocular torticollis).

Simple Tests for Squints

Observation of the *corneal light reflexes* is a simple easily applied test. Even a young baby will look at a small light such as that of an ophthalmoscope or a pocket torch. If each eye is properly fixing the light, the reflections of the light from the corneal mirrors will be on the same, more or less central, part of each cornea (Fig 10-4a). This can best be judged by noting the position of the reflex in relation to the underlying pupil. If one eye is not directed to the light the corneal reflex of that eye will be displaced, e.g. temporally if the eye is convergent (Fig 10-4b).

The cover test is the most certain single test but it can be difficult to do with babies or young infants (Fig 10-5). The cover-uncover test applied to each eye in turn not only reveals or confirms the presence of a squint, but shows whether it is alternating or monocular (p. 103).

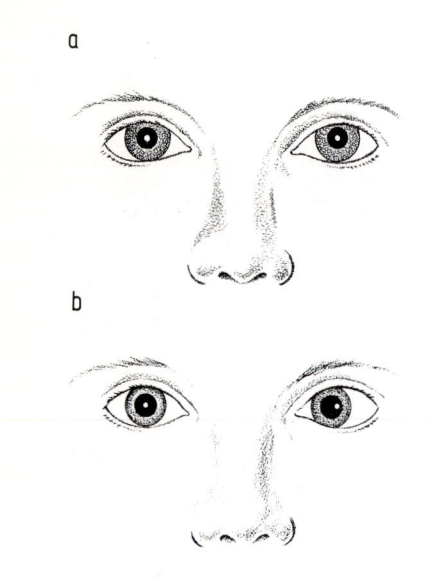

Fig 10-4 Corneal light reflexes.

a With normal binocular fixation the reflections are symmetrical in the two eyes.

b With a left convergent squint the reflection from the left cornea is temporal to the centre of the pupil.

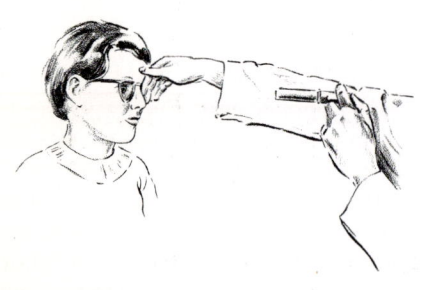

Fig 10-5 Cover test. The subject fixes the light of the pocket torch while her eyes are covered and uncovered.

Treatment

The treatment of squints can be complex and of long duration, but the essentials are (1) the search for ocular defects (corneal scar, cataract, retinoblastoma, macular lesion), (2) refraction and glasses to correct significant refractive errors, (3) occlusion to overcome any amblyopia and secure alternation, and, in some, (4) surgical adjustments of one or more extraocular muscles of one or both eyes in one or more stages.

The aims of treatment are threefold. The prevention or cure of amblyopia is usually possible with early treatment, but will fail if treatment is delayed. The cosmetic aim of remedying disfigurement can always be achieved at any age. The establishment or restoration of binocular vision is possible with early treatment in some but by no means all; failure in this third aim is of much less importance than failure in the other two.

Some Definitions

A *squint* or *strabismus* (heterotropia) is that condition in which the visual axis of one eye (the *squinting eye*) is not directed to the object being looked at by the other eye (the *fixing eye*). (The visual axis is the line from the fovea to the point of fixation.)

The *angle of squint* is the angle (in degrees or prism dioptres) through which the visual axis of the squinting eye is deviated from what it should be if the eye was correctly directed to the point of fixation.

A *concomitant squint* is one in which the angle of squint is much the same in all directions of gaze and whichever eye is fixing.

An *incomitant squint* is one in which the angle of squint alters with different directions of gaze and with a change of fixation between the two eyes (p. 28). It results from paralysis of one or more of the extraocular muscles and is often called a *paralytic squint*.

A *unilateral squint* (monocular squint) is one in which one eye is habitually the squinting eye; hence, a right or a left squint. An *alternating squint* is one in which either eye is the squinting eye.

The direction of the squint may be *convergent* (esotropia) when the squinting eye turns in, *divergent* (exotropia) when it turns out, or *vertical* when it turns up (hypertropia) or down (hypotropia).

A *latent squint* (heterophoria) is one in which the tendency to squint is controlled by the fusion mechanism except under conditions of fatigue, illness, or increasing age when it may become *manifest*. It is revealed by artificially preventing binocular vision, most simply by the cover test.

AMBLYOPIA

In its present day usage the term amblyopia means defective vision resulting from failure of development of vision in a child due to interference with use of the eye during the critical period when cortical visual connections normally become fixed. An amblyopic eye is colloquially known as a lazy eye.

Amblyopia can occur only in a child (up to the age of six or seven years), and it can be treated only in childhood. To be treated in childhood it must be diagnosed in childhood. And to be diagnosed it must be specifically looked for, since with normal vision in one eye the amblyopic child's visual behaviour is normal. This is why **the vision of each eye in all infants should be tested by the time they are four years old.**

Amblyopia is common. The prevalence of amblyopia in all children is about 5%. The vision of amblyopic eyes varies from slightly impaired (6/9) to grossly defective (less than 6/60). The degree of visual defect is largely determined by the age of onset; the younger the child when normal seeing is interfered with, the more profound will be the loss of vision. The likelihood of recovery of vision with treatment is largely determined by the duration; the longer the amblyopia has been present, the less effective will treatment be.

The commonest cause of unilateral amblyopia is a monocular squint. Almost as common is amblyopia due to unequal refractive errors in the two eyes (anisometropia). Because, unlike most squinting children, there is no manifest abnormality which leads to eye examination, this *hidden amblyopia* is only detected when the vision of both eyes is deliberately tested and compared. In both these groups there is a strong hereditary factor; infants with an amblyopic parent or sibling should be tested earlier, at say three years of age.

A few children are amblyopic as a result of unilateral corneal opacities or congenital cataract. A unilateral congenital cataract is not usually treated because this only converts the eye into one handicapped by a large unilateral refractive error which cannot be corrected with spectacles while the other unaffected eye is being used, due to the difference in size of the retinal images of the two eyes.

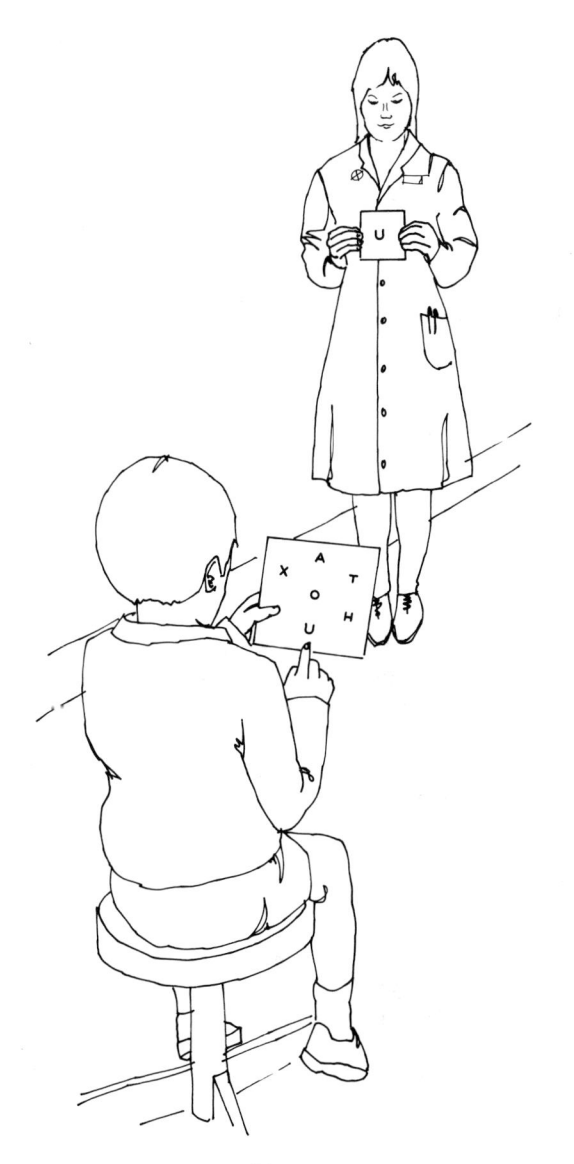

Fig 10-6 Letter matching test.

Amblyopia can be bilateral as a result of bilateral obstacles to normal seeing, e.g. congenital cataracts.

Detection

Several methods of estimating the vision of a small child are reliable enough for *screening* purposes since it is not so much the absolute level of visual acuity which is required as a comparison of the vision of the two eyes.

The most useful tests are the letter matching test (Fig 10-6) and the illiterate E test (p. 67).

These are possible with most four year olds and many three year olds, especially when the single cards are used at the shorter distance of 4m (p. 67).

Referral for formal ophthalmic investigation is indicated if the difference in the levels reached by a pair of eyes is two lines or more on a test chart, or if the vision of either eye is worse than 6/12 or 4/8 for children less than four years or worse than 6/9 or 4/6 for children between four and five years.

Treatment

This is based on the simple idea of forcing the child to use his or her amblyopic eye. All that is necessary is correction with spectacles of any significant refractive error and *occlusion* of the other normally used eye. Since this is essentially a learning process it must be consistent and continued until normal seeing is well established. The duration of treatment depends on the duration of the amblyopia. With prompt treatment a few weeks may suffice, with long delayed treatment more than a year may be needed, or indeed treatment may fail. Measures to eliminate the original cause are also needed to prevent recurrence of the amblyopia when occlusion is stopped.

Chapter 11

FAILING VISION IN OLD PEOPLE

Normal changes in vision with age
Cataract
   Senile cataract
     Nuclear cataract
     Cortical cataract
       Cuneiform
       Posterior cupuliform
     Mature cataract
     Hypermature cataract
   Symptoms
   Examination
   Treatment
     Cataract extraction
     Indications for operation
     Briefing the patient
Senescent macular degeneration

In this chapter 'failing' means a slow deterioration of vision as compared with the abrupt loss of vision which in old people results from retinal and cerebral vascular accidents, giant cell arteritis, acute angle closure glaucoma, and retinal detachment. 'Old' vaguely signifies 65 years plus — 'the sixth age of the lean and slippered pantaloon with spectacles on nose. . . .'

Normal Changes in Vision with Age
A diminution of keenness of sight is, like a similar change in hearing, common and is accepted as inevitable by most old people. This acceptance can prevent a person seeking advice for a pathological and remediable change. While some change with age is normal, reduction of sight of a handicapping degree is not. For example, difficulty in reading is always pathological. Physiological changes with age result in slightly reduced visual acuity (e.g. from 6/4 to 6/6 or 6/9), altered colour vision so that blues are subdued and reds enhanced, delayed and reduced dark adaptation, and impaired recovery from dazzling glare (this is important for night driving).

Pathological Visual Deterioration in Old People
The three commonest causes of failing vision in old people are cataract, chronic open angle glaucoma, and senescent macular degeneration. Cataract and senescent macular degeneration will be dealt with here; the glaucomas warrant a separate chapter (p. 174).

CATARACT

A cataract is an opacification of the lens, partial or complete; any loss of complete transparency of the lens is a cataract. The loss of transparency is due to the accumulation of water and/or denaturation of the lens protein.

Cataracts may be classified according to age of onset (congenital, developmental, adult, senile), aetiology (traumatic, associated with a systemic disorder, secondary to an ocular disorder, senile), or location and form of the opacity (nuclear, cortical, posterior polar). Most cataracts are either senile, congenital, traumatic, or related to a systemic or an ocular disorder.

Senile Cataract
This term includes all forms of cataract which occur in the absence of any congenital disorder, causative ocular disease, ocular trauma, or associated systemic disorders. It usually occurs in the elderly but it can occur earlier, for example at 40 years of age, and so the term senile is not altogether apt. Like greying of the hair, some degree of senile opacification of the lens is almost inevitable but the age at which this occurs varies greatly from person to person.

Diabetes causes more frequent occurrence, earlier onset, and more rapid progress of senile cataracts. True diabetic cataracts are very rare and occur in young growth-onset diabetics.

Forms of Senile Cataract
1 Nuclear Cataract
The central portion of the lens becomes opaque. It interferes more with vision in bright light when the pupil is smaller (and therefore the patient may be helped by regularly using mydriatic drops to moderately dilate the pupil). Nuclear cataract is often preceded by nuclear sclerosis in which the nucleus of the lens becomes harder and denser and has increased refractive power (nuclear hyperrefringence). This results in myopia and hence the new-found ability to read without glasses which some old people experience — 'second sight'. Ophthalmoscopically the opacity is seen as a dark disc in the centre of the red fundus reflex (Fig 11-1). When examining the fundus, a better view is often obtained by dilating the patient's pupil and looking through the unaffected periphery of the lens.

2 Cortical Cataract
(a) *Cuneiform cataract*
Radial, white, irregular wedge-shaped opacities develop within the periphery of the cortex. This is the commonest form of senile cataract.

It is seen ophthalmoscopically as spokes silhouetted against the red reflex (Fig 11-2).

(b) *Posterior cupuliform cataract*
A thin layer of more or less uniform opacity develops in the axial part of the cortex, immediately in front of the posterior lens capsule.

When the red reflex is examined with the ophthalmoscope, this opacity gives rise to a central disc of mottled darkness (Fig 11-3).

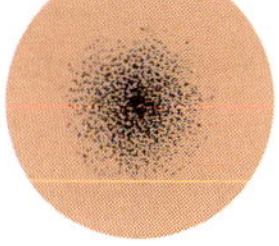

CATARACT

Fig 11-1 Nuclear cataract silhouetted in the red reflex.

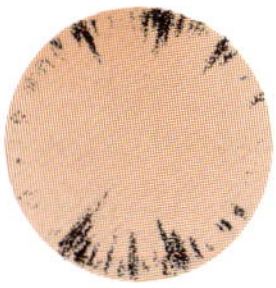

Fig 11-2 Peripheral wedge-shaped opacities of a commencing cuneiform cataract silhouetted in the red reflex.

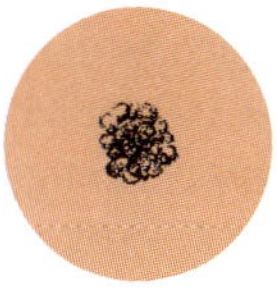

Fig 11-3 Posterior cupuliform cataract silhouetted in the red reflex.

3 Mature Cataract

When the whole lens becomes opaque the cataract is mature or 'ripe'. Before this stage the cataract is described as immature. Useful vision will be lost before a cataract is mature and assessment of maturity used to be used as a guide to the choice of surgical treatment and not for the purpose of deciding on the need for surgical treatment. Total absence of the red reflex does not necessarily mean that a cataract is mature because there may be some clear cortex in front of an opacity which fills the diameter of the lens.

4 Hypermature Cataract

In a few untreated mature cataracts the opaque cortex becomes liquified and the lens capsule and zonule become fragile. Secondary glaucoma or iritis may occur as complications of hypermaturity and so this should be forestalled by extracting the cataract.

Symptoms of Cataract

Gradually increasing loss of vision is the major symptom. When the cataract is nuclear, acuity may be worse in bright light. Vision may fluctuate because of variations in the water content of the lens. Alterations in refraction, which can be corrected by altering spectacles, may occur. Occasionally monocular diplopia results from axial opacities. There is no pain.

The rate of development of a cataract is very variable; for example, maturity can occur in a few months or never. In many people the lens opacities do not increase for years at a time.

Examination

Senile cataracts are commonly accompanied by other independent disorders of the eye and therefore the most important part of the examination of a cataract patient is a search for co-existing ocular abnormalities, for example, chronic glaucoma, macular degeneration, vascular retinopathy. It must never be assumed that because a cataract is present, it is the sole cause of the reduced vision. With experience it becomes possible to judge whether a given lens opacity is sufficient to account for the visual loss which is present. The *pin-hole test* is very useful in determining this; if visual acuity is improved with a pin-hole, macular function is probably normal. A record of the visual acuity made prior to the development of the cataract can be very helpful, for example in making known the existence of amblyopia. Unfortunately, patients' general hospital records usually lack this information.

Once the lens has become so opaque that the fundus cannot be seen ophthalmoscopically, only indirect tests, such as the accuracy of light projection, are available for the assessment of the integrity of the deeper parts of the eye. Therefore all patients with cataracts should be seen and fully examined at an early stage in the development of their lens opacities. The attitude that it is just an early cataract which does not yet require treatment and therefore does not warrant ophthalmological examination, is wrong.

Treatment

There is no effective medical means for prevention or treatment of cataract. Mydriatic drops can be a temporary help for axial lens opacities and a hand-magnifying glass may be a temporizing expedient.

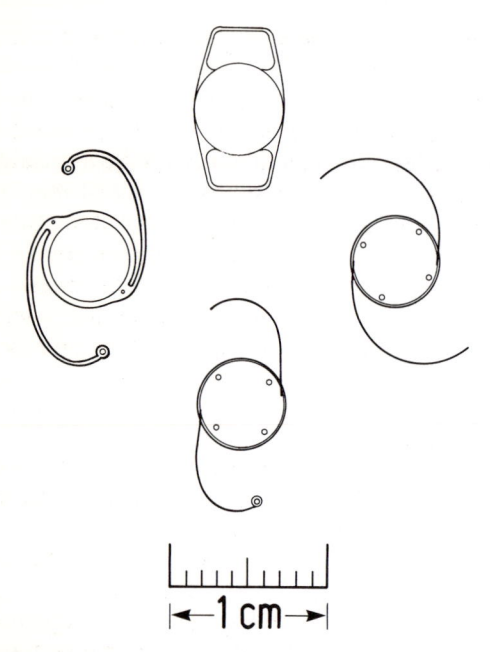

Fig 11-4 Four of the many designs of posterior chamber intraocular lenses.

Treatment is surgical and until recently there were two basic methods of *cataract extraction* (in adults). In both the globe is opened by an incision through the corneo-scleral junction in its upper half and this is sutured after removal of the lens.

Extra-capsular extraction
A central piece of anterior lens capsule is torn away, the solid nucleus expressed from the eye and the soft cortical lens matter removed by irrigation, leaving the posterior lens capsule and zonule intact. This older method of extraction is more suitable for mature cataracts, because clear lens fibres are sticky and more difficult to remove; some patients still believe that they will have to 'wait for the cataract to ripen' before it can be operated on.

Intra-capsular extraction
The lens is removed intact within its capsule and therefore the anterior face of the vitreous is exposed to the iris and through the pupil to the anterior chamber. The enzyme alphachymotrypsin is often used to free the attachment of the zonule to the lens capsule and thereby facilitate removal of the lens without tearing the capsule when this is pulled on in the act of extracting the lens. A grip on the tense but fragile lens capsule is obtained with special forceps, with a suction device or with a cryo-probe which is frozen to the lens.

Now the operation of choice in suitable patients is
Extraction with insertion of an intraocular lens.
Many types of intraocular lens (IOL) have been designed and used since 1949. Currently those most favoured are lenses designed to be placed behind the iris in the posterior chamber (Fig 11-4). In these, projections, of which there is a great variety, support and fix the plastic optic portion in position. After a microsurgical extracapsular removal of all the lens from within its capsule the IOL is inserted into the capsular bag (Fig 11-5) or failing that in front of the collapsed capsule and zonule, with the IOL supports engaged in the sulcus between ciliary body and iris.

When a posterior chamber lens cannot be used, for example as a secondary IOL implant after a previous intracapsular extraction, an anterior chamber lens is placed in front of the iris. With these the supports engage in the angle of the anterior chamber. Any contact between lens and the posterior corneal surface must be prevented because this leads to loss of corneal endothelium and the likelihood of consequent permanent corneal oedema (bullous keratopathy).

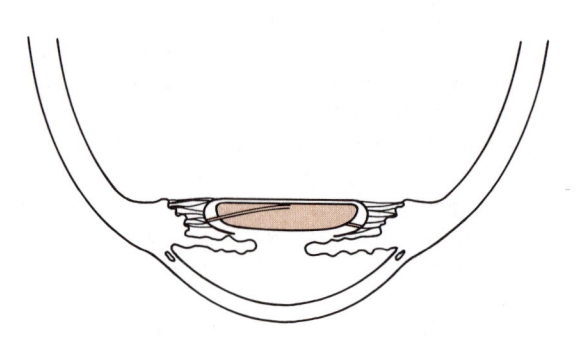

Fig 11-5 One type of posterior chamber IOL placed within the 'capsular bag' after extracapsular removal of a cataract.

Indications for Operation

Cataract extraction is by far the most frequently performed ocular operation and the following discussion is given in some detail to provide an insight into the approach of an ophthalmologist. It also illustrates the truism that deciding when and how to operate is often more difficult than doing the operation.

The decision whether or not to remove a cataract is rarely straightforward, not only because, as in most surgery, risks have to be taken but because aphakic vision is not normal vision.

The likelihood of a successful surgical result is about 90%. In addition to complications at the time of operation and during the immediate postoperative period, cataract surgery is associated with the development of retinal detachment in a significant minority and this becomes greater as the years following operation accumulate. Although cataract operation in old people entails very little risk to life, it does give rise in some patients to general complications such as psychological upsets ranging from a confusional psychosis to a more common change that can best be described as a sudden ageing. In short, although mortality can be almost ignored, general morbidity associated with cataract operations in the aged cannot be ignored.

Aphakic vision with spectacles has very real shortcomings. Although central vision as tested on a test-type may be 6/5, this is accompanied by distortion of objects (for example, doorways may seem to curve inwards and tables to slant away from the horizontal), misjudgements of the position of objects (for example, steps; crockery on a table), apparent movements of objects on turning the head or eyes, a 'jack-in-the-box' disappearance and reappearance of objects as they move between 60° and 30° from the peripheral into the central field, and alteration of colour values.

These disconcerting abnormalities of seeing usually diminish over a period of six to eight weeks and most patients learn to adapt to and accept persisting imperfections. Some people, however, take longer and need encouragement. The benefits of operation are more readily appreciated and the drawbacks better tolerated by patients whose vision had been appreciably impaired before surgery; this is an argument against too early operation in certain types of people. These defects of aphakic vision can be greatly lessened by the use of a contact lens instead of spectacles, although this may not be a practical proposition for some old people. And they are fully eliminated by insertion of an IOL, which is why this is now the favoured treatment.

Another inevitable consequence of aphakia is the total loss of accommodation but this is nothing new to the majority of patients who have their lenses removed.

Monocular aphakia when the other eye has reasonable vision poses a difficult optical problem. Because the retinal image in the aphakic eye with glasses is 30% larger than the image in the phakic eye, it is not possible to use the two eyes together because of the diplopia which occurs. Either the aphakic eye is not corrected, in which case all that has been gained by operation is enlargement of the peripheral field of vision, or the operated eye is corrected with spectacles and a lens is used to blur the vision of the other eye sufficiently to eliminate the confusion from the two unequal images. The disparity in retinal image size (aniseikonia) is reduced to 10% by contact lenses and some patients are able to overcome this difference and enjoy binocular vision when a contact lens is worn. Since there is minimal disparity with an IOL good binocular vision is likely.

The indications for cataract extraction can be better assessed against this background of what may be gained and what may be lost.

The right time for cataract surgery depends as much on the individual patient as on the state of his or her eyes. An active, intelligent patient will require surgery sooner than a person with limited interests who never did much reading.

It is worth emphasizing that many senile cataracts remain stationary for long periods and progress only slowly, and in fact only a small proportion of people with lens opacities do eventually require surgical treatment. Many patients think they can retard the progression of their cataract by 'saving their eyes'. There is no evidence that this is so and they should be specifically told this to prevent them needlessly curtailing their visual activities. Another misconception is the belief that surgical relief from a cataract can be given only when the cataract is 'ripe' and some patients have resigned themselves to a period of waiting with a growing handicap.

The need for operation is usually determined by the vision of the *better* eye. With adequate vision in the other eye, the presence of even a mature cataract in one eye is not in itself a sufficient indication for operation. There are, however, good reasons for advising surgery for uniocular cataract. Apart from local ocular reasons, such as hypermaturity of the cataract, these are: the aim of restoring binocular vision or a wider field of vision with an IOL; the desirability of doing the operation before local changes in the eye, as in some diabetics, or failing health, adversely affect the chances of success; and to enable an apprehensive patient to get the operation behind him or her.

As a generalization, operation on the worst eye is indicated when the vision of the better eye has failed to the stage that reading is becoming difficult or, in some cases, driving is no longer possible or distance vision is inadequate for the patient's occupation. Commonly this stage is reached when the distance vision is reduced to 6/18 or less and the near vision is worse than N6. In many cases it is possible to say that the patient can have the operation when he or she needs it. Indeed with understanding and sensible patients it is good practice to let the patient decide, after explanation and discussion, when he or she will have the operation. Nevertheless, in spite of being told how little they would gain from surgery, some patients have difficulty in understanding the wisdom of inaction when they know that an operation would probably restore the vision of a cataractous eye.

The decision about a cataract operation is often complicated by other ocular pathology and judgement can be difficult. The accompanying changes in the eye may have caused the cataract, for example chronic iridocyclitis, following glaucoma surgery; they may both be related to a common cause, for example diabetes; or they may be coincidental, for example macular degeneration. In some of these situations the risks of surgery are increased, whereas in others vision is likely to be poor even if the operation is successfully accomplished. In some of the latter group it is possible to predict that little improvement would result from removal of the cataract. In others this is not possible and surgery becomes more of a gamble than usual. However it is often the sort of gamble where the patient has little to lose and most patients will understand this and try. With older patients it is wise to be sure that they fully understand and do not expect too much because they can become depressed if their unfounded hopes are not realized.

Occasionally operation is suggested in a disorientated patient whose vision is grossly defective in the hope that the restoration of vision will ameliorate the mental state, but the general experience has been that this does not occur.

Patients who have had one eye successfully operated on are often keen to have the cataract removed from their second eye. In fact, old people may gain little from a second operation if they already have adequate vision from their first operation. A number of older folk have difficulty in understanding that if they have normal corrected vision in one eye they will not see any better with two eyes, although they may with IOLs regain binocular vision.

Briefing the patient

Patients often dread an eye operation both for understandable psychological reasons and on account of the pain they mistakenly anticipate they will have to endure. It surprises and relieves patients to be told that they need not expect any real pain in the eye post-operatively.

Some restriction of a patient's freedom is still required post-operatively but the days of prostrate immobility with both eyes covered are past. It encourages patients to know that they will be out of bed the day after operation and that both eyes will be covered for probably only the first day. The usual time in hospital is two to four days and in some centres cataract extraction is done as an outpatient procedure.

If an IOL is not inserted patients are told that since cataract extraction involves the removal of the lens from the eye, vision will only be restored by a lens worn as spectacles or as a contact lens, but they are liable to forget this and in the post-operative period assume that the operation has failed because the sight of the operated eye is not clear. A reminder of the need for glasses, or better, demonstration of potential vision with a lens held before the eye, can prevent this unnecessary disappointment.

Unless the patient is one-eyed, spectacles or a contact lens are rarely prescribed earlier than six weeks after the operation because during this time the refraction of the eye is often not stabilized. If there are operative complications this period of waiting for glasses can be much longer. Temporary plastic spectacles can be most useful during this waiting period.

Disappointing vision after cataract extraction may be due to an imperfect surgical result or to other ocular pathology, such as macular degeneration or diabetic retinopathy.

Some patients with an excellent result need to be told to use their eye freely and many are relieved to learn that a cataract cannot recur. However after extra-capsular extraction of a cataract with or without insertion of an IOL, the remaining lens capsule may thicken and thereby reduce vision. This is remedied by *capsulotomy* in which a central hole is made in the capsule by a surgical incision or, more recently, by photodisruption with a 'YAG' laser. The neodymium: yttrium/aluminium/garnet (Nd:YAG) laser is a pulsed instrument which acts by formation of a plasma at its focal point with explosive expansion of tissue. It can also be used to perform an iridotomy, e.g. in the treatment of angle closure glaucoma (p. 177).

SENESCENT MACULAR DEGENERATION (SMD)

Senescent or age related macular degeneration is common. It is the commonest cause of inability to read in old people. (Until recently SMD in fact stood for senile macular degeneration with its less kind connotations.)

Central visual acuity diminishes gradually over some years with involvement of one eye preceding the other by months or years. Peripheral vision is not affected.

Ophthalmoscopically, at the macula there are fine specks and streaks of pigment intermingled with minute areas of reduced pigmentation (Fig 11-6). Colloid bodies are often present and there may be small yellow exudates. Small haemorrhages occasionally occur.

There is little parallelism between the ophthalmoscopic appearances and the degree of visual loss; a minimal pigmentary disturbance may accompany severe visual loss or conspicuous ophthalmoscopic changes may be associated with only moderate visual impairment.

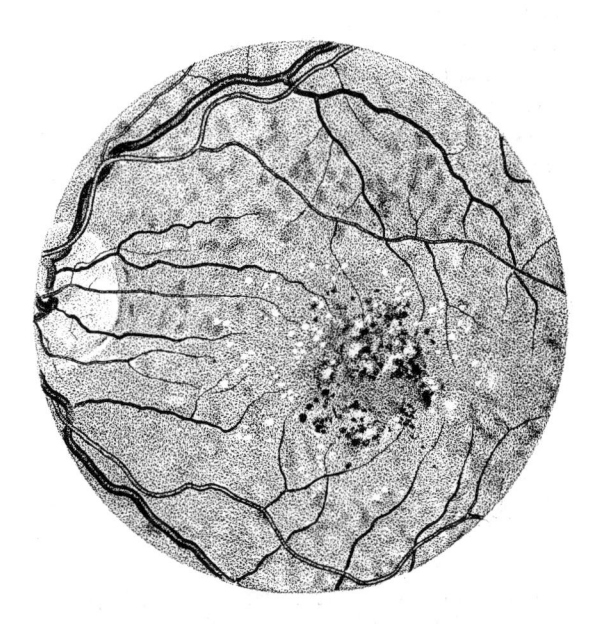

Fig 11-6 Senescent macular degeneration. The macular area is speckled with tiny areas of both reduced and increased pigmentation. Colloid bodies surround the macula.

Less common is *disciform degeneration of the macula* in which an exudate occurs between Bruch's membrane and the retinal pigment epithelium. This is usually followed by haemorrhage from choroidal new-formed vessels into the same space with rapid, permanent loss of macular function (Fig 11-7). In a few patients this destructive bleeding stage can be forestalled by photocoagulation of the subretinal neovascular membrane when this happens to be at a safe distance from the fovea (p. 146). This has to be done promptly after the earliest disturbance of vision such as the subtle distortion detected with an Amsler grid (p. 101).

SMD is probably not a single condition. In some it is due to ageing changes in Bruch's membrane which are accompanied by degeneration of the retinal pigment epithelium with displacement of pigment and by degeneration of the retinal receptors.

When there is a uniocular cataract, the macular degeneration may be less advanced in the eye with the cataract and this fact can be significant in reaching a decision as to whether cataract extraction is worth trying.

Since the cause is not fully known, there is no effective treatment. Systemic vasodilators, hormones, iodides, vitamins, etc. have been used but all are valueless. Magnifying spectacles, called low vision aids (LVA), or a hand-magnifying glass may help some patients to continue reading for a while.

Almost all patients understandably expect that their visual failure will progress to blindness and the most important part of the management of these patients is to assure them that this is not so, that they will retain their peripheral vision and therefore always be able to get about unaided. Another common misconception is that use of the eye as in reading and sewing will hasten the deterioration. Patients need to be told that this is not so and that there is nothing to be gained by 'saving their eyes'; although reading may be difficult, they will not 'strain their eyes' by doing this or anything else that their failing sight will allow them to do.

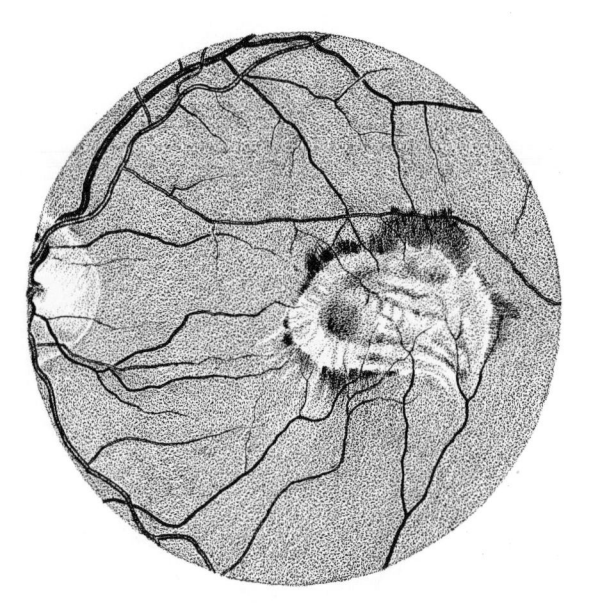

Fig 11-7 Disciform macular degeneration. Fluid and haemorrhage have raised the central retina into an irregular mound. This is fringed with blood which has come through the pigment epithelium to lie between it and the neural retina.

PART FOUR

CASUALTY OFFICER OPHTHALMOLOGY

Doctors working in hospital accident and emergency centres and those in general practice are confronted with a variety of acute eye problems. It is reasonable to expect them, when faced with a patient presenting with an eye injury, with a painful eye, with a red eye or with sudden loss of vision, 'to be able to undertake immediate diagnostic procedures, institute first aid treatment, decide on their competence to treat the patient without referral, and, if justifiably confident, explain to the patient the condition, its prognosis, and the proposed management, and initiate treatment' (p. 222).

This section deals mainly with those eye injuries and diseases in which the early management, including referral to an ophthalmologist, is significant. It includes those conditions in which the prognosis may be adversely affected if the appropriate treatment is not started within about 24 hours and those for which the patient seeks immediate relief of his or her symptoms.

Likely *presenting complaints* come under the headings of
1   injuries,
2   painful red eyes, or
3   sudden loss of vision

Non-acute presenting complaints which come under the heading of
4   watering of the eye
will also be considered.

Clinical Approach

In any branch of clinical medicine it is neither sensible, necessary, nor economically possible to carry out all possible interrogations and examinations. On the other hand there is a bare skeleton of clinical procedure which cannot be reduced without risk of serious oversight. Each casualty officer and general practitioner has to fashion for him or herself his or her own ophthalmic clinical skeleton and then programme him or herself to follow it routinely, fleshing it out where and when necessary.

Always start by taking a *history* and avoid the temptation to examine the eye before doing so. Record the relevant details, especially those which could be of medico-legal significance. Sift the facts from the patient's interpretation of the facts and his or her suppositions. Frequently the history gives a lead to the diagnosis. Hesitate to diagnose conjunctivitis unless there has been a conjunctival discharge. Pain and watering without a history of a foreign body or other injury suggest the possibility of a dendritic ulcer. Itching suggests an allergic reaction. If the patient felt something strike his or her eye when hitting metal on metal, e.g. while using a hammer and chisel, assume that there is an intraocular foreign body until proved otherwise. Exposure to ultraviolet light, e.g. a welding flash, is not often volunteered by a patient. Enquire about previous attacks; a number of eye diseases tend to recur, for example, uveitis, dendritic ulcers, marginal corneal ulcers, episcleritis, allergic reactions.

In all cases determine and record the *visual acuity* of each eye separately (with distance glasses if worn) before the eyes are examined. This will prevent more inexcusable mistakes in diagnosis than any other test and of course it may be of medico-legal importance. The pinhole test is particularly useful in distinguishing between lowered acuity due to refractive errors or opacities in the ocular media and that due to lesions of the retina or optic nerve. If the vision is normal and remains normal immediate referral to an ophthalmologist is rarely necessary.

The first step in *examination* is to look at the face, the eyelids and then the eyes in a good light. Adequacy of lighting cannot be over-emphasized. If there is much pain and spasm of the eyelids instillation of one drop of a sterile anaesthetic, e.g. proxymetacaine (proparacaine) eyedrops, will ease the patient and facilitate examination. Follow naked eye inspection by examination with focal illumination and then, if indicated and available, slit-lamp microscopy. Next use the ophthalmoscope to examine the red reflex and the fundus.

If there is evidence of a perforating wound proceed no further with examination; protect the eye with a sterile eye pad, warn the patient to gently close his or her lids and to refrain from shutting his or her eye tightly, and seek immediate specialist care. If there is uncertainty about a corneal surface lesion instil one drop of sterile fluorescein eye-drops 1% or 2% or insert the end of a fluorescein impregnated strip of filter paper inside the lower lid and after half a minute wash out the fluorescein with generous amounts of sterile normal saline. Deficiencies of corneal epithelium stain bright green (foreign body, ulcer, abrasion, erosions) while damaged conjunctival

CLINICAL APPROACH   197

epithelium stains yellow (thereby revealing the area of conjunctiva affected in a chemical injury such as from lime).

If a sudden loss of vision is unexplained and the anterior segment of the eye (including the pupillary reactions) and its tension are normal, dilate the pupil for ophthalmoscopy with a drop of tropicamide eye-drops 0.5% or cyclopentolate eye-drops 0.5%.

Chapter 12

INJURIES

Lid laceration
Facial fractures
Conjunctival foreign body
Conjunctival laceration
Chemical injuries
Actinic keratoconjunctivitis
Solar retinopathy
Corneal abrasion
Corneal foreign body
    Removal
Corneal perforation
    Iris prolapse
    Cataract
Intraocular foreign body
Contusion
    Lid haematoma
    Subconjunctival ecchymosis
    Traumatic hyphaema
    Iris injuries
    Dislocation of the lens
    Concussion cataract
    Vitreous haemorrhage
    Choroidal ruptures
    Retinal oedema

INJURIES

Lacerations of an eyelid are less frequent than they used to be now that more people are restrained by seat belts from smashing into car windscreens. Even gross injuries do well provided they are repaired with meticulous accuracy. Lid tissue heals well because of its vascularity and it is a good rule not to excise wound edges and to remove only most severely crushed tissue. Vertical lacerations involving the lid margin require care in their repair to avoid notching of the lid margin, which is prevented by overcoming horizontal tension in the lid and by using fine sutures with precision.

Occasionally an upper lid is torn away so that the cornea is exposed. First aid covering of the cornea must be obtained with temporary sutures to hold the torn tissues over the eye and the whole region covered with tulle gras and a generous dressing.

The significance of a small tear or cut of the inner portion of the lower lid is easily overlooked. A superficial-looking laceration in this region may have severed the lacrimal canaliculus and if this is not repaired without delay permanent epiphora is likely because late repair is difficult. A stout nylon thread is used to bridge the cut ends and to maintain patency of the canaliculus for about six weeks while it is healing.

Facial fractures which implicate the margins and walls of the orbits may involve the eye itself or its muscles. An ophthalmologist is a permanent member of the team dealing with facio-maxillary injuries and his or her advice should be sought early when assessing this type of injury. A fracture with depression of the floor of the orbit into the maxillary sinus may occur with other facial fractures or, as a result of a blow to the eye, it may occur as an orbital 'blowout' fracture without the anterior orbital margin being broken. If not corrected the dropped enophthalmic eye may be disfiguring and there may be permanent limitation of movement of the eye with ensuing diplopia. Repair of this fracture displacement is much easier if undertaken within two weeks of the injury.

A *conjunctival foreign body* which is not flushed out by the reflex lacrimation which it stimulates is most commonly found on the under surface of the upper lid where it is caught in the small groove which runs parallel and close to the lid margin. This situation explains both the gritty foreign body type of discomfort which occurs with each blink as the particle scratches the cornea and the frequent success in removing the foreign body by the time honoured manoeuvre of pulling the upper lid by its eyelashes out and down over the lower lid and then letting go. A foreign body lodged subtarsally is seen by everting the upper lid (p. 109) and is removed by wiping gently with the tip of the finger.

A patient's subjective localization of just where a foreign body is 'in his eye' is commonly misleading and should not be allowed to interfere with a systematic search of the conjunctival sac and the cornea. The complaint of 'something in the eye' in itself may be misleading. A foreign body type of pain frequently occurs in the absence of any foreign body as in corneal ulcers (e.g. dendritic, marginal), corneal erosion (e.g. actinic keratitis), and corneal abrasions. Do not accept at face value a patient's complaint of something in his or her eye.

Two bodies which are not strictly foreign but which act in this way and abrade the cornea are conjunctival concretions and ingrowing eyelashes. A *concretion* is the result of slow accumulation of debris in a crypt of the lower tarsal conjunctiva. Most are small soft cream spots of no significance but occasionally one becomes calcareous and projects above the surface. It then feels rough to the finger tip and can be readily removed with a sharp needle under surface anaesthesia.

Lashes which grow inwards towards the cornea *(trichiasis)* follow severe inflammation of the lid margins (blepharitis) or scarring of the lids, e.g. from trachoma (Fig 12-1). An ingrowing lash is commonly light coloured and may not be seen unless oblique focal illumination is used. Epilation will give temporary relief. Permanent relief requires destruction of the lash follicle, for example with electrolysis.

In themselves *lacerations* of the bulbar *conjunctiva* are not of great importance. Suturing is not necessary if the conjunctiva is in more or less normal position and the wound does not gape more widely than a few millimetres. More extensive wounds are simply sutured with fine silk or gut to coapt the edges. Conjunctiva heals quickly and non-absorbable sutures can be removed in four or five days. The importance of

INJURIES

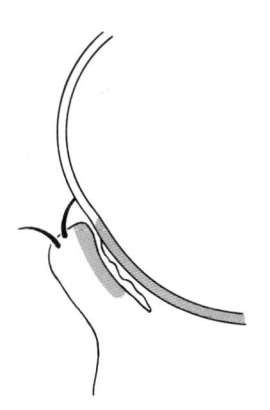

Fig 12-1 Trichiasis. A misdirected eyelash rubs on the cornea.

conjunctival lacerations is that they may signify deeper damage. Often a small laceration of the sclera is not obvious and this should be looked for specifically whenever the conjunctiva has been breached. The force which tore the conjunctiva may have contused internal ocular structures such as the retina and this should also be investigated. As always, in any eye injury it is mandatory to test and record visual acuity; if this is normal and remains normal it is unlikely that there is serious injury requiring immediate attention.

First aid treatment is the same for all *chemical injuries* caused by irritants in liquid or powder form being splashed or blown into an eye. It consists in urgent and prolonged washing with water (or irrigation with saline if available). Forceful separation of the eyelids, although most painful, is essential to allow flushing of the chemical from the conjunctiva and cornea while the head is plunged into a basin of water or the face is held under a running tap. Alkalies, such as lime and ammonia, cause the worst of the commonly seen chemical eye injuries because they continue to act for some time after their introduction and the damage they cause is not limited to the outside of the eye. Staining with fluorescein will allow assessment of the extent of surface damage and if more than one quarter of the cornea stains, if the cornea is distinctly grey, or if the opposing tarsal and bulbar conjunctiva extensively stain, specialist advice should be sought. In the case of lime burns, if expert attention is not immediately available the eye should be anaesthetized (e.g. proxymetacaine (proparacaine) eye-drops 0.5%) and a search made for particles of lime which should be painstakingly picked out with fine forceps. Instillation of a saturated solution of glucose will form an insoluble calcium gluconate with any fragments which are missed and thus inactivate them.

Actinic keratoconjunctivitis, due to exposure to ultraviolet light, may follow careless therapeutic exposure, careless exposure to a welding arc (arc flash) or exposure to intense reflected sunlight (snow blindness). It can always be prevented by sensible use of protective goggles. There is a latent period of several hours between exposure and onset of symptoms of intense photophobia, foreign body pain, and lacrimation. There is general conjunctival hyperaemia and corneal epithelial oedema with punctate epithelial loss. The temptation to use anaesthetic eye-drops should be resisted because the relief they give is transient and they delay epithelial regeneration. Phenylephrine eye-drops 0.125% three-hourly, analgesics, and avoidance of light usually make the discomfort bearable until it subsides in about twelve hours.

Solar retinopathy or eclipse blindness is due to a burn of the foveal retina from absorption of infrared wavelengths when the sun is looked at, as during observation of an eclipse or during cultic sun gazing. The resulting central scotoma is permanent. Looking at the sun through ordinary sun glasses or over-exposed photographic films will not prevent damage. The only safe way to see an eclipse is to form an image of the sun on a black surface with a pinhole made in a piece of cardboard.

A twig, a baby's finger nail, a poorly fitting or too long retained contact lens, and many other objects may beat the protective reflexes and strip some epithelium from the cornea to give a *corneal abrasion*. The pain suggests to the patient that a foreign body is in the eye which becomes red, especially in the circumcorneal (ciliary) region, and waters. The loss of epithelium can be detected as an imperfection of the mirror surface of the cornea by using oblique focal illumination or more dramatically by staining with sterile fluorescein. Healing is rapid (12 to 24 hours) unless infection causes the abrasion to become a corneal ulcer. Treatment consists of antibiotic drops (e.g. chloramphenicol eye-drops), a short acting cycloplegic (e.g. cyclopentolate eye-drops 0.5% or 1%) to reduce iris and ciliary spasm, and firm padding of the eye to splint the lids. Anaesthetic drops should not be repeated because they delay healing. An occasional abrasion breaks down at intervals months later, possibly due to imperfect attachment of the epithelial cells to their underlying basement membrane. Such *recurrent erosions of the cornea* most characteristically cause a foreign body type of pain when the lids are first opened in the morning.

Foreign bodies, such as a wind-blown particle of grit, a minute fragment from a grindling wheel or the tool being ground, a bird-seed husk, commonly lodge on the *cornea.* A superficial foreign body may be dislodged by squirting it with a jet of sterile normal saline from a syringe after anaesthetizing the cornea. More often the foreign body is impacted in the epithelium or deeper and requires direct removal.

To *remove a corneal foreign body* anaesthetize the cornea with two or three drops of proxymetacaine (proparacaine) 0.5% eye drops or other suitable local eye anaesthetic. If anaesthetic eye-drops are not available injectable lignocaine with or without adrenalin is satisfactory. Good oblique illumination of the cornea is essential and a binocular magnifying loupe is needed by all but the young. It is easier if the patient lies down and you work from the head end of the couch. Use a sterile sharp instrument to neatly cut around and then prise out the foreign body; a sterile disposable number 20 hypodermic needle with a small syringe barrel as handle is ideal. Ask the patient to open both his eyes and to fix a suitable mark with his uninjured eye so as to keep his eyes steady. Separate the lids of the affected eye with finger and thumb of your non-dominant hand. Attempts to scrape the foreign body off the cornea with the tip of the needle will damage a larger area of epithelium than elevating the foreign body after freeing by cutting around it; with moderate force there is little danger of perforating cornea which is tough. However, do not hesitate to refer the patient to someone with more experience if you are not entirely confident of your ability.

Small fragments of iron, as from an emery wheel, become ringed around by rust. A *rust ring* should be removed but if this is difficult, leave it till the following day when it will be found that the stained corneal tissue has softened and can be more readily excised. A small sterile dental burr twirled in the fingers is useful for removing a difficult rust ring.

After removal of the foreign body, instil antibiotic eye-drops and, unless the foreign body was quite superficial, a short-acting cycloplegic such as cyclopentolate 1% eye-drops. Close the eye with a firmly applied eye pad. Ask the patient to attend the following day to ensure that infection has not occurred. This would be indicated by a definite greyness of the surrounding cornea or by the eye becoming more painful and more red. It demands immediate referral.

Most *perforating wounds* are obvious and all such injuries should be referred for specialist attention without delay. Prompt repair is desirable for two reasons. First, the risk of intraocular infection decreases the sooner a corneal laceration is sealed and the shorter interval there is before prophylactic antibiotics are administered subconjunctivally. Secondly, oedema of the cornea occurs adjacent to the cut and this swelling makes it more difficult to get accurate coaptation of the wound edges with the fine direct sutures which are used.

The first aid treatment of all perforating wounds of an eye consists of lightly padding the injured eye and also covering the uninjured eye to reduce eye movements.

Quite small corneal perforations are self-sealing and their gravity may be unrecognized. A suggestive history should not be ignored. There will usually have been loss of some aqueous with consequent reduction in the depth of the anterior chamber when compared with that of the fellow eye. The depth of a corneal wound can be readily seen with a slit-lamp to determine whether or not it involved the full thickness of the cornea.

When the cornea is cut a portion of the iris is commonly washed into and out of the wound by the escaping aqueous. This *prolapsed iris* lies on the surface of the cornea and/or sclera as a small black nodule which has been mistaken for a foreign body by those who are not aware of the possibility. When there is an iris prolapse the pupil is always distorted, the usual change in shape being to a pear-shaped pupil with the apex towards the prolapse (Fig 12-2). If the iris plugs the hole in the cornea the aqueous does not continue leaking from the eye and the anterior

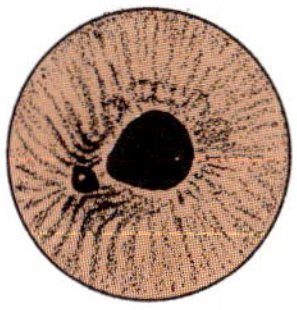

Fig 12-2 Iris prolapse through a small perforating corneal wound.

chamber, although shallow, is then not absent. If the prolapse is small and recent the iris may be replaced within the eye. In other cases the portion which has been within the wound and outside the eye is abscised before the laceration is sutured in a watertight fashion and the anterior chamber reformed with sterile Ringer's solution or air.

The injury which cuts a cornea often cuts the lens capsule as well and then *cataract* formation is inevitable. When the opening in the lens is wide the soft cortical substance of the lens spills into the anterior chamber and into the wound. This increases the technical difficulties of repair and worsens the prognosis for a useful seeing eye.

A retained *intraocular foreign body* is frequent enough to be known by the initials IOFB. The commonest sort is a small chip, 1-4mm in size, struck from a metal tool and which, travelling at high velocity, neatly penetrates the eye. The classic source is the head of a hammer or a cold chisel, but it can happen whenever metal is struck with metal and protective goggles are not worn. The wound of entry, which may be through sclera rather than cornea, can be hard to see. And the patient's symptoms are usually deceptively minor. After the initial pain and the feeling of having been struck in the eye there may be very little discomfort. When a patient complains of something in the eye it is wise to ask specifically what he or she was doing when he or she felt something hit his or her eye, and if he or she was hitting metal on metal to assume that the eye harbours an IOFB until this is excluded.

Visual acuity is commonly disturbed but can be normal. A wound as small as 1mm can usually be spotted with careful inspection. There may be a hole or tear of the iris, distortion of the pupil, a hyphaema, or a lens opacity. If the anterior part of the eye looks normal, dilatation of the pupil may reveal vitreous bleeding or even a metallic foreign body lying on the retina. If any doubt remains an x-ray of the orbit will always confirm or exclude a metallic IOFB.

If an IOFB of iron or steel is not removed a slowly developing chemical change called siderosis occurs which ultimately destroys the vision. Removal is therefore necessary and the sooner the better because it is technically easier (using an electro-magnet) if done before the foreign body becomes firmly embedded in the scar tissue which surrounds it.

Contusions of the eye are common and their effects are many and varied. The following are some of the injuries which can result from a blow on the eye.

In the common black eye or *haematoma of the eyelids* the important thing is to exclude damage to the eye itself. The bruising clears without treatment in a week or so. A *subconjunctival ecchymosis* due to direct injury does not usually extend backwards as far as the conjunctival fornix, whereas subconjunctival blood which spreads forwards from the orbit, as in orbital fractures, has no such posterior limit. Most subconjunctival ecchymoses are spontaneous and are not due to injury. They look alarming but rarely signify any local or systemic abnormality. The blood absorbs within a week or so and throughout it retains an arterial colour because of the high oxygen tension in the vascular conjunctiva.

A *traumatic hyphaema* (blood in the anterior chamber) is a frequent result of a blunt injury. The haemorrhage comes from the iris and the red cells sediment to the bottom of the anterior chamber (Fig 12-3). Unless blood fills the whole

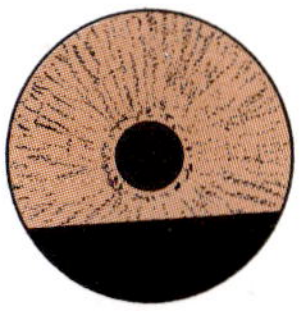

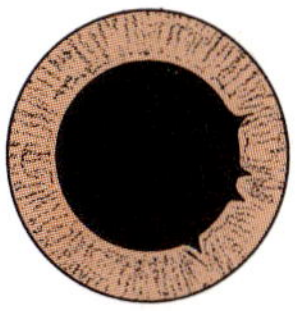

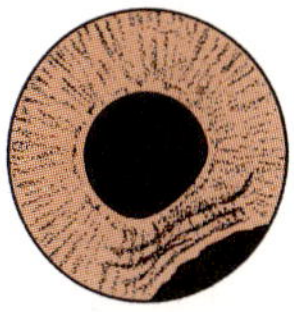

Fig 12-3 Hyphaema. The red cells of blood in the anterior chamber gravitate downwards to form a fluid level.

Fig 12-4 Traumatic mydriasis and four ruptures of the iris sphincter.

Fig 12-5 Iridodialysis.

anterior chamber it is usually absorbed in a few days. Sometimes secondary bleeding occurs, most commonly about three days after injury, and this is likely to be more extensive and to cause secondary glaucoma. Because of this possibility a patient with a traumatic hyphaema should be admitted for observation and also to ensure that the injured eye is immobilized as much as possible by covering both eyes. Although use of a mydriatic-cycloplegic drug would seem reasonable treatment, experience has shown that these eyes do better if drugs which act on the pupil are not used. Cortico-steroid eye-drops reduce the traumatic inflammation.

Other manifestations of injury to the iris are *traumatic mydriasis,* in which the pupil is dilated and does not react, perhaps permanently, *rupture of the iris sphincter* so that there are notches in the pupil margin (Fig 12-4), and *iridodialysis* in which part of the iris is torn away from its attachment to the ciliary body and the pupil consequently becomes D shaped (Fig 12-5).

The *lens* may be *dislocated* and drop to the bottom of the vitreous but usually its suspensory zonule is only partially ruptured. This is called a *subluxation* of the lens and, because the lens no longer firmly supports the iris, it gives rise to a characteristic jelly-like tremulousness of the iris when the eye is moved which is called iridodonesis. A concussion cataract may follow a severe blow.

Bleeding into the *vitreous* can follow a non-perforating injury which ruptures vessels in the ciliary body, choroid, or retina. Blood is absorbed slowly from the vitreous and until it has cleared enough for the retina to be seen the possibility of an associated retinal detachment should be kept in mind. *Choroidal ruptures* which, after the blood has cleared, are seen as ragged white lines of exposed sclera often concentric with the optic disc, interfere surprisingly little with the function of the eye.

Traumatic *oedema of the retina,* sometimes called by the old name of commotio retinae, occurs under the point of impact and opposite to this in the contrecoup position. The macula is frequently involved and herein lies the threat to central vision, because if the macular retina is oedematous for more than a day or two permanent vacuolation and cystic degeneration with pigmentary speckling is likely. Immobilization of the injured eye may hasten the disappearance of the oedema and this means padding both eyes for a few days. Corticosteroids given systemically for the same time may also limit the oedema.

Chapter 13

PAINFUL RED EYES

Conjunctivitis
  Acute bacterial
  Follicular
    Trachoma
    Inclusion conjunctivitis
  Ophthalmia neonatorum
  Viral
  Allergic
    Contact dermatitis
Inflammation of the eyelids
  Stye
  Meibomian cyst
  Blepharitis
  Dacryocystitis
Inflammation of the cornea
  Corneal ulcer
  Marginal corneal ulcers
  Dendritic ulcer
  Disciform keratitis
  Herpes zoster ophthalmicus
  Punctate epithelial erosions
  Keratoconjunctivitis sicca
    Sjögren's syndrome
  Interstitial keratitis
Episcleritis
Iridocyclitis
  Acute iritis
    Sympathetic ophthalmitis

PAINFUL RED EYES

The five major causes of ocular pain and redness are conjunctivitis, keratitis, episcleritis, iritis, and acute angle closure glaucoma. This chapter considers the first four of these conditions while angle closure glaucoma is included in the chapter on glaucoma (p. 176). The differential diagnosis of 'the acute red eye' is so important that it warrants tabulation of those features which are most helpful in distinguishing the five causal conditions. Inflammations of the eyelids are also dealt with since they too can give rise to local pain and redness.

DIFFERENTIAL DIAGNOSIS OF THE RED EYE

	Conjunctivitis	Corneal lesion, e.g. abrasion foreign body, ulcer	Acute iritis	Acute angle closure glaucoma	Episcleritis
Symptoms	Discomfort	Pain, photophobia	Pain, photophobia	Severe pain	Aching pain; tenderness localized to affected area
Discharge	Mucopurulent	Watery discharge	Watery	Slight watering	Slight watering
Vision	**Never impaired**	May be impaired	**Impaired**	Severely **impaired**; haloes	Normal
Hyperaemia	Generalized	Ciliary (may be localized to region nearest to lesion)	Ciliary	Ciliary (surprisingly little in early stages)	Predominantly area affected
Cornea	Normal	Alteration of surface reflection; ± opacity	Normal	Steamy, loss of lustre	Normal
Pupil	Normal	May be irritative miosis	**Small** and may be irregular	**Dilated** and non-reacting	Normal
Ocular tension	Normal	Normal	May be secondary glaucoma	Raised	Normal

CONJUNCTIVITIS

Conjunctivitis is an inflammation of a mucous membrane and therefore in most types there is hyperaemia and thickening of the conjunctiva and an exudation of mucus (catarrhal) or of mucus and inflammatory cells (mucopurulent).

The bacteria which cause the common *acute infectious conjunctivitis,* sometimes aptly called by patients 'a cold in the eye', range from the more common staphylococcus and diplococcus pneumoniae to the less common organisms of the haemophilus group and the now rare neisseria gonorrhoeae. Infection is almost always bilateral. The patient experiences discomfort in the form of smarting and grittiness, moderate photophobia in the severest forms, but not true pain. He or she is aware of the discharge which characteristically causes the lids to be stuck together or at least crusted on awakening. The hyperaemia in conjunctivitis is generalized in contrast to the predominantly ciliary hyperaemia of corneal or intraocular inflammation (Fig 13-1).

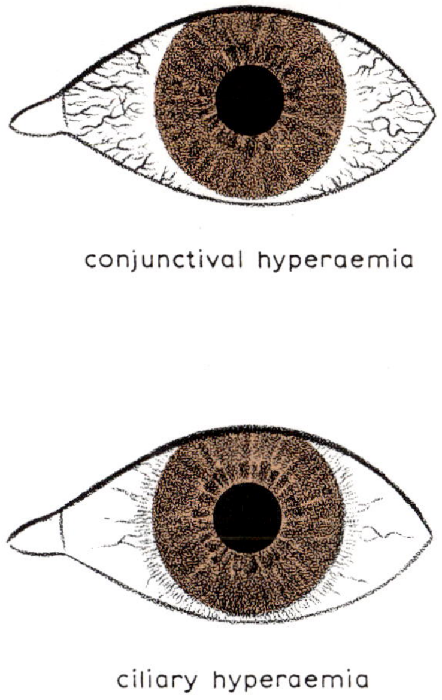

Acute bacterial conjunctivitis responds within a day or so to treatment with an appropriate antibiotic applied locally to the eye. Because of this and a lack of diagnostic confidence, some practitioners tend to treat all cases presenting as an acute red eye with local antibiotics on the grounds that if it gets better it was conjunctivitis and if it does not it is something else which requires the skills of a specialist. Although this reliance on a therapeutic trial is often successful because conjunctivitis is commoner than the other more serious causes of the acute red eye, it is however bad practice. Valuable time may be lost in starting the correct treatment for dangerous conditions such as corneal ulceration, acute iritis, angle closure glaucoma. Diagnosis is not difficult if it is remembered that conjunctivitis does not cause real pain, that it does not lower vision, that it does not alter pupil size or movement, and that there is almost always a mucous or mucopurulent discharge.

In choosing an antibiotic for local ocular use it is preferable to select one that is not commonly used systemically so that it will matter less if resistant strains of the organism should emerge or if the patient should become sensitized to the antibiotic. A wide spectrum of action is also desirable. On these grounds chloramphenicol or proprietary mixtures of neomycin, polymyxin, and bacitracin can be recommended. Eye-drops are used hourly in severe cases or 3-hourly in less severe. An eye ointment instilled at bedtime will prevent the lids from becoming glued together overnight. It is wise to continue treatment for about two days after the symptoms have resolved to forestall a recurrence or the infection becoming chronic. The eye should not be covered because this would prevent the escape of discharge.

Other infectious agents which cause conjunctivitis are the *Chlamydia and viruses*. In this type of infection follicles commonly form as a result of proliferations of lymphoid tissue in the subepithelial adenoid layer of the conjunctiva. They are seen on the palpebral conjunctiva as quite small slightly raised pale areas which may be arranged in rows parallel to the lid margin. Two members of the genus Chlamydia (obligate intracellular organisms sensitive to antibiotics and intermediate between bacteria and viruses) are important causal agents of *follicular conjunctivitis*. They are those causing *tr*achoma and *i*nclusion *c*onjunctivitis, which are very closely related if not the same and are known as the TRIC agents.

Trachoma is a disease of great antiquity and is probably still the major cause of seriously

Fig 13-1 The two types of 'acute red eye'.

impaired vision throughout the world. It is very rare in countries with a temperate climate and when it does occur it is in a mild form. It is a chronic follicular conjunctivitis chiefly affecting the upper lid which becomes deformed from scarring, and there is secondary scarring and opacification of the cornea. It responds to local or systemic broad-spectrum antibiotics and sulphonamides.

Inclusion conjunctivitis is a benign acute follicular conjunctivitis which does not result in corneal or lid scarring. The chief reservoir for the agent is the genital tract and transmission is commonly venereal. The possibility of transmission in non-chlorinated swimming pools led to the name swimming-bath conjunctivitis. Infection during birth gives rise to one form of ophthalmia neonatorum.

Ophthalmia neonatorum is an acute conjunctivitis occurring in the newborn. In times past, when much blindness resulted from secondary corneal ulceration in gonorrhoeal ophthalmia neonatorum, any discharge from the eyes within three weeks of birth was made a notifiable disease. This, the only dangerous conjunctivitis in the newborn, is now rare and responds well to antibiotic treatment provided this is prompt and intensive.

Numerous *viruses* can cause conjunctivitis. Some of the adenoviruses, which primarily inflame the mucosa of the upper respiratory tract, may produce an acute follicular conjunctivitis and with some types the cornea is also involved in the form of a superficial punctate keratitis. Keratoconjunctivitis is common in measles and explains the photophobia of this disease. Reiter's disease or syndrome may be of viral origin and consists of a sterile urethritis, polyarthritis, and mild conjunctivitis or iritis.

Allergic conjunctivitis commonly causes itching and occurs in a number of forms. Hypersensitivity of the conjunctiva to exogenous antigens is responsible for the hyperaemia, chemosis (conjunctival oedema), and profuse watering of hay fever, for the more chronic inflammation of the conjunctiva and adjacent skin in sensitivity to such locally applied drugs as penicillin, pilocarpine, atropine, antihistamines, or to cosmetics, and probably for the condition known as spring catarrh or vernal conjunctivitis. This last condition occurs in children and young adults and may be worse during the summer. Large gelatinous vegetations form on the upper tarsal conjunctiva where they look like cobblestones or on the bulbar conjunctiva surrounding the limbus. Treatment of allergic conjunctivitis involves removal of the antigen if possible and the use of vasoconstrictor and/or corticosteroid eye-drops. Great care is necessary when using local corticosteroids in the eye because a rise of intraocular pressure occurs in about one-third of people and in some this is high enough to cause glaucomatous loss of vision if the drops are used for any length of time *(steroid glaucoma)* (Plate 2, p. 121).

Contact dermatitis commonly affects the skin of the eyelids with minimal involvement of the conjunctiva. The response may be a moist eczema or a dry thickening and stiffening of the skin. Itching is likely. An individual may become sensitized to almost any drug applied locally to the eyes and a host of other substances such as industrial chemicals, detergents, and cosmetics can be responsible. Treatment requires identification of the cause, which may not be easy, and its removal. Local application of corticosteroids to the inflamed skin gives speedy relief.

INFLAMMATION OF THE EYELIDS

Patients may present with inflammatory conditions of the eyelids because of the superficial pain or discomfort and the redness of the lid which they cause. Some are accompanied by a localized conjunctivitis. The three commonest conditions are a *stye*, an internal stye or tarsal cyst, and blepharitis.

A *stye* is a boil involving an eyelash follicle rather than a hair follicle elsewhere. There is tense swelling and some redness of the affected part of the lid which causes considerable pain until the little abscess points beside an eyelash and the pus escapes. Local heat, preferably dry to avoid maceration of the skin, as by resting the closed lids on a cloth pad on a hot-water-bottle, may ease the pain and perhaps more quickly 'bring it to a head'. A local antibiotic eye ointment is commonly used but the only value in this is to forestall possible satellite infections of nearby lash follicles. Epilation of the involved lash if it can be identified may hasten the discharge of pus. Repeated styes may be due to the spread of the infecting staphylococci by the patient's fingers from his or her nose. Bacteriological identification of this as a carrier site and an attempt to eradicate the organisms from the anterior nares with locally applied antibiotics should be undertaken in such patients.

An *internal stye, tarsal cyst,* or *chalazion* is a chronic granuloma of a tarsal (Meibomian) gland which is usually symptomless and manifests as a small hard spherical lump within the lid which can usually be better felt than seen. Occasionally secondary infection occurs with pain and lid oedema and eventual discharge, usually on the conjunctival surface of the lid. Small asymptomatic tarsal cysts require no treatment and may in time spontaneously resolve. When necessary, treatment consists of surgical incision vertically through the conjunctival surface and evacuation of the contents by curettage.

Blepharitis is dandruff of the eyelid margin. In this stubborn inflammation the eyes look red-rimmed with flakes and scales among the eyelashes. Burning discomfort and itching wax and wane and encourage rubbing of the eyelids. Occasionally there is secondary staphylococcal infection which causes ulcerative blepharitis and when this happens eyelashes may be permanently lost or grow askew with resulting trichiasis. Blepharitis can be controlled but rarely cured. Treatment entails daily or twice daily cleansing of the lid margins of scales and crusts with cotton wool applicators moistened in a bland alkaline lotion, judicious application of a proprietary eye ointment containing an antibiotic and corticosteroid, and control of the associated seborrhoeic condition of the scalp.

An *acute dacryocystitis* (inflammation of the lacrimal sac) occurs suddenly as a painful, tense swelling below the medial canthus overlying the lacrimal fossa. If it is untreated an abscess may form and rupture through the overlying skin. There is usually a previous history of watering of the eye due to a preceding chronic dacryocystitis and consequent obstruction of the nasolacrimal duct. Sometimes the acute inflammation follows a mucocoele of the lacrimal sac in which, as a result of the loss of patency of the nasolacrimal duct, the sac slowly becomes distended and filled with mucous material which can be made to regurgitate through the canaliculus by finger pressure on the swelling. Acute dacryocystitis is treated with systemic antibiotics and, if an abscess has formed, by surgical drainage. Chronic obstruction of the lacrimal passages requires surgical correction, for example by dacryocystorhinostomy in which a new mucosal-lined opening is fashioned between the tear sac and the middle meatus of the nose.

INFLAMMATION OF THE CORNEA

Keratitis (inflammation of the cornea) is more commonly the result of an exogenous infection or injury than of an endogenous hypersensitivity reaction. Lesions which start superficially first disrupt the corneal epithelium and therefore when it is localized this type of superficial keratitis is traditionally called a corneal ulcer.

Corneal ulcers are caused by bacteria, such as the pneumococcus, staphylococcus, streptococcus, gonococcus, and pseudomonas aeruginosa (pyocyaneus), by viruses such as herpes simplex, and by fungi. Normal corneal epithelium resists bacterial invasion and some break in the form of a scratch, a foreign body, or damage from a conjunctivitis therefore usually precedes corneal ulceration. The sensible preventive use of antibiotics and meticulous technique in removing corneal foreign bodies should prevent most bacterial corneal ulcers. On the other hand an ulcer may be induced by removing a corneal foreign body with an inadequately sterilized needle or through using contaminated eye-drops. The ulcer distorts the smooth mirror surface of the cornea as can be seen by looking at the reflection from a focused light. It is grey due to the loss of corneal transparency from oedema and infiltration with inflammatory cells (Fig 13-2). When centrally located it impairs vision. The accompanying hyperaemia is chiefly of the ciliary type and may be localized to an area nearest to the ulcer if this is close to the periphery of the cornea. It causes pain of the foreign body type which may be severe, photophobia, and watering. Toxins diffuse through the cornea into the aqueous to cause an irritative iritis. When moderately severe this manifests as a miosis and in the most severe cases the cells of the inflammatory exudate from the iris sediment at the bottom of the anterior chamber to form a sterile *hypopyon* (Fig 13-2).

Aggressive treatment with appropriate antibiotics if started promptly will usually overcome the infection. Maximum sustained concentration of antibiotics in the cornea is achieved by subconjunctival injection, e.g. gentamicin 20mg in 0.5ml sterile water after local anaesthesia. Atropine eye-drops are used to relax the spastic iris sphincter muscle. In severe cases inpatient treatment is desirable.

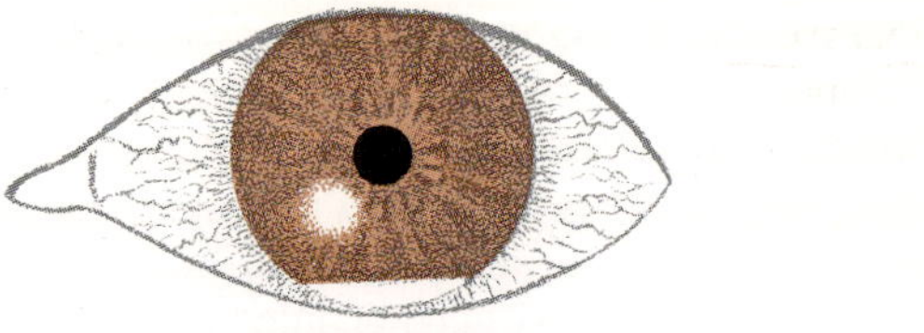

Fig 13-2 Acute bacterial corneal ulcer with a hypopyon. The pupil is constricted because of the associated iritis.

Multiple *marginal corneal* cellular infiltrates and ulcers just inside the limbus occur most frequently in middle-aged women (Fig 13-3). They may be due to staphylococcal infection or to an intracorneal antigen-antibody reaction involving staphylococcal exotoxin. Although painful, they are benign and respond well to treatment with antibiotic and corticosteroids. Another type of marginal corneal inflammation occurs in acne rosacea.

In countries favoured with a high standard of living the most common and most damaging corneal ulcers are now those due to the virus of *herpes simplex*. This invades the corneal epithelium where it causes minute vesicles which rupture to form punctate ulcers. Commonly the vesicles are confluent in a branching pattern and give rise to the diagnostically characteristic *dendritic ulcer* (Fig 13-4). Larger geographic or amoeboid areas may be involved. The patient experiences foreign body irritation and may present with the complaint of something in his or her eye. This is a trap for the unwary clinician who accepts the patient's assumption without question. There is watering and, if the lesion is central on the cornea, blurred vision. In the early stages conjunctival hyperaemia may be minimal.

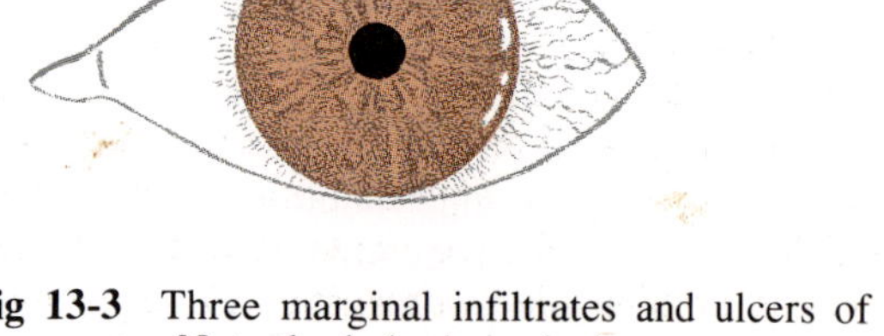

Fig 13-3 Three marginal infiltrates and ulcers of the cornea. Note the irritative miosis.

Recurrence of the lesions in the same eye is common and this may be triggered by a fever, stress, or too much sun.

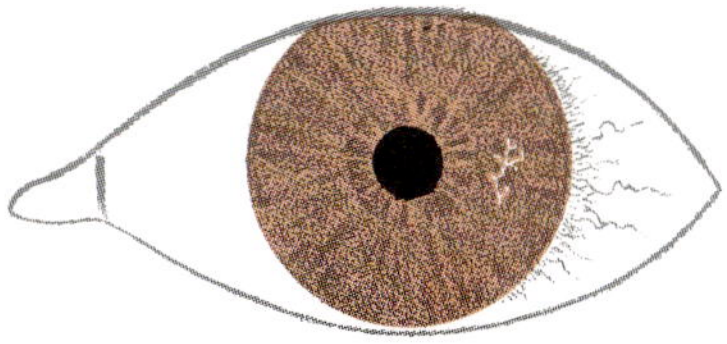

Fig 13-4 Dendritic ulcer of the cornea.

In some eyes the corneal stroma is involved, one distinctive type being *disciform keratitis* in which there is oedematous thickening and opacification of a more or less central disc of cornea. This reaction is probably an immunological response resulting from the meeting of virus from the epithelium with antibody which diffuses into the stroma from the limbal blood vessels. Another important type of stromal involvement results from the *improper use of corticosteroids*. These are dangerous in the presence of herpetic infection because, although the eye may become more comfortable and less red, they permit the ulcer to extend and deepen and eventually perforate the cornea with consequent loss of aqueous and collapse of the anterior chamber.

Treatment of dendritic ulcers is not straightforward or predictable and the responsibility for it is therefore usually better assumed by an ophthalmologist. The aim is to destroy the virus while it is confined to the corneal epithelium and this is achieved either by mechanical removal of the affected epithelium or by the use of locally applied antiviral agents. The preparation commonly used is idoxuridine (IDU; 5-iodo-2'-deoxyuridine) which is a thymidine analogue and interferes with DNA synthesis. This has to be instilled as drops hourly by day and 2-hourly by night or as an eye ointment 3-hourly. It was the first effective viral antibiotic used in medicine. Two more recently introduced antiviral drugs which may be effective when IDU is not are adenine arabinoside (vidabarine) 3% eye ointment and acyclovir ('Zovirax') 3% eye ointment.

Cautious minimal applications of topical corticosteroids, usually under an antiviral cover, are used to suppress the hypersensitivity reaction in disciform keratitis. Corneal grafting may be necessary for recalcitrant stromal lesions or for residual corneal scarring when this has greatly reduced vision.

Herpes zoster ophthalmicus involves the eye in about half the patients and when it does its major impact is on the cornea. Severe neuralgic pain in the distribution of the ophthalmic division of the fifth nerve may precede the skin eruption by several days. Ocular involvement is more likely when there are vesicles on the tip of the nose in the cutaneous distribution of the nasociliary nerve which also innervates the cornea. Swelling of the eyelids is usual but does not necessarily mean that the globe is affected. When involved the cornea is anaesthetic and oedematous with punctate ulcers and stromal opacities. There is usually also an iridocyclitis with KP (p. 211). The inflammation lasts for weeks and may leave permanent damage. Treatment is with systemic acyclovir together with local steroids and atropine.

Other viruses which cause corneal inflammation are the adenovirus type 8, measles, smallpox, and vaccinia. The first two cause a superficial punctate keratitis in which there are minute epithelial erosions and in some cases subepithelial opacities.

Punctate epithelial erosions, which are more readily seen after staining with fluorescein, also occur with severe staphylococcal conjunctivitis, in exposure keratitis, e.g. following facial nerve paralysis, in neurotrophic keratitis due to lesions of the ophthalmic division of the trigeminal nerve (in this condition painless and if untreated progressing to extensive ulceration), in actinic keratitis, e.g. arc flash and 'snow blindness', from careless use of aerosol hair sprays, and in keratitis sicca.

Keratoconjunctivitis sicca is the result of grossly reduced tear production either from atrophy of the lacrimal glands, as in Sjögren's syndrome, or from conjunctival scarring blocking their ducts and destroying the unicellular glands, as occurs in erythema multiforme, pemphigus, and trachoma. Tear secretion is estimated by Schirmer's test in which a 4mm wide strip of filter paper is inserted into the inferior conjunctival fornix and bent down over the lower lid margin.

The length of paper wetted by the tears in say 4 minutes is observed. When tears are deficient there is usually increased secretion of conjunctival mucus.

Sjögren's syndrome consists of keratoconjunctivitis sicca, reduced salivary and mucous membrane secretions, and rheumatoid arthritis or one of the collagen diseases. It may be the result of auto-immune destruction of the involved glands. Patients experience burning ocular discomfort but the diagnosis is too frequently overlooked. As well as punctate erosions of the desiccated conjunctival and corneal epithelium, minute filaments of mucus in twisted strands may form on the cornea (filamentary keratitis). Symptomatic treatment with artificial tears, e.g. hypromellose eye-drops (saline with hydroxypropylmethycellulose 0.5% to prolong its retention in the eye), gives relief but installation may have to be very frequent, for example half hourly.

Interstitial keratitis should be synonymous with stromal keratitis and non-specific, but traditional usage has tended to restrict its use to the now rare endogenous deep keratitis which occurs about puberty in children afflicted with congenital syphilis. Both corneas become cloudy and later pink due to the ingrowth of deep stromal blood vessels (Fig 13-5). Antiluetic treatment and local corticosteroids often reduce the amount of residual scarring but, if not, and corneal grafting is undertaken, the result is likely to be good.

Episcleritis is a 'collagen' inflammation of episcleral tissues which may be associated with rheumatic conditions and is essentially a scleral rheumatic nodule. There is a localized area of both deep and superficial conjunctival hyperaemia which can ache severely and is almost always tender to palpation through the eyelid with the tenderness localized to the area of inflammation. Recurrences are likely. Topical corticosteroids and oral salicylates may suppress the inflammation until it eventually abates.

IRIDOCYCLITIS

Iridocyclitis is an inflammation of the anterior portion of the uveal tract and is also known as *anterior uveitis*. Iris and ciliary body are usually both implicated, but at times an *iritis* (inflammation of the iris) and at other times a *cyclitis* (inflammation of the ciliary body) may predominate. *Choroiditis* is a *posterior uveitis*.

Acute iridocyclitis causes severe aching in and about the affected eye, intense photophobia, watering, and often some blurring of vision. The eye is red due to ciliary hyperaemia and there may be general conjunctival hyperaemia as well. The pupil is constricted due to direct irritation of the two iris muscles, the stronger of which, the sphincter, wins. Adhesions of the posterior surface of the iris to the anterior lens capsule, *posterior synechiae,* are likely and when mydriatic drops are used to dilate the pupil it can move only in those parts which are not adherent to the lens with the result that the pupil becomes irregular (Fig 13-6). Occasionally in neglected cases the whole pupillary margin becomes adherent to the lens and, because aqueous cannot then pass forwards through the pupil, the mid-portion of the iris becomes ballooned forwards (iris bombé) and there is a severe secondary glaucoma (Fig 13-7). The inflammatory exudate from the inflamed tissues enters the aqueous. The proteins abnormally present in the aqueous scatter enough light from a slender pencil of light crossing the anterior chamber for it to be visible with a slit-lamp microscope as an aqueous flare (Fig 5-4). Leucocytes of the exudate also reflect light as they float into a beam of light like motes of dust in a shaft of sunlight which penetrates a darkened room. Occasionally the cellular exudate is sufficiently dense to form a hypopyon. In some types of iridocyclitis the corneal mesothelium becomes oedematous and sticky so that microscopic clumps

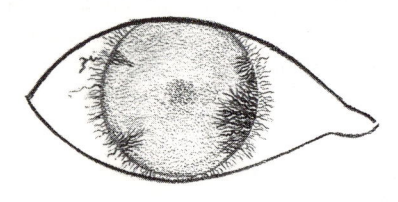

Fig 13-5 Interstitial keratitis. The whole cornea is like opaque ground glass and deep blood vessels are growing into the stroma in places.

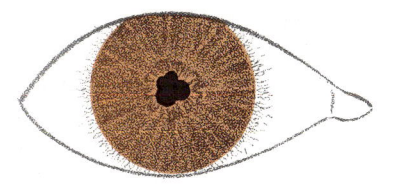

Fig 13-6 Acute iridocyclitis. The pupil is small and irregular because posterior synechiae had formed before mydriatic eye-drops were used.

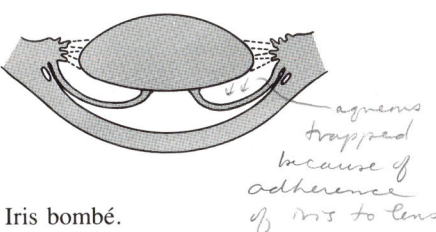

Fig 13-7 Iris bombé.

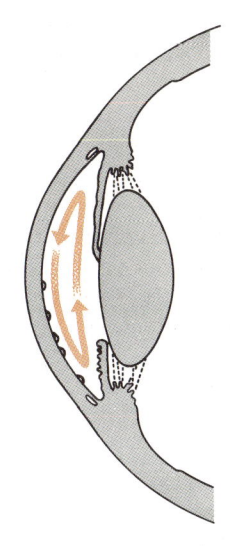

Fig 13-8 A vertical section showing a posterior synechia above, five KP on the corneal mesothelium, and the flow-pattern of the normal thermal circulation of the aqueous humour.

of inflammatory cells form on the posterial surface — *keratic precipitates,* familiarly known as KP (Fig 13-8). Untreated, acute iridocyclitis eventually subsides but is likely to leave irreparable visual damage. Iridocyclitis also occurs as an insidious chronic condition with few or no symptoms other than progressive loss of vision.

Exogenously caused uveitis may follow injury, including surgery, or perforation of a corneal ulcer. Most cases are endogenous and in most the cause is unknown. Over the years various aetiologies have been believed and a sequence of ineffective treatments adopted. Syphilis, tuberculosis, focal sepsis, viral infection, metabolic disorders, allergy, and autoimmunity have all been implicated and probably a few cases are in fact caused by each of these factors. Sometimes iridocyclitis is associated with ankylosing spondylitis, sarcoidosis, gonorrhoea, or Still's disease, while toxoplasmosis is the commonest known cause of choroiditis in temperate countries.

Sympathetic ophthalmitis is a rare specific form of uveitis which occurs only after a perforating wound of the eye. Uveitis in the injured eye is followed from three weeks to years later by a similar severe uveitis in the other eye. For this reason an injured eye with little hope of regaining useful vision is removed within three weeks of injury to forestall its fellow eye becoming involved.

The chief objective in treating acute iridocyclitis is to suppress the inflammation so long as this is not necessary to combat an infection, as is usually the case. Corticosteroids achieve this objective and are used in whatever dose is needed to quieten the inflammation. In increasing order of potency the drug is administered by local eye-drops, hourly if necessary, by subconjunctival injection, and occasionally systemically. An old and still important objective is to dilate the pupil to prevent the formation of posterior synechiae and by resting the inflamed iris and ciliary body to ease the pain. Atropine sulphate eye-drops 1% two or three times daily is the most effective mydriatic and cycloplegic. Analgesics for pain and dark glasses or an eye pad for photophobia may be required. Local heating of the closed eye is an old adjunct to treatment which may give comfort. Complications will demand further measures, such as oral acetazolamide if there is secondary glaucoma.

Chapter 14

THE WATERING EYE

Lacrimation
Epiphora
    Eversion of the punctum
    Obstruction of lacrimal passages
    Congenital obstruction

Overflow of tears on to the skin can be due to either overproduction of tears, when it is called lacrimation, or to faulty drainage, when it is called epiphora.

Apart from emotional causes, *lacrimation* is a reflex secretion of tears initiated by irritation of the conjunctiva, cornea, or iris, or by photophobia, and is not directly treated. It is a presenting symptom of congenital glaucoma.

Epiphora results from displacement of the lower lid or obstruction of the lacrimal passages anywhere from punctum to nasolacrimal duct. *Eversion of the lower lacrimal punctum* so that it is not directed posteriorly on to the conjunctiva prevents the tears from gaining access to the lacrimal passages. If the punctum can be seen without pulling the lower lid slightly away from the globe it is not in its correct position. This is a common result of ageing which is correctable with simple plastic surgery. The common senile ectropion of the lower lid due to slackening of the orbicularis muscle also displaces the punctum with consequent epiphora, which is worsened by the lacrimation provoked by exposure of the conjunctiva.

Patency of the lacrimal passages is *assessed* by trying to inject saline from a syringe through a blunt-ended lacrimal cannula which is delicately introduced by way of the lower punctum into the canaliculus. The fluid should pass freely into the subject's nose. If fluid does not enter the nose and flows out of the upper canaliculus there is an obstruction beyond the lacrimal sac. If there is no flow, the lower canaliculus itself is blocked.

The *punctum and canaliculus* are occasionally blocked by a foreign body such as an eyelash or suffer post-inflammatory stenosis. Improperly managed lacerations of the lid involving the canaliculus inevitably result in epiphora.

Obstruction in the *nasolacrimal duct* is common in women in middle life. It may follow chronic dacryocystitis or may give rise to acute dacryocystitis or to a mucocoele of the lacrimal sac (p. 207).

Congenital obstruction of the nasolacrimal duct in infants is common and manifests as a watery eye soon after birth. Secondary infection gives rise to mucoid discharge. It is due to delayed canalization and usually resolves spontaneously, especially if encouraged by gentle finger-tip pressure on the lacrimal sac and if antibiotic eye-drops are used to suppress any infection. If the condition persists for more than about six months, probing of the duct under general anaesthesia effectively overcomes the blockage.

Chapter 15

SUDDEN LOSS OF VISION

Vitreous opacities
   Haemorrhage
   Inflammatory
Pre-retinal haemorrhage
Choroidal haemorrhage
Retinal artery occlusion
   Amaurosis fugax
Retinal vein occlusion
Choroido-retinitis
   Macular
   Juxtapapillary
Retinal detachment
Central serous retinopathy
Pigment epithelial detachment
Ischaemic optic neuropathy
Optic neuritis
Homonymous hemianopia
Migraine
Discovery of long-standing defective sight

SUDDEN LOSS OF VISION

As would be anticipated, rapid painless loss of sight is most often due to a vascular occlusion or a haemorrhage somewhere in the visual pathway. Other less frequent causes are an inflammatory lesion involving the optic nerve or the choroid and retina, and retinal detachment.

A *vitreous haze* or cloud which diminishes vision will degrade the ophthalmoscopic red reflex and partly obscure the retina. It may be due to haemorrhage (p. 145) or to inflammation (p. 142). In either case prompt assessment and treatment is desirable.

A *pre-retinal haemorrhage* (Fig 6-31) which blacks out central vision by blanketing the macular retina will absorb more rapidly if it does not break into the vitreous. The chances of its doing this are lessened if the eyes are immobilized for some days by covering them or by using opaque glasses with only a small central pin-hole aperture before the unaffected eye.

Detachment of the macular pigment epithelium from Bruch's membrane by haemorrhage (a *choroidal haemorrhage* (Fig 6-34)) is a sudden, central vision-destroying episode in disciform macular degeneration (p. 194). There is no treatment at this stage and even after absorption of the blood the visual loss is permanent.

Occlusion of a retinal artery is a classic eye emergency because in the few cases in which treatment might be effective it has to be started within at most three or four hours. When the central retinal artery is occluded there is immediate total loss of vision and abolition of the direct pupillary reaction to light. If the superior or the inferior retinal artery is blocked an altitudinal half field is totally lost. When a branch artery is obstructed the corresponding sector of the visual field is lost. Ophthalmoscopically the infarcted area within an hour or so becomes cloudy and pale, with a 'cherry-red spot at the macula' if the central area of the retina is involved (Fig 15-1) (p. 142). When there is a cilio-retinal artery the retina which it supplies is spared (Plate 9, p. 125). The retinal arteries are usually quite narrowed and the blood column in some may be fragmented so that segments of blood alternate with apparently empty spaces (railway-trucking). At times sludging of the almost stationary red cells in the veins gives their blood columns a shimmering

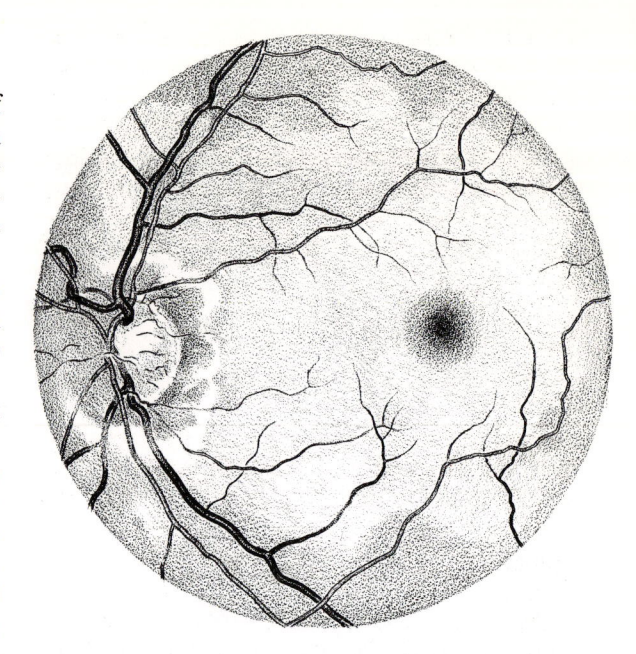

Fig 15-1 Central retinal artery occlusion. The fundus is pale due to cloudy swelling of the neural retina except at the macula where transparency is preserved.

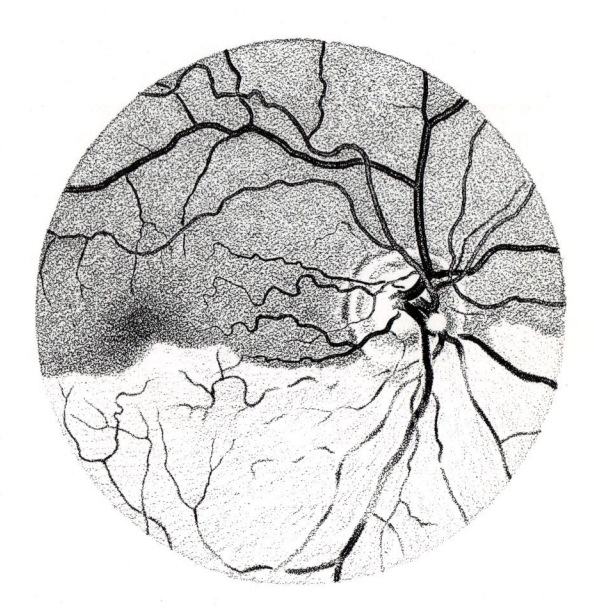

Fig 15-2 Platelet embolus impacted in the inferior branch of the central retinal artery. The infarcted retina is cloudy and pale.

SUDDEN LOSS OF VISION

granular appearance and sometimes reverse flow may be seen. If not spontaneously present these changes may be induced by gentle finger pressure on the eye through the lid while looking with the ophthalmoscope; the increase in intraocular pressure further embarrasses the already impaired retinal circulation.

The abrupt reduction in retinal artery blood flow can be due to an embolus, or to thrombosis or vaso-spasm occurring in relation to an arterial degenerative or inflammatory lesion. Most cases occur in older atherosclerotic hypertensive people and the precise mechanism is not known. Giant cell arteritis can affect the central retinal artery rather than the posterior ciliary arteries and some of these occlusions are potentially treatable. Very occasionally a migrainous vaso-spasm affects the retinal artery and if not relieved this can last long enough to cause death of the inner retinal neurones. Platelet, fibrin, or, very rarely, calcific emboli from the heart or from atheromatous lesions in the aorta or carotid are ophthalmoscopically visible unless it is the intraneural part of the artery in which they are impacted (Fig 15-2).

Treatment aims at relieving vaso-spasm or dislodging an embolus to a more peripheral vessel branch. Firm intermittent massage of the globe with the two index fingers as the patient looks downwards may achieve this and should be done immediately the diagnosis is made. Pressure is applied for 20-30 seconds and then, after a brief interval, repeated. The object is to express aqueous from the eye and thereby lower the intraocular pressure which is of course the extravascular pressure. More effective reduction of intraocular pressure is achieved by anterior chamber paracentesis in which a small cut is made through the cornea just inside the temporal limbus with a small cutting needle or knife so that aqueous suddenly escapes from the eye. When the retinal circulation is marginal, lying the patient flat without pillows sometimes increases perfusion sufficiently to keep the retina going; in such cases the eye blanks out when the patient sits up. Inhalation of 5% carbon dioxide and 95% oxygen by face mask for 5-10 minutes may induce retinal vasodilatation. Intravenous infusions of low molecular weight dextrans (Rheomacrodex) and intravenous administration of heparin may be indicated in cases which partially respond, while systemic steroids are given urgently if there is any possibility of arteritis being implicated.

Amaurosis fugax is an old name given to repeated transient episodes of visual loss of one eye. These may be due to giant cell arteritis or very rarely to migraine but most are due to carotid artery insufficiency as a result of atherosclerotic lesions in the neck. In a majority the immediate cause is temporary occlusion of a retinal artery by platelet or cholesterol emboli, while in others it is the reduction in blood pressure and flow in the ophthalmic artery consequent on a severe narrowing or total occlusion of the internal carotid artery. The blood pressure in the ophthalmic artery can be simply measured by *ophthalmodynamometry*. In this the intraocular pressure is increased by compressing the globe with the footpiece of a spring-loaded plunger, or more precisely by creating a controlled negative pressure within a small suction-cup applied to the outside of the eyeball, while the arteries on the optic disc are watched with an ophthalmoscope. The pressure required to just produce a fully collapsing pulsation of the vessels corresponds to diastolic pressure, while systolic pressure is that which just keeps the vessels fully collapsed throughout the cardiac cycle.

In a few patients eventually an attack occurs which does not pass off and the picture of retinal artery occlusion occurs. Symptoms of cerebral ischaemia may accompany the visual symptoms and in a few patients a hemiplegia may ensue. In one study, 16% of patients with amaurosis fugax eventually suffered permanent loss of sight and/or a stroke. Full medical assessment is obviously necessary with a view to possible carotid endarterectomy. Aspirin, 300mgm daily, may reduce the frequency of attacks of amaurosis fugax, presumably by inhibiting platelet aggregation. Systemic steroids are immediately used if there is any evidence of giant cell arteritis.

Occlusion of a retinal vein is more common than retinal artery occlusion. The onset of symptoms is less dramatic and total loss of vision is rare. Occlusion is often less than total and may affect the central retinal vein or a venous branch (Plate 10, p. 125). Ophthalmoscopically the whole of the territory drained by the involved vein becomes spattered with superficial and deep retinal haemorrhages (Fig 15-3). In central vein occlusion haemorrhages cover the fundus out to the periphery. The obstructed veins are usually

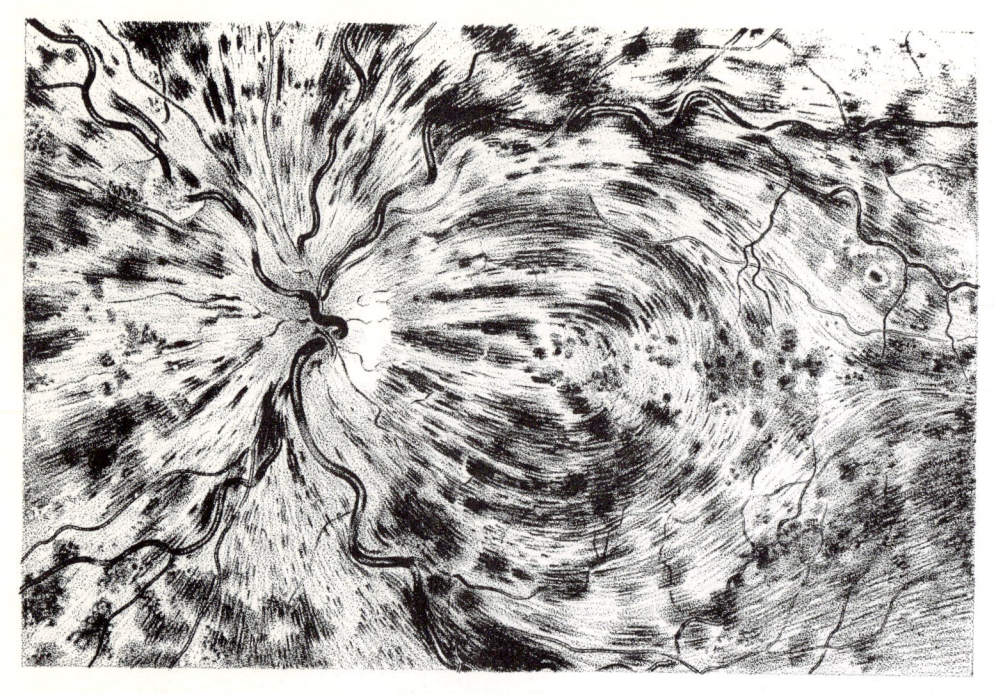

Fig 15-3 Partial occlusion of the central retina vein in a left eye. The course of the retinal nerve fibres is vividly revealed by the superficial haemorrhages lying between them.

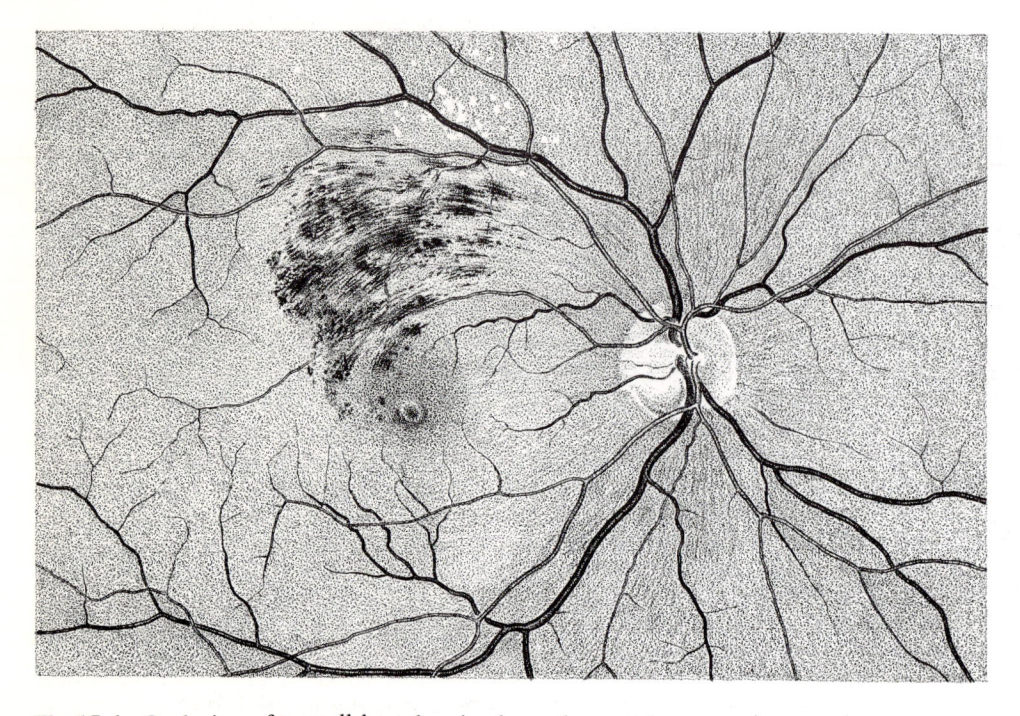

Fig 15-4 Occlusion of a small branch vein above the macula.

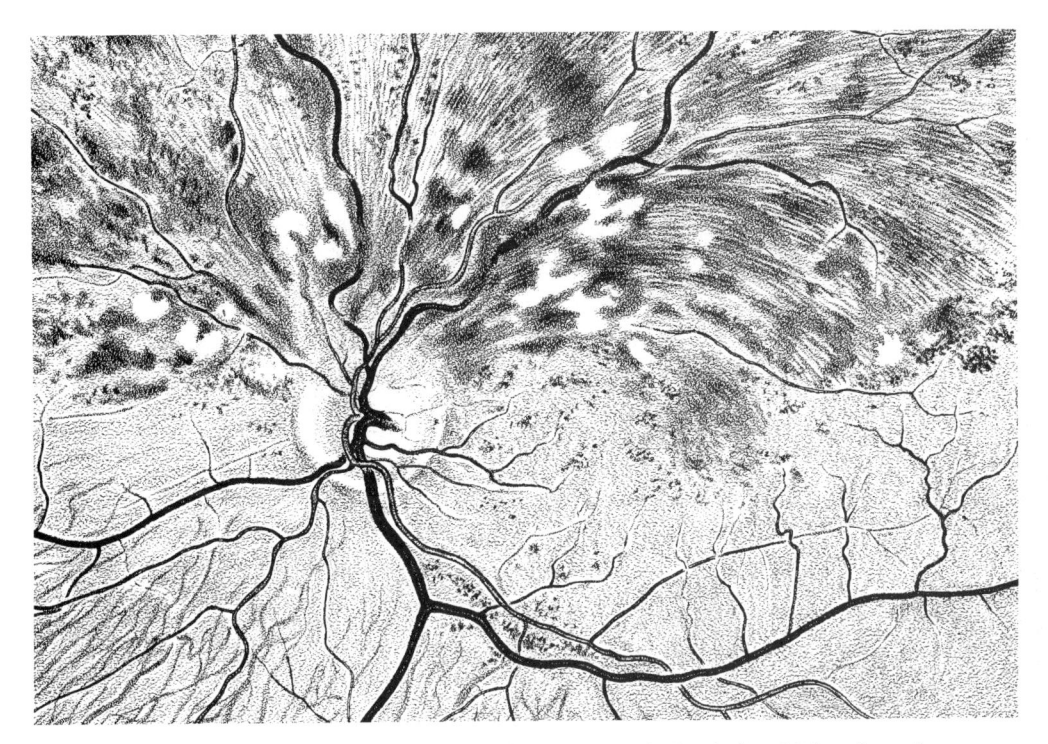

Fig 15-5 Occlusion of the superior branch of the central retinal vein in which soft exudates are prominent.

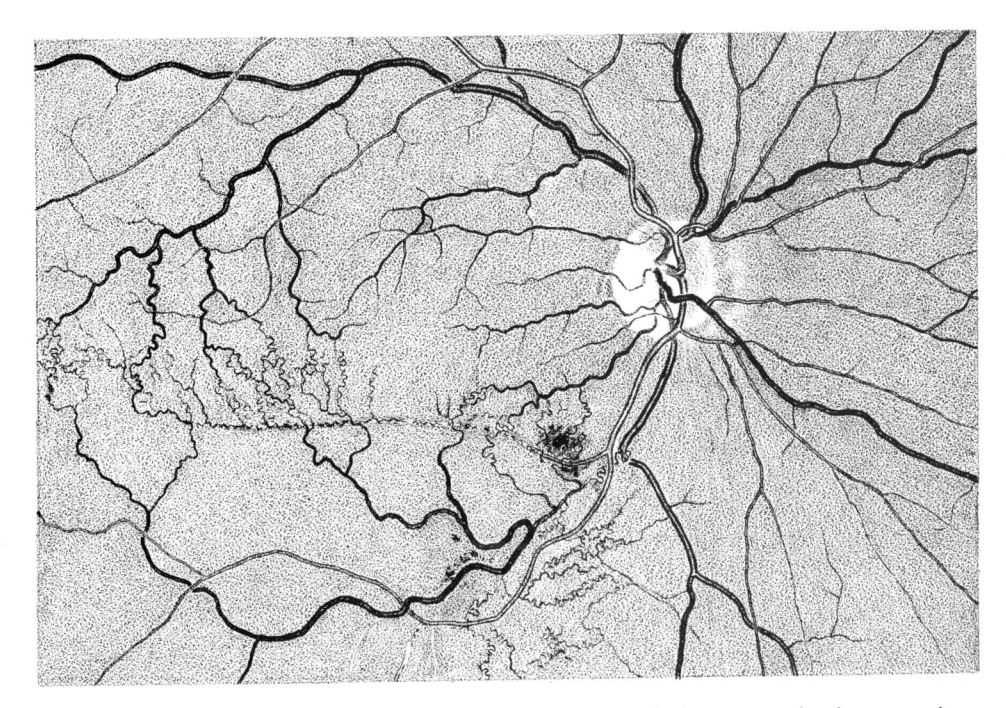

Fig 15-6 Venous collateral vessels after occlusion of the inferior temporal vein at a major arteriovenous crossing.

obviously distended, dark, and tortuous, except in small branch vein occlusions (Fig 15-4). The retina is oedematous but, in central vein occlusion, the optic disc is not greatly swollen. Macular oedema may develop or increase some time after the onset of symptoms with worsening of central vision. Soft exudates commonly appear (Fig 15-5). Absorption of haemorrhages takes many months and may reveal collateral vessels bypassing the venous obstruction (Fig 15-6).

Most retinal vein occlusions occur at sites where the vein shares a common adventitial sheath with an artery, that is at arterio-venous crossings and at the lamina cribrosa. The primary lesion is probably an arterial sclerosis which impedes venous flow; hypertensive arteriolar sclerosis at arterio-venous crossings and in the optic nerve, or atherosclerosis in the optic nerve. Venous occlusion also occurs with retinal phlebitis, glaucoma (a secondary glaucoma also occurs as a result of central retinal vein occlusion), and hyperviscosity of the blood as in polycythaemia and dysproteinaemia.

The effectiveness of most forms of *treatment* is not known. Conditions such as glaucoma, hypertension, diabetes, hyperlipidaemia, polycythaemia, and macroglobulinaemia which might play a part should be treated. Medical treatment, e.g. with acetazolamide tablets, which will lower raised IOP, even if the increase is small, is probably one of the most useful measures that can be taken. It follows that in retinal vein occlusion IOP as well as BP should be measured. Systemic steroids may be indicated for phlebitis. In the later stages retinal photocoagulation may be needed to forestall or treat pre-retinal or iris neovascularization which develops in a proportion of those cases of occlusion of the central retinal vein in which there is extensive non-perfusion of retinal capillaries.

When a focus of *choroidoretinitis* (p. 142) happens to occur near to the macula and central vision is threatened, an attempt is made to suppress the inflammation with systemic steroids. If it is thought to be due to toxoplasmosis, chemotherapy with pyrimethamine or cotrimoxazole may help. When a focus of posterior uveitis is adjacent to the optic disc the condition is called *juxtapapillary choroiditis* (Fig 8-4). The appearance of pale oedema of that part of the disc beside an area of soft white opacification of the retina seen through a hazy vitreous has been confused with papilloedema due to raised intracranial pressure, but the definite visual loss due to optic nerve involvement aids in the distinction. Although the visual prognosis is good, systemic steroids may hasten recovery.

The mode of visual loss with a *retinal detachment* is variable (Fig 6-27). Commonly the patient experiences, over the course of hours or days, a shadow or curtain in front of his or her eye, depending on whether the separation of the neural retina from the pigment epithelium starts inferiorly or superiorly. When the detachment reaches the macula, central vision is abruptly lost. The earliest symptom may be flashes or twinkling lights due to mechanical stimulation of the retina as it floats and moves. For some patients floaters or a blackout due to a vitreous haemorrhage is the presenting feature. On ophthalmoscopy detached retina is slightly pale, often gently wrinkled if well forward into the vitreous, and its vessels are dark and tortuous.

Treatment is successful in about 80% of retinal detachments, but if not, a detachment usually increases in extent to eventually become total and all sight is lost. The results of treatment are better if it can be undertaken within a few days of the onset of a detachment. Immobilization of the eye as much as possible by pin-hole spectacles or by padding both eyes often leads to rapid, if temporary, reduction of a detachment and therefore this is the first aid management in most cases.

A quite different type of retinal detachment, *central serous retinopathy,* occurs most often in middle aged males (Plate 16, p. 128). The macular retina is elevated by serous fluid which leaks from the choriocapillaris through a small break in Bruch's membrane. Displacement of the retina causes micropsia and hypermetropia. The translucent bulge in the retina is not easily seen with an ophthalmoscope but a common clue is the glint of a narrow line of light reflected from the retinal surface where the slope changes around the edge of the lesion. Recovery in weeks or months is usual.

In yet another condition, *retinal pigment epithelium detachment* (PED), both layers of the retina are locally detached from the underlying Bruch's membrane by serous fluid. With an ophthalmoscope they are seen as inconspicuous greyish mounds from one-quarter to two or three disc diameters in size which persist for months. If close to the fovea vision is reduced. In about one-third of older patients a choroidal neovascular membrane develops under a PED and then disciform macular degeneration is likely (p. 194).

In *ischaemic optic neuropathy* (p. 167) the loss of visual function is usually worse than the ophthalmoscopic appearances would suggest (Plate 12, p. 126). The pallid oedema of the optic disc may not occur or may be very slight in some eyes which have suddenly lost even perception of light. An ESR should be urgently done whenever an old person suffers a sudden visual failure for which there is no immediate explanation and, if it is elevated, giant cell arteritis should be assumed to be the cause and systemic corticosteroids, e.g. prednisolone 60mgm per day, immediately started.

In *optic neuritis* (p. 166) the ophthalmoscopic picture also varies. The disc may be normal, as in retrobulbar neuritis when the lesion is more than about 1cm from the globe, or oedematous when the nerve close to the eye is involved, that is when there is papillitis (Plate 4, p. 122). A younger age group is affected and central vision is more severely affected than is peripheral visual function. Systemic steroids are sometimes used to hasten recovery.

When a *homonymous hemianopia* suddenly occurs patients may or may not know that something has happened to their sight, but it is rare for them to realise that they have lost the same half of both visual fields. Commonly they are unable to interpret their experience or, if they do, they believe that they have lost the sight of the eye on the side of the field loss. Those with a right hemianopia find it difficult to read along a line of print while those with a hemianopia on the left side tend to lose the start of the next line of print. The field loss will usually be readily demonstrated by confrontation testing. Visual acuity as tested with test types is not affected. A sudden onset is presumptive evidence of a vascular lesion in the middle cerebral artery territory in the parietotemporal region or in the posterior cerebral artery territory in the occipital lobe. Associated changes, such as hemiplegic signs, accompany middle cerebral artery occlusion. Hemianopia occurs alone in occipital lesions due to posterior cerebral artery occlusion, but in basilar artery occlusion there are also changes due to brain stem ischaemia.

Transient attacks of blurred vision or blackouts are commonly due to *vertebro-basilar insufficiency,* that is an atherosclerotic narrowing of these arteries by at least 80% so that blood flow through them is marginally sufficient. Sooner or later one of these ischaemic attacks may not be transient but be permanent; however, this is by no means inevitable. Referred pain in an eye, and occasionally flickering light, may accompany the episode.

The sudden disturbance of vision which can occur as part of the *migraine* symptom complex is disconcerting to the patient until its aetiology is understood. Zigzag lights are seen in a homonymous field and are followed by a shimmering obscuration of vision which spreads towards fixation (scintillating scotoma). Usually this lasts about 15 minutes and is followed by the migrainous headache. But in some people or in some attacks there is no pain and then the diagnosis is not so obvious.

Occasionally the complaint of sudden loss of vision is *unfounded*. It is due to the patient, usually an old person, suddenly discovering loss of vision which had been present for some time. An eye may gradually lose sight from a cataract or open angle glaucoma without the patient being aware of it until by chance the sight of the other eye is temporarily occluded.

Epilogue

OBJECTIVES IN UNDERGRADUATE OPHTHALMOLOGY

A tangible way of defining the role of ophthalmology in an undergraduate medical curriculum is to state the educational objectives or goals for students in this field. Educational objectives can take the form of a list of things a student should be able to *do* at the end of his or her training; in this way they differ from the traditional curriculum, which broadly outlines the things a student ought to *know*.

The goals which follow have in large measure determined the contents of this book. They can be referred to from time to time as a learning guide and a means of self assessment.

At the end of his or her undergraduate training in ophthalmology a student should

1. have gained sufficient basic understanding of the subject so that he or she will be able to follow accounts of new developments written for non-specialists;
2. be able to elicit a history of a patient's ocular and visual symptoms and relevant general health and be able to suggest possible causes of the patient's experiences and observations;
3. be able to test a patient's visual function, i.e. measure and record the distant and near visual acuity, the visual fields (to confrontation), and colour vision;
4. be able to test a patient's pupillary function;
5. be able to test and record a patient's binocular function, i.e. observe if nystagmus occurs, test eye movements, test for the presence of a latent or manifest squint, and analyse a diplopia to determine the weak muscle(s);
6. be able to measure a patient's intraocular pressure with a Schiötz tonometer;
7. be able to examine a patient's eyes with focal illumination and with an ophthalmoscope and be able to describe and interpret his or her findings and to indicate whether they are normal or abnormal;
8. when he or she sees abnormal appearances in the fundus be able to interpret the ophthalmoscopic changes in terms of probable pathological changes and be able to state the relationship, if any, between them and any general disease process;
9. be able to make a decision as to whether the optic disc is normal, oedematous, glaucomatous, or atropic;
10. given a patient with a possible eye injury (e.g. foreign body, chemical injury, contusion, laceration) or with sudden reduction of the sight of an eye, be able to undertake immediate diagnostic procedures, institute first aid treatment, decide on his or her competence to treat the patient without referral and, if justifiably confident, explain to the patient the condition, its prognosis and the proposed management, and initiate treatment;
11. given a patient with a painful red eye, be able to make a decision as to the likely cause, decide on his or her competence to treat the patient without referral and, if justifiably confident, explain to the patient the condition, its prognosis and the proposed management, and initiate treatment;
12. given a patient seeking advice on a non-cute ocular symptom, i.e. altered function, abnormal sensation, or altered appearance, be able to decide on the probable cause and importance of the complaint and on the necessity for referral, including the degree of urgency involved.

FURTHER READING

Ophthalmology is rich in books and journals, so rich as to bewilder a newcomer. The next step for those seeking further information is probably one of the single-volume major textbooks such as:

Spalton, D. J., Hitchings, R. A., Hunter, P. A. *Atlas of Clinical Ophthalmology.* Gower Medical Publishing, London. 1984. (Distributed by Churchill Livingstone, Edinburgh in Europe and by J. B. Lippincott, Philadelphia in North America.)

Newell, F. W. *Ophthalmology: Principles and Concepts.* 6th Edn. C. V. Mosby, St Louis. 1986.

Miller, S. J. H. *Parsons, Diseases of the Eye.* 17th Edn. Churchill Livingstone, Edinburgh. 1984.

Beyond these are the multi-volume reference books and the separate monographs on a host of ophthalmic topics.

Duke-Elder, S. *System of Ophthalmology.* Fifteen Vols. Henry Kimpton, London. 1958-76.

Although dated, this magnificent narrative encyclopaedia provides information not otherwise easily available and is a standard by which to judge other books. The late Sir Stewart Duke-Elder was a master of English prose; he wrote in a postscript to his previous seven-volume *Textbook of Ophthalmology* that a textbook '. . . should aspire to integrate the facts of science rather than record them, to be vigilant for knowledge but no less vigilant for the truth of knowledge, to ease the transition from the groping past to the dissatisfied present and on to the uncertain future, and at the same time to preserve through the transition the essential continuity of all that is good by weaving it into a coherent philosophy . . .'. A vintage publication with no current counterpart.

Duane, T. D. (Ed.). *Clinical Ophthalmology.* Five Vols. Harper and Row, Philadelphia. 1987.

This multi-author compendium in a loose-leaf format is updated each year.

There is almost an embarrassment of valuable books on individual topics. These are written primarily for ophthalmologists, both those in training and those with experience. It may help others to list for each subject one of the books which is likely to be more accessible to a non-ophthalmologist.

Anatomy:

Warwick, R. *Eugene Wolff's Anatomy of the Eye and Orbit.* 7th Edn. H. K. Lewis, London. 1976. (Needs to be supplemented by a more current text on ocular fine structure such as Fine, B. S., Yanoff, M. *Ocular Histology: A Text and Atlas.* 2nd Edn. Harper and Row, New York. 1979.)

Physiology:

Moses, R. A., Hart, W. M. (Eds). *Adler's Physiology of the Eye. Clinical Application.* 8th Edn. C. V. Mosby, St Louis. 1987.

Colour Vision:

Hurvich, L. M. *Colour Vision.* Sinauer Associates, Sunderland, Massachusetts. 1981.

Perception:

Frisby, J. P. *Seeing: Illusion, Brain and Mind.* Oxford University Press, Oxford. 1979.

Optics:

Michaels, D. D. *Visual Optics and Refraction; a clinical approach.* 3rd Edn. C. V. Mosby, St Louis. 1985.

Pathology:

Garner, A., Klintworth, G. K. (Eds). *Pathobiology of Ocular Disease. Parts A and B.* Marcel Dekker, New York. 1982.

Orbit:

Jones, I. S., Jakobiec, F. A. *Diseases of the Orbit.* Harper and Row, New York. 1979.

Infections:

Fedukowicz, H., Stetson, S. *External Infection of the Eyes.* 3rd Edn. Appleton-Century-Crofts, New York. 1985.

Virus Diseases:

Easty, D. L. *Virus Disease of the Eye.* Year Book Medical Publishers, Chicago. 1985.

Cornea:

Grayson, M. *Diseases of the Cornea.* 2nd Edn. C. V. Mosby, St Louis. 1983.

Sclera:

Watson, P. G., Hazelman, B. L. *The Sclera and Systemic Disorders.* W. B. Saunders, London. 1976.

Uveitis:

Kraus-Mackiw, E., O'Connor, G. R. *Uveitis: Pathophysiology and Therapy.* Thieme-Stratton, New York. 1983.

Retina:

Wise, G. N., Dollery, C. T., Henkind, P. *The Retinal Circulation.* Harper and Row, New York. 1971. (There is no newer equivalent to this old classic.)

Michaelson, I. A., Benezra, D. *Textbook of the Fundus of the Eye.* 3rd Edn. Churchill Livingstone, Edinburgh. 1980.

Gass, J. D. M. *Stereoscopic Atlas of Macular Diseases: Diagnosis and Treatment.* 3rd Edn. C. V. Mosby, St Louis. 1987.

Bloome, M. A., Garcia, C. A. *Manual of Retinal and Choroidal Dystrophies.* Appleton-Century-Crofts, New York. 1982.

Glaucoma:

Cairns, J. E. (Ed.). *Glaucoma.* Grune and Stratton, London and Orlando, Florida. 1986.

Tumours:

Shields, J. A. *Diagnosis and Management of Intraocular Tumours.* C. V. Mosby, St Louis. 1983.

Strabismus:

Von Noorden, G. K. *Burian and Von Noorden's Binocular Vision and Ocular Motility: Theory and Management of Strabismus.* 3rd Edn. C. V. Mosby, St Louis. 1985.

Eye Movements:

Leigh, R. J., Zee, D. S. *The Neurology of Eye Movements.* F. A. Davis, Philadelphia. 1983.

Neuro-ophthalmology:

Burde, R. M., Savino, P. J., Trobe, J. D. *Clinical Decisions in Neuro-ophthalmology.* C. V. Mosby, St Louis. 1985.

Medical Ophthalmology:

Rose, F. C. (Ed.). *The Eye in General Medicine.* Chapman and Hall, London. 1983.

Paediatric Ophthalmology:

Wybar, K., Taylor, D. *Pediatric Ophthalmology: Current Aspects.* Marcel Dekker, New York. 1983.

Surgery:

Roper-Hall, M. J. *Stallard's Eye Surgery.* 6th Edn. John Wright, Bristol. 1980.

At most, these suggestions are a guide as to where to start. At least, they or alternatives should be available in a local medical library.

Index

Abduction, 26
Abnormal retinal correspondence, 182
Accelerated hypertension, 160
Accommodation, 7, 20, 29, **36**, **43**, 89, 116, 182
Accommodative squint, 182
Acetazolamide, 177, 178, 211, 220
Acne rosacea, 208
Actinic keratoconjunctivitis, 94, **199**, 209
Acyclovir, 209
Adduction, 26
Adenine arabinoside, 209
Adenovirus, 206, 209
Adie's pupil, 34, 106
Adrenal insufficiency, 166
Adrenalin eye drops, 178
After image, 55, **64**, 83
Age changes, 188
Agnosia, 92
Airy's rings, 49
Albinism, 103
Alkali burn, 199
Allergy, 95, 206
Alpha chymotrypsin, 19, 190
Alternating squint, 103, 182, 184
Amacrine cell, 11, 12
Amaurosis fugax, 217
Amblyopia, 48, 80, 182, **185**
Ametropia, 44
Amsler grid, 94, **101**
Anaemia, 143, 146, 166, 167, 171
Angiography, fluorescein, **16**, 142, 143, 150, **155**, 169
Angioid streaks, 147
Angle
  of anterior chamber, 2, **21**, 175
  of squint, 87, 184
Aniseikonia, 191
Anisocoria, 106
Anisometropia, 185
Ankylosing spondylitis, 211
Anomaloscope, 72
Anomalous trichromat, 73
Anterior chamber, 2, **21**, 113, 114
  depth, 21, 110, 175, 176, 180, 200
  paracentesis, 217
Antibiotic-corticosteroid eye ointment, 207, 208
Antibiotic
  eye drops, 199, 200, 205, 208
  ointment, 205, 207
Aphakia, 44, 45, 47, 191
Aphakic vision, 191
Applanation tonometry, 107, 174

Aqueous
  flare, 110, 113, 210
  humour, 3, 7, **21**, 113, 174
  vein, 6, 114
Arc flash, 199, 209
Arcuate scotoma, **12**, 93, 102, 178
Arcus senilis, 98
Areas 17, 18 and 19, 32, 33, 79
Argyll Robertson pupil, 34, 106
Arterio-venous crossing, 16, **135**, 159, 220
Artery
  anterior ciliary, 6, 8
  central retinal, 15
  cilioretinal, 16, 216
  long posterior ciliary, 8
  posterior ciliary, 6, 14
  retinal, 15, 16
Artificial tears, 210
Aspirin, 217
Asthenopia, 95
Astigmatism, 44, 45
Atherosclerosis, 136, 167, 217, 220, 221
Atropine eye drops, 7, 9, 208, 211
Autokinetic movement, 55
AV
  crossing, 16, **135**, 159, 220
  ratio, 137
Axoplasmic flow, 143, 151, 168

Banking of vein, 136
Basal-cell carcinoma, 97
Basilar artery insufficiency, 93, 221
Bell's palsy, 23
Bell's phenomenon, 23, 39
Benign intracranial hypertension, 166
Beta movement, 65
Bezold-Brücke phenomenon, 71
Bifocal spectacles, 44
Binocular vision, **80**, 83, 87, 182
Bipolar cell, 11, 12
Bitemporal hemianopia, 32, 93, 102
Bjerrum's screen, 59
Black eye, 201
Blepharitis, 97, 109, 198, **207**
Blind spot, 12, 165
Blonde fundus, 10, 141
Blood-ocular barriers, 17
Blood pressure, 158, 159
Blood-retina barrier, 16
Blowout fracture, 198
Bone corpuscle pigmentation, 137, 148
Bowman's membrane, 5, 113, 114
Brightness, 55, 57, 60, 71

Bruch's membrane, 7, 144, 146, 194
Buphthalmous, 180

Calcarine cortex, 32
Calific embolus, 136
Camera obscura, 3, 42
Canal of Schlemm, 2, **6**, 175
Canthus, 22
Cardinal directions, 28, 103
Carotid
  artery insufficiency, 139, 217
  endarterectomy, 217
Caruncle, 23
Cataract, 19, 51, 120, **188**
  concussion, 202
  congenital, 103, 182, 185, 188
  cortical, 188
  cuneiform, 188
  extraction, 190
  hypermature, 189
  mature, 189
  nuclear, 188
  posterior cupuliform, 188
  ripe, 189
  senile, 188
  traumatic, 188, 201
Cat's eye reflex, 144
Cavernous sinus thrombosis, 166
Central scotoma, 93, 166, 170, 199
Central vision, 92, 165, 170, 193
Cerebellar lesions, 105
Cerebral
  abscess, 166, 171
  ischaemia, 217, 221
  palsy, 182
  tumour, 166
Chalazion, 207
Chemical injury, 199
Chemosis, 206
Cherry-red spot, 142, 216
Chiasma, 31, 93, 101, 170, 171
Chlamydia, 205
Chloramphenicol eye drops, 199, 205
Cholesterol embolus, 136
Choriocapillaris, 6
Choroid, 2, 6
Choroidal
  crescent, 13
  haemorrhage, 146, 216
  malignant melanoma, 148
  naevus, 148
  pigment, 6, 10, 141
  rupture, 202
  tubercle, 142
Choroiditis, **142**, 167, 171, 210, 220

INDEX

Choroidoretinitis, **142**, 171, 220
Chromatic aberration, 47, 50
Ciliary,
  body, 2, 7
  ganglion, 19
  hyperaemia, 8, 205, 208
  injection, 8, 205, 208
  muscle, 2, 7, 43
  processes, 7, 174
  vasculitis, 167,
Cilium, visual receptor, 13
Circinate retinopathy, 143
Circle of Zinn, 14
Cog-wheel movements, 39
Collagen diseases, 143, 210
Collarette, 114
Collector channels, 6, 174
Colloid bodies, 7, **144**, 156, 193
Coloboma, 3, 145
Colour
  coding, 78
  matching, 72
  mixture, 71
  vision, 55, **70**, 188
    defects, 73, 89, 158
Column
  ocular dominance, 79
  orientation, 79
Commotio retinae, 202
Complementary colours, 71
Complex cell, 77, 79
Concave lens, 45, 116, 120
Concealment of vein, 135
Concomitant squint, 184
Cones, 11, 12, 14, 56
Confrontation testing, 101, 221
Confusion, 87
  bars, 67
Congenital obstruction naso-lacrimal duct, 25, 213
Congruous field defect, 32
Conical cornea, 47
Conjugate movement, 28
Conjunctiva, 24, 109
  bulbar, 24, 114
  palpebral, 24
Conjunctival
  concretion, 198
  foreign body, 198
  fornix, 24
  hyperaemia, 9, 24, **205**
  laceration, 198
  lymphoid follicles, 24, 205
  sac, 24
Conjunctivitis, 94, 97, 196, 204, **205**
  acute infectious, 205
  allergic, 95, 206
  follicular, 205
  inclusion, 206

swimming-bath, 206
vernal, 206
viral, 206
Constricted pupil, 34, 106, 110, 208, 210
Contact dermatitis, 206
Contact lens, 47, 191, 199
  diagnostic, 21, 112, 175
Contour interaction, 67
Contrast, 12, 55, 61, 75
  sensitivity tests, 69
Contusion, 201
Convergence, 29, 89
  micropsia, 87
  sensory, 58
Convergent squint, 183
Convex lens, 42, 44, 45, 116
Cornea, 2, **4**, 109, 113, 114
Corneal
  abrasion, 94, 199, 204
  endothelium, 5
  epithelium, 5, 113, 114
  exposure, 198
  foreign body, 200, 204
  graft, **5**, 209, 210
  inflammation, 208
  light reflex, 51, 52, 87, **102**, 118, 183
  mesothelium, 5, 113, 114
  nerve, 5, 114
  oedema, 5, 49, 176, 199
  perforating wound, 200
  reflex, 99
  rust ring, 200
  sensation, 99
  stroma, 5, 113, 114
  tear film, 25, 113, 114
  ulcer, 94, 204, **208**
    dendritic, 94, 196, **208**
    marginal, 208
Corresponding retinal areas, 83, 84
Cortical blindness, 34
Corticosteroid
  eye-drops, 174, 202, 206, 209-211
  systemic, 167, 202, 211, 217, 220, 221
Cotrimoxazole, 220
Cotton wool spot, 143, 151, 155, 160
Cover test, 88, **103**, 183
Craniopharyngioma, 171
Craniostenosis, 171
Critical fusion frequency, 65
Crocodile tears, 25
Crowding phenomenon, 67
Cryo-probe, 190
CSF pressure, 15, 165, 168
Cupping, 130, 170, 177
Cyclitis, 210
Cyclopentolate eye drops, 7, 120, 197, 200

Cycloplegic eye drops, 200, 202
Cylindrical lens, 45

Dacryocystitis, 207, 213
Dacryoscystorhinostomy, 207
Dark adaptation, 55, **59**, 74, 188
Deep retinal haemorrhage, 146
Dendritic corneal ulcer, 94, 196, **208**
Depression of eye, 26
Dermatitis, 95, 207
Descemetocoele, 5
Descemet's membrane, 5, 113, 114
Detachment, retinal, 10, 20, 57, 93, 140, **144**, 145, **147**, 155, 191, **220**
Deuteranopia, 73
Deviation of vein, 135
Devic's disease, 166
Dextran iv, 217
Dextrodepression, 28
Dextroelevation, 28
Dextroversion, 28
Diabetes, 94, 151, 152, 167, 171, 188, 220
Diabetic retinopathy, 152
Diamox, 177, 178, 211
Dichromat, 73
Differential threshold, 55, 57, **61**
Diffraction, 47, **48**, 68, 113
Digitalis, 93
Dilatation of pupil, 9, 116, **120**, 176, 188, 208, 211
  contraindications, 120
Dilated pupil, 34, 106, 110, 176, 202
Dipivalyl adrenalin eye drops, 178
Diplopia, 86, **94**, 189, 191, 198
  analysis of, 105
Disc
  diameter (dd), 13, 120
  oedema, 132, **164**
Discharge, 97, 205
Disciform macular degeneration, 146, 194, 216
Disjunctive movement, 28
Disparity, 85
Disseminated lupus erythematosis, 143
Disseminated sclerosis, 64, 70, 74, 94, 166, 171
Distance vision, 92, 99
Divergence, 29
Divergent squint, 96, 182-184
Doll's head phenomenon, 38, 39
Dot and blot haemorrhages, 146, 152, 155
Double vision, **86**, **94**, 189, 191, 198
  analysis of, 105
Drainage operation, 179
Drusen
  optic disc, 164
  retinal, 144

Dry eyes, 95
Dual visual systems, 54
Duochrome test, 51
Dysproteinaemia, 220

E test, 67, 99, 185
Eale's disease, 140
Eccentric Fixation, 182
Echothiophate eye drops, 178
Eclipse blindness, 199
Ectropion, 96, 213
Edinger-Westphal nucleus, 34
Educational objectives, 222
Egocentric direction, 81
Electro-oculography, 74
Electroretinography, 74
Elevation of eye, 26
Emboli, retinal, 136, 217
Embryology, 3
Emmetropia, 44, 116
Encephalitis, 166
Enophthalmos, 96, 198
Entropion, 94
Epicanthic folds, 97, 183
Epicapsular lens stars, 4
Epikeratophakia, 48
Epiphora, 25, 213
Episcleral vein, 6, 8, 174
Episcleritis, 196, 204, **210**
Epithelioma, 97
Erythema multiforme, 209
Eserine eye drops, 178
Esotropia, 184
Eversion of lacrimal punctum, 213
Exophthalmos, 94, 96
Exotropia, 184
Extorsion, 26
Extra-ocular muscle, 2, 26, 82
  paresis, 28
Exudate
  hard, 143, 144, 151-158, 160
  soft, 143, 151, 155, 160, 165, 220
Eyedrops
  adrenalin, 178
  antibiotic, 199, 200, 205, 208
  artifical tears, 210
  atropine, 7, 9, 208, 211
  chloramphenicol, 199, 205
  corticosteriod, 174, 202, 206, 209-211
  cyclopentolate, 7, 120, 197, 200
  cycloplegic, 200, 202
  dipivalyl adrenalin, 178
  echothiophate, 178
  eserine, 178
  fluorescein, 196
  hypromellose, 210
  idoxuridine, 209
  miotic, 120, 176, 178

mydriacil, 120
mydriatic, 118, 120, 176, 188, 189, 202, 210, 211
mydrilate, 120
neomycin-polymyxin-bacitracin, 205
neosynephrine, 120
parasympatholytic, 7, 9, 44, 46
parasympathomimetic, 8, 9
phenylephrine, 9, 120, 199
phospholine, 178
physostigmine, 8, 178
pilocarpine, 8, 120, 178
proparacaine, 108, 196, 199, 200
proxymetacaine, 108, 196, 199, 200
steroid, 174, 202, 206, 209-211
sympathomimetic, 9
timolol, 178
tropicamide, 9, 120, 197
vasoconstrictor, 206
Eye movements, 26, 36, 80, 88, 103
Eyeball size, 3, 180
Eyelid, 22
  laceration, 198, 213
Eyestrain, 95

Facial
  fracture, 198
  palsy, 23, 96
False projection, 82
Farnsworth colour tests, 73
Fat embolus, 136
Fechner's law, 63
Field defects, 101
Fifth nerve lesion, 209
Filtering operation, 179
Fixing eye, 184
Flame haemorrhage, 146
Flicker, 55, 65
Floaters, 93, 220
Fluorescein
  eye drops, 196
  staining, 110, 114, 196, 199
  angiography, **16**, 142, 143, 150, **155, 169**
Foetal fissure, 3
Following movements, 37
Foreign body pain, 94, 198
Form vision, 55, **65**, 92
Fourth nerve lesion, 29
Fovea, 2, **14**, 68, 120
Foveal reflex, 14, 120
Frontal motor cortex, 38
Fundus, 2, 115
  colour, 10, 140
Fungus, 208
Fusion, 36, 80, 85, 87, 182

Ganglion cell, 11, 75
  layer, 11

X and Y, 75
Gaze
  centre, 38, 39
  palsy, 38
Gentamicin injection, 208
Giant cell arteritis, 167, 217, 221
Glasses, 45, 48, 182, 191
Glaucoma, 174
  acute angle closure, 49, 93, 120, **176**, 204
  angle closure, 175
  congenital, 95, 171, 174, **180**
  low tension, 174, 175, 178
  open angle, 70, 131, 139, 174, **177**, 220
  primary, 174
  secondary, 174, 175, 189, 202, 210, 220
  steroid, 174, 206
Glaucomatous
  cupping, 131, 170, 177
  optic atrophy, 132, 171
Globe size, 3, 180
Glycerine, 177
Gonioscopy, **21**, 114, 175, 178
Goniotomy, 180
Gonococcus, 205, 206, 208, 211
Grating, 66, 68
  sinusoidal, 69, 77
  tests, 70
Grönblad-Strandberg syndrome, 147

Haloes, 49, 93, 176
Haploscope, 84
Hard Exudate, 143, 144, 151-158, 160
Hay fever, 206
Headache, 95
Hemianopia, 31, 102, 221
Hemiplegia, 32, 102, 217, 221
Henle's layer, 14
Hering's
  experiment, 83
  law, 28
Herpes
  simplex, 208
  zoster ophthalmicus, 209
Heterochromia iridis, 110
Heterophoria, 88, 103, 184
Heterotropia, 184
Hidden amblyopia, 185
Homonymous, 31
  hemianopia, 33, 93, 102
Horizontal cell, 11, 12
Horner's syndrome, 24, 35, 95, 106
Horopter, 83
Hue, 55, 70
Hutchinson's pupil, 106
Hydrocephalus, 171
Hyperacuity, 69

INDEX

Hypercolumn, visual cortex, 76, 79
Hypercomplex cell, 77
Hyperlipidaemia, 97, 98, 220
Hypermetropia, 44, 182
Hypertension, 151, 158, 166, 220
Hypertensive,
  retinopathy, 158, 160
  vessel changes, 159
Hypertropia, 184
Hyphaema, 8, 110, **201**
Hypoparathyroidism, 166
Hypopyon, 110, 208, 210
Hypotropia, 184
Hypromellose eye drops, 210

Idoxuridine eye drops, 209
Image formation, 42
Incomitant squint, 28, 184
Incongruous field defect, 32
Incremental threshold, 61
Indentation tonometry, 107, 174
Ingrowing eyelash, 198
Inhibition, 55, 75
Inner
  nuclear layer, 11
  plexiform layer, 11
Insulin, 152
Interference, 48
Internal limiting membrane, 13
Internuclear ophthalmoplegia, 38
Intorsion, 26
Intracranial
  aneurysm, 94, 171
  pressure, 15, 164, 168
Intraocular
  foreign body (IOFB), 95, 201
  lens, 47, 190
  pressure (IOP), 3, 107, 168, 174
IOL, 47, 190
Iridectomy, 177
Iridocyclitis, 210
Irido-dialysis, 110, 202
Iridodonesis, 8, 110, 202
Iridotomy, laser, 177
Iris, 2, **8**, 114
  bombé, 110, 175, 210
  colour, 9, 49
  dilator muscle, 9, 35
  epithelium, 8
  pigment, 9
  prolapse, 200
  sphincter
    muscle, 9, 34, 115
    rupture, 202
  vessels, 8, 114
Iritis, 9, 113, 189, 204, **210**
IRMA, 154
Ischaemic optic neuropathy, 102, **167**, 171, 221

Ishihara test, 73, 170
Isopter, 59, 179
Itching, 95

Juxtapapillary choroiditis, 167, 220

Keith, Wagener, Barker classification, 159
Keratic precipitates (KP), 110, 211
Keratitis, 208
  aerosol, 209
  disciform, 209
  exposure, 209
  filamentary, 210
  interstitial, 210
  neurotrophic, 209
  superficial punctate, 94, 206, 209
Keratoconjunctivitis
  actinic, 94, **199**, 209
  measles, 206, 209
  sicca, 209
Keratoconus, 47
Keratometry, 52
Keratoscopy, 51
Keratotomy, radial, 48

Lacrimal
  canaliculi, 24, 213
  canaliculus laceration, 198
  fossa, 22
  gland, 24
  obstruction, 213
  passages, 24
  punctum, 23, 24, 213
  sac, 24
Lacrimation, 25, 213
Laevodepression, 28
Laevoelevation, 28
Laevoversion, 28
Lagophthalmos, 96
Lamina cribrosa, 4, 130, 177
Lantern test, 73
Laser, 48
  argon, 157, 177, 179
  YAG, 177, 193
Latency, 55
Latent squint, 88, 103, 184
Lateral geniculate body (LGB), 32, 76
Lateral rectus paralysis, 28, 94, 182
Lazy eye, 185
Lead poisoning, 171
Learning guide, 222
Leber's optic neuritis, 166, 171
Lens, 2, **19**, 115, 120
  capsule, 19, 43, 189, 190, 193
  cortex, 20, 115
  dislocation, 202
  epithelium, 19
  extraction, 19, 190

  intraocular, 47, 190
  nucleus, 19, 115
  opacity, 19
  subluxation, 202
  sutures, 20, 115
  vesicle, embryonic, 4
Letter matching test, 67, 185
Leukaemia, 136, 146
Levator palpebrae muscle, 23
Lid, 22
  retraction, 96
  eversion, 109
Light
  adaptation, 55, 59
  reflex
    corneal, 51, 87, 102, 118, 183
    foveal, 14, 120
    pupillary, 34, 106
    vessel, 16, 137, 159
Lignocaine, 200
Light-near dissociation, 106
Limbal hyperaemia, 8
Limbus, 4
Lime burn, 199
Low vision aid (LVA), 194
Luminance, 55, **58**
Lustre, 86
Lysozyme, 25

Macroglobulinaemia, 139, 166, 220
Macula, 14, 120, 141
Macular
  degeneration, 146-148, **193**, 202
  fan, 15, 143, 160
  oedema, 142, 156, 157, 202
  sparing, 33
  star, 15, 143, 160
Maculopathy, diabetic, 70, 156, 157
Maddox
  rod test, 88
  wing test, 89
Magnification in ophthalmoscopy, 116
Magnifying glass, 189, 194
Manifest squint, 88, 103, 184
Mannitol iv, 177
MAR, 65
Marcus Gunn sign, 106
Marginal corneal ulcer, 208
Media, ocular, 92
Median longitudinal bundle (MLB), 38, 105
Meibomian
  cyst, 97, 207
  gland, 23
Melanoma, 148
Meningioma, 171
Meningitis, 166, 171
Metamerism, 72
Metamorphopsia, 93

229

Methyl alcohol poisoning, 171
Meyer's loop, 32
Microaneurysm, retinal, 139, 150, 154, 156
Microcystic macular oedema, 142
Micropsia, 87, 93
Migraine, 93, 95, 217, 221
Minimum angle of resolution (MAR), 65
Miotic eye drops, 120, 176, 178
Molteno drain, 179, 180
Monochromat, 73
Monocular squint, 184
Mossy haemorrhage, 146
Motor pathways, 36
Movements, ocular, 26, 36, 80, 88, 103
Mucocoele, lacrimal sac, 207, 213
Müller's
 cell, 11, 13
 muscle, 24
Multiple sclerosis, 64, 70, 74, 94, 166, 171
Muscae volitantes, 52, 93
Muscle
 ciliary, 2, 7, 43
 extraocular, 2, 19, 26, 82
 iris
  dilator, 9, 35
  sphincter, 9, 34, 115
 levator palpebrae, 23
 Müller's, 24
 oblique, 22, 26
 orbicularis oculi, 23
 rectus, 19, 22, 26
Myasthenia gravis, 94, 95
Mydriacil eye drops, 120
Mydriasis
 diagnostic, 9, 118, 120, 176, 197
 pathological, 34, 94, 106, 110, 176, 202
 therapeutic, 8, 9, 188, 189, 208, 211
Mydriatic eye drops, 118, 120, 176, 188, 189, 202, 210, 211
Mydrilate eye drops, 120
Myelinated nerve fibres, 142
Myokymia orbicularis, 97
Myopia, 44, 48, 147, 188
Myopic choroido-retinal atrophy, 145
Myotonic pupil, 34, 106

Narrow angle, 21, 175
Nasolacrimal duct, 25, 207, 213
Near vision, 68, 92, **99**
Negative lens, 116, 120
Neomycin-polymyxin-bacitracin eye drops, 205
Neosynephrine eye drops, 120

Neovascularization, retinal, 139, 145, 151-153, 155, 158, 220
 choroidal, 146, 194
Nerve
 fibre
  bundle defect, 12, 93, 178
  layer, 12
 fifth cranial, 6, 209
 fourth cranial, 26, 37
 optic, 2, 19
 parasympathetic, 7, 9, 24, 34, 44
 seventh cranial, 23, 24
 sixth cranial, 26, 37, 94
 sympathetic, 9, 35
 third cranial, 7, 26, 34, 37, 94, 95
Neural retina, 11
Neuromyelitis optica, 166
Night blindness, 56, 93
Non-proliferative diabetic retinopathy, 153
Nuclear
 hyper-refringence, 188
 sclerosis, 188
Nystagmus, 36, 103
 ataxic, 105
 end-position, 105
 fixation, 105
 jerky, 103, 105
 latent, 105
 optokinetic, 39, 105
 pendular, 103
 physiological, 60
 vertical, 38, 105
 vestibular, 37, 38, 105

Oblique muscle, 22, 26
Occipital motor cortex, 38
Occlusion
 retinal
  artery, 137, 142, 162, 171, **216**
  vein, 155, 162, **217**
 therapeutic, 184, 186
Ocular,
 hypertension, 174, 175, 178
 tension, 99, 107, 174
 torticollis, 183
Oculocentric direction, 80
Opaque nerve fibres, 142
Open angle, 21, 175
Ophthalmia neonatorum, 206
Ophthalmodynamometry, 217
Ophthalmoscope, 112, 115
Ophthalmoscopy, 115-120
Opponent-pairs process, 72
Optic
 atrophy, 32, 132, 134, 165, 166, **170**
 canal, 19, 22
 chiasma, 31, 93, 101, 171

cup, embryonic, 3, 7-9
disc, 2, **13**, 119, **130**
 colour, 14, 133, **170**
 cup, 13, **130**, 164, 177
 elevation, 132, 164
 haemorrhage, 133, 165, 177
 hyperaemia, 133, 165
 margin, 130, 132, 165
 oedema, 132, 139, 162, **164**, 221
 pallor, 134, 170
neuritis, 102, **166**, 221
neuropathy, 102, 167, 171, 221
nerve, 2, **19**, 31, 64, 75
 glioma, 171
 sheath, 2, 19, 168
 radiation, 32, 102
 stalk, embryonic, 3
 tract, 32, 102
 vesicle, embryonic, 3
Optical section, 112, 113
Optokinetic nystagmus, 39, 105
Ora serrata, 10, 20
Orbicularis oculi muscle, 23
Orbit, 22
Orbital,
 fracture, 198
 tumour, 96, 166, 171
Orthophoria, 88
Orthoptist, 87
Outer,
 nuclear layer, 11
 plexiform layer, 11
Oxycephaly, 166

Paget's disease, 171
Pain, 94
Palpebral
 ligament, 23
 opening, 22
Papillitis, 132, 164, **166**, 171, 221
Papilloedema, 14, 132, 160, **164**, 171
Papilloma, 97
Papillo-macular bundle, 12
Parallactic movement, 116, 130, 132
Paralytic squint, 184
Parastriate area, 33
Parasympatholytic eye drops, 7, 9, 44, 46
Parasympathomimetic eye drops, 8, 9
Parinaud's syndrome, 39
Pathological cupping, 131, 177
Pemphigus, 209
Perception, 54
Perforating wound, 94, 196, 200
Perimeter, 59
Peripapillary atrophy, 145
Peripheral
 iridectomy, 177
 vision, 92

INDEX

Peristriate area, 33
Pernicious anaemia, 167, 171
Phenylephrine eye drops, 9, 120, 199
Phi movement, 55, 65
Phospholine eye drops, 178
Photochromatic interval, 61
Photocoagulation, 10, 143, 157, 194, 220
Photogenic epilepsy, 65
Photophobia, 95, 180
Photopic vision, 54, 55, 59
Photopigment, 12, 54, **56**, 71, 78
Photopsia, 93
Photoreceptor, 11-13
Physiological
  cupping, 130
  diplopia, 86, 94
Physostigmine eye drops, 8, 178
Pickwickian syndrome, 166
Pigment
  crescent, 13, 130, 141
  epithelium, **10**, 14, 56, 140, 148, 194
  detachment, 220
Pigmentary degeneration of the retina, 137 **148**, 170, 171
Pilocarpine eye drops, 8, 120, 178
Pinguecula, 97
Pin-hole
  camera, 42
  glasses, 216, 220
  test, 47, 99, 189, 196
Pituitary tumour, 32,, 93, 171
Platelet embolus, 136
Plerocephalic papilloedema, 164
Plica semilunaris, 23
Plus lens, 119
Pneumococcus, 205, 208
Pointillism, 71
Polarized light, 49
Polycythaemia, 139, 166, 220
Pontine reticular formation, 38
Posterior chamber, 21
Pre-retinal haemorrhage, 145, 155, 157, 216
Presbyopia, 44
Pretectal nuclei, 32, 34, 39
Primal colours, 72
Primary
  colour, 71
  optic atrophy, 170
  position, 26
Proliferative diabetic retinopathy, 153
Proparacaine eye drops, 108, 196, 199, 200
Proptosis, 96
Protanopia, 73
Protective goggles, 48, 199
Proxymetacaine eye drops, 108, 196, 199, 200

Pseudoisochromatic plates, 73
Pseudomonas, 208
Pseudopapilloedema, 14, 132, 164, 168
Pseudophakia, 47
Pseudo-squint, 97, 183
Pterygium, 97
Ptosis, 24, 94, 95
Pulfrich pendulum effect, 63
Pulsation
  retinal,
    vein, 15, 134, 165
    artery, 15, 134
Punctate epithelial erosions, 209, 210
Pupil, 2, 4, 8
  constricted, 34, 106, 110, 208, 210
  dilated, 34, 106, 110, 176, 202
  immobile, 34, 106, 176, 202
  irregular, 34, 110, 200, 210
Pupillary
  block, 176
  membrane, 4, 114
  pathways, 34
  reflexes, 34, 106
Purkinje-Sanson images, 51
Purkinje shift, 60
Pyocyaneus, 208
Pyrimethamine, 220

Quadrantanopia, 32, 102
Quantum, 57
Quinine poisoning, 171

Radial keratotomy, 48
Railway-trucking, 216
Rapid eye movements (REM), 37
Reading glasses, 44
Reading type, 68, **99**
Receptive field, 12, **75**
Rectus muscle, 19, 22, 26
Recurrent corneal erosion, 200
Red
  eye, 98, **204**
  reflex (RR), 119, **120**, 188
Reduced eye, 43
Reflecting surfaces, 51
Reflex
  accommodation, 36
  corneal, 99
    light, 51, 52, 87, **102**, 118, 183
    foveal, light, 14, 120
    pupillary, 34, 106
    red, 119, **120**, 188
    vessel, light, 16, 137, 159
Refraction, 7, 43, 46
Refractive
  error, 44, 182, 185
  index, 43
Reiter's disease, 206

Renal hypertension, 159
Resolving power, 65
Retina, 2, **9**
Retinal (retinaldehyde), 56
Retinal
  artery, 15
    embolus, 136, 217
    irregularity, 134, 138, 155, 159
    narrowing,
      generalized, 137, 159, 216
      segmental, 134, 159
    occlusion, 137, 142, 162, 171, **216**
    sheathing, 136, 155
  capillaries, 16, 139
    abnormal, 139, 150, 154, 156
  cloudy swelling, 142
  detachment, 10, 20, 57, 93, 140, **144**, 145, **147**, 155, 191, **220**
  dialysis, 147
  exudate, 142
  haemorrhages, 146, 151
  hole, 20, 146
  microaneurysm, 139, 150, 154, 156
  neovascularization, 139, 145, 151-153, 155, 158, 220
  oedema, 142, 155, 157, 160, 202
  phlebitis, 220
  photograph, 115, 118, 157
  pigment epithelium, **10**, 14, 56, 140, 148, 194
    detachment, 220
  rivalry, 83, 85
  vasculitis, 136, 140, 167
  vein, 15, 16
    dilatation, 136, **139**, 155, 164, 217
    occlusion, 155, 162, **217**
    sheathing, 155
Retinitis
  pigmentosa, 137, **148**, 170, 171
  proliferans, 140
Retinoblastoma, 144, 182
Retinopathy, 139, 150
  carotid insufficiency, 139
  central serous, 220
  of prematurity, 140
  venous stasis, 139
Retinoscopy, 46
Retrobulbar neuritis, 166, 221
Retolental fibroplasia, 140
Ring scotoma, 102, 170
Rheomacrodex, 217
Rheumatoid arthritis, 210
Rhodopsin, 56
Rodent ulcer, 97
Rods, 10-13, 54, 56

Saccadic movements, 37,

INDEX

Salicylates, 210
Sarcoidosis, 211
Saturation, 71
Schiötz tonometer, 108
Schirmer's test, 99, **209**
Sclera, 2, **4**, 113
Scleral
   crescent, 13, 130, 145
   foramen, 4, 12
   laceration, 4, 199
   rigidity, 174
   ring, 13
   spur, 6, 178
Scotoma, 31, 93
   arcuate, **12**, 93, 102, 178
   central, 93, 166, 170, 199
   scintillating, 221
Scotopic vision, 54, 55, 59
Second sight, 45, 188
Secondary optic atrophy, 170
Senescent macular degeneration (SMD), 148, 193
Sensation, 54
Sensitivity, 57
Seventh nerve lesion, 23, 96, 209
Shade, 71
Sheathing, 136, 155
Siderosis, 201
Simple cell, 76
Simultaneous
   contrast, 61
   perception, 87
Sixth nerve lesion, 28, 94
Size constancy, 87
Sjögren's syndrome, 210
Slit-lamp microscope, 112
Smallpox, 209
Smooth pursuit movements, 37, 88
Snellen chart, 66, 99
Snow blindness, 199, 209
Soft exudate, **143**, 151, 155, 160, 165, 220
Solar retinopathy, 199
Spatial
   frequency, 69, 77
   induction, 65
   summation, 55, 58
Spectacles, 44, 45, 48, 182, 191
Spectral
   absorption curve, 56, 57
   luminosity curve, 56, 60
   sensitivity, 60
Spectrally opponent cells, 78
Sphenoidal ridge meningioma, 102
Spherical aberration, 47, 50
Spring catarrh, 206
Squamous cell carcinoma, 97
Squint, 28, 48, 80, 87, 96, 144, **182**
   accommodative, 182

   alternating, 103, 182, 184
   concomitant, 184
   convergent, 183, 184
   divergent, 96, 183, 184
   incomitant, 28, 184
   latent, **88**, 103, 184
   manifest, 88, 103
   monocular, 103, 182, 184
   paralytic, 184
   unilateral, 103, 182, 184
   vertical, 183, 184
Staphylococcus, 205, 207, 208
Stereopsis, 80, **85**, 87
Stereoscope, 84
Stereoscopic vision, 80, 83, **85**, 87
Steriod
   eye drops, 174, 202, 206, 209-211
   glaucoma, 174, 206
   systemic, 167, 202, 211, 217, 220, 221
Stills' disease, 211
Strabismus, 182, 184
Streptococcus, 208
Striate area, 32
Stye, 97, 207
Subarachnoid haemorrhage, 146, 166
Subconjunctival
   drug injection, 200, 208, 211
   ecchymosis, 201
   haemorrhage, 98, 201
Subhyaloid haemorrhage, 145
Subretinal haemorrhage, 146
Successive contrast, 65, 70
Superficial
   punctate keratitis, 94, 206, 209, 210
   retinal haemorrhage, 146, 160
Suppression, 85, 87, 182
Suspensory zonule, 2, 7, **19**, 43
Swinging flashlight test, 106, 166
Sylvian aqueduct syndrome, 39
Sympathetic ophthalmitis, 211
Sympathomimetic eye drops, 9
Synaptic layer, 11
Synechia
   anterior, 175
   posterior, 8, 110, 175, **210**
Synoptophore, 84, 87
Syphilis, 34, 102, 142, 170, 171, 210, 211

Tangent screen, 59
Tarsal
   cyst, 207
   gland, 23
Tarsus, 22
Tear meniscus, 25
Tears, 24, 25
   artifical, 210

Temporal
   arteritis, 167
   induction, 65
   pallor, 134, 170
   summation, 55, 58
Tenon's capsule, 24
Tension, 107, 174
Tessellated fundus, 10, 141
Test type, 46, **66**
Tetartanopia, 73
Third nerve lesion, 24, 34, 94, 95
Threshold, 55, 57
Thyroid eye disease, 94, 96, 166, 171
Tigroid fundus, 10, 141
Timolol eye drops, 178
Tint, 71
Tonometry, **107**, 174
Tobacco amblyopia, 102, 170, 171
Toric, 45
Torticollis, ocular, 183
Tortuosity of retinal vessels, 138
Toxaemia of pregnancy, 159
Toxoplasma, **142**, 211, 220
Toxocara, 142
Trabeculae, 6, 174, 177
Trabecular meshwork, 6, 174, 177
Trabeculectomy, 179
Trabeculoplasty, laser, 179
Trachoma, 198, 205
Tracking systems, 36
Trauma, 198
Trephine operation, 179
Trial
   frame, 46
   lenses, 46
TRIC agents, 205
Trichiasis, 94, 198
Trichromatic colour
   mixing, 71
   vision, 71
Tritanopia, 73
Trochlea, 22
Tropicamide eye drops, 9, 120, 197
Troxler effect, 60
Tuberculosis, 142, 171, 211

Ultraviolet light, 97, 196, 199
Unilateral squint, 103, 182, 184
Urea iv, 177
Uvea, 6
Uveitis, 6, 167, **210**

Vaccinia, 209
Vasoconstrictor eye drops, 206
Vein
   aqueous, 6, 114
   anterior ciliary, 8
   central retinal, 15
   episcleral, 6, 8, 174

INDEX

retinal, 15, 16
vortex, 6, 8
Venous collaterals, 139, 219, 220
Venous stasis retinopathy, 139
Vernier acuity, 69
Vergence, 28, 29, 36, 88
Version, 28
Vertebro-basilar insufficiency, 221
Vertical squint, 183, 184
Vestibular
  eye movements, 37, 88
  nuclei, 38
Visual
  acuity, **65**, **99**
  angle, 65
  axis, 26, 184
  cortex, 32, 76
  direction, 55, 80
  field, **31-33**, **58**, **101**
  pathway, 31
  pigment, 10, 12, **56**, 72
  persistence, 64
  receptor, 12
Visually evoked response, 74
Vitamin A, 10, 56, 166
Vitamin B deficiency, 167, 171
Vitrectomy, 158
Vitreous, 2, **20**, 113, 115
  haemorrhage, 120, **145**, 155, 157, 202, 216, 220
  opacity, 52, 93, 120, 142, 145, 216
  shrinkage, 20, 147, 155
Vortex vein, 6, 8

Watering eye, 25, **213**
Wavelength, 55, 56
Weber's law, 63
Welding flash, 196, 199, 209

Xanthelasma, 97

Yoke muscles, 28

Zonule, lens, 2, 7, **19**, 43